Basic Monitoring in Canine and Feline Emergency Patients

Basic Monitoring in Canine and Feline Emergency Patients

Edited by

Elizabeth J. Thomovsky, DVM, MS, DACVECC
Paula A. Johnson, DVM, DACVECC
Aimee C. Brooks, DVM, MS, DACVECC

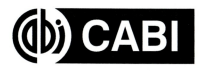

CABI is a trading name of CAB International

CABI
Nosworthy Way
Wallingford
Oxfordshire OX10 8DE
UK

CABI
WeWork
One Lincoln St
24th Floor
Boston, MA 02111
USA

Tel: +44 (0)1491 832111
Fax: +44 (0)1491 833508
E-mail: info@cabi.org
Website: www.cabi.org

Tel: +1 (617)682-9015
E-mail: cabi-nao@cabi.org

© CAB International 2020. All rights reserved. No part of this publication may be reproduced in any form or by any means, electronically, mechanically, by photocopying, recording or otherwise, without the prior permission of the copyright owners.

A catalogue record for this book is available from the British Library, London, UK.

Library of Congress Cataloging-in-Publication Data

Names: Thomovsky, Elizabeth J., editor. | Johnson, P.A. (Paula A.), editor. | Brooks, Aimee C., editor.
Title: Basic monitoring in canine and feline emergency patients / edited by: Elizabeth J. Thomovsky, Paula A. Johnson, Aimee C. Brooks.
Description: Wallingford, Oxfordshire, UK ; Boston, MA : CABI, [2020] | Includes bibliographical references and index. | Summary: "This book discusses the various basic monitoring techniques available for emergency patients. The book elaborates on and explains monitoring techniques that can be easily performed in basic ER clinics and primary care clinics"-- Provided by publisher.
Identifiers: LCCN 2019039193 (print) | LCCN 2019039194 (ebook) | ISBN 9781789242997 (paperback) | ISBN 9781789243000 (ebook) | ISBN 9781789243017 (epub)
Subjects: LCSH: Veterinary emergencies. | Veterinary critical care. | Patient monitoring. | Point-of-care testing. | Dogs--Wounds and injuries--Treatment. | Cats--Wounds and injuries--Treatment. | Dogs--Diseases--Treatment. | Cats--Diseases--Treatment.
Classification: LCC SF778 .B37 2020 (print) | LCC SF778 (ebook) | DDC 636.089/6025--dc23
LC record available at https://lccn.loc.gov/2019039193
LC ebook record available at https://lccn.loc.gov/2019039194

References to Internet websites (URLs) were accurate at the time of writing.

ISBN-13: 978 1 78924 299 7   (paperback)
       978 1 78924 300 0   (ePDF)
       978 1 78924 301 7   (ePub)

Commissioning Editor: Alexandra Lainsbury
Editorial Assistant: Emma McCann
Production Editor: Marta Patiño

Typeset by SPi, Pondicherry, India
Printed and bound in the UK by Severn, Gloucester

Contents

Contributors		vii
Preface		ix
1	Physical Examination and Point-of-care Testing Paula A. Johnson	1
2	Blood Pressure Monitoring Daniel S. Foy	26
3	Electrocardiography Jessica L. Ward	45
4	Pulse Oximetry Kristen A. Marshall and Aimee C. Brooks	71
5	Venous and Arterial Blood Gas Analysis Aimee C. Brooks	85
6	Capnography Laura A.M. Ilie	110
7	Applications of Serial Focal Ultrasound Techniques in the Hospitalized Small Animal Patient Danielle M. Hundley	129
8	Electrolyte Monitoring Elizabeth J. Thomovsky	156
9	Coagulation Elizabeth J. Thomovsky and Aimee C. Brooks	177
10	Manometer-based Monitoring Adesola Odunayo	199
Index		209

Contributors

Aimee C. Brooks, DVM, MS, DACVECC
Purdue University College of Veterinary Medicine, West Lafayette, Indiana, USA

Daniel S. Foy, MS, DVM, DACVIM (SAIM), DACVECC
College of Veterinary Medicine, Midwestern University, Glendale, Arizona, USA

Danielle M. Hundley DVM, MS, DACVECC
VCA Midwest Referral and Emergency Center, Omaha, Nebraska, USA

Laura A.M. Ilie DVM, MS, DACVECC
Veterinary Specialty Center, Buffalo Grove Illinois, USA

Paula A. Johnson, DVM, DACVECC
Purdue University College of Veterinary Medicine, West Lafayette, Indiana, USA

Kristen A. Marshall, DVM, MS, DACVECC
Department of Small Animal Clinical Sciences, University of Tennessee, Knoxville, Tennessee, USA

Adesola Odunayo, DVM, MS, DACVECC
Department of Small Animal Clinical Sciences, University of Tennessee, Knoxville, Tennessee, USA

Elizabeth J. Thomovsky, DVM, MS, DACVECC
Purdue University College of Veterinary Medicine, West Lafayette, Indiana, USA

Jessica L. Ward, DVM, DACVIM (Cardiology)
Iowa State University, Ames, Iowa, USA

Preface

As instructors in veterinary schools, all of the authors have faced the same dilemma – the student who cannot find the correct resource to answer a particular question. While we all acknowledge the importance and value of *looking something up*, sometimes in multiple resources, this book is an attempt to create a repository of information in one resource.

The intended audience, therefore, is the veterinary student or the veterinary practitioner who would like a fairly succinct approach to understanding the monitoring equipment that they are using on their patients. This book does not attempt to provide comprehensive details of treatment and diagnosis of disease but rather how to use the available monitoring equipment to gather information about a case.

In our attempt to provide information about a monitor, we have also attempted to provide the relevant physiology upon which the monitor is based (or which is needed to understand the output from the monitor). And most importantly of all, since no monitor is perfect and all monitors have inherent weaknesses, this book attempts to point out how to properly use each monitor to avoid some of these weaknesses as well as provide some guidelines to rational interpretation of the results that are acquired. We hope that we have succeeded in our goals.

Elizabeth J. Thomovsky,
15 January 2020.

1 Physical Examination and Point-of-care Testing

PAULA A. JOHNSON*

Purdue University College of Veterinary Medicine, West Lafayette, Indiana, USA

The efficient, accurate, and timely assessment of emergent patients is necessary to have successful outcomes. This chapter will review physical examination (PE) and point-of-care blood testing (POCT), important first-line tools that guide therapeutic decision making in an emergency and critical care setting. The specific point-of-care tests to be covered include packed cell volume/total protein (PCV/TP), blood glucose (BG), ketone values, and blood lactate. Point-of-care instrumentation is available, which also reports such parameters as electrolytes, blood gas values, acid–base, and coagulation. Discussion of these parameters as well as other point-of-care assessments, including blood pressure and point-of-care ultrasound, are covered elsewhere in this book.

1.1 Basic Physiology and Anatomy

Physical examination

As technology has evolved, more diagnostic instrumentation that allows for quick or instantaneous test results is readily accessible; as a result, the physical exam has seemingly decreased in its importance and utility. However, no technology can replace the value of the physical exam, defined as 'an examination of the bodily functions and condition of an individual,' for the practicing clinician. The physical exam is a skill that has to be nurtured, practiced, and fine-tuned by repetition and experience over time. In fact, the more experienced the clinician, the more important the information that can be gleaned from the exam. The benefits associated with performing thorough physical exams are numerous. Those benefits include its immediate availability, use of basic senses (seeing, hearing, touching, and smelling), and, with the exception of a stethoscope, lack of need for any special instrumentation. Additionally, it is cost-effective, provides a wealth of information regarding the patient's clinical status in a short period of time, and can be utilized for serial monitoring to identify changes or trends in a patient's condition or response to therapy.

Point-of-care blood testing

Blood glucose

As the primary source of fuel for energy production in most cells in the body, the availability and regulation of glucose is necessary to sustain life. In most cases, glucose is present in ample amounts in mammals although sometimes the ability to deliver the glucose to the needed locations can be challenging. An example would be a diabetic patient who has ample circulating glucose but is unable to provide that glucose to the mitochondria within the cells.

The concentration of glucose within the body is controlled within a set range during the resting state. Table 1.1 lists the reference range for BG in canines and felines at rest. Normal BG levels are primarily maintained by the hormone insulin that serves to transport glucose into the cells for conversion to adenosine triphosphate (ATP) by the stages of aerobic metabolism (glycolysis, transport through the tricarboxylic [TCA] cycle, and passage through the electron transport chain). Thus, insulin's major effect is to lower the BG concentration. BG levels are further regulated and the effects of

---

* Corresponding author: johns357@purdue.edu

Table 1.1. Normal reference range for blood glucose during the resting state in dogs and cats.

Species	Normal reference range (mg/dL)
Canine	80–120
Feline	80–140

insulin opposed by the counter-regulatory hormones glucagon, cortisol, epinephrine, and growth hormone. These hormones can stimulate further glucose release into the bloodstream to maintain or increase BG levels. When glucose is not maintained under tight control, hypoglycemia or hyperglycemia can occur. Both conditions can be affiliated with morbidity and mortality.

The brain is an obligate glucose user and has reduced or minimal capabilities to liberate its own glucose from glycogen stores or to use protein as an energy source. Therefore, the brain relies on *systemic delivery* of glucose to maintain normal metabolic function. Thus, when *hypoglycemia* occurs, not only are the majority of clinical signs associated with insufficient glucose delivery to the brain (neuroglycopenia), but they also occur within a relatively short period of time. If the hypoglycemia is not corrected quickly or is allowed to persist for an extended period of time, these neurologic-related clinical signs may persist beyond the time of correction and may progress to include cortical blindness and peripheral nerve demyelination.

Hyperglycemia can be tolerated for longer periods of time with the more minor increases in BG (<200 mg/dL) typically not leading to clinical signs and hence able to be tolerated for longer periods of time. Severe hyperglycemia (>200 mg/dL) is associated with clinical signs and is not tolerated for long periods. The most common clinical signs in the case of hyperglycemia are associated with fluid losses. This is due to the fact that significant hyperglycemia causes fluid to shift into the vascular space from the cells. Large quantities of glucose molecules act as an effective osmole and draw water from the cells into the vasculature. These fluid shifts lead to cellular dehydration. At the same time, the glucose molecule will similarly retain water with it in the renal tubules, leading to polyuria. Significant polyuria can cause enough fluid and concurrent electrolyte loss via the urinary system to lead to further cellular dehydration and electrolyte deficiencies (especially hypokalemia and hyponatremia). Typically, glucosuria (and volume loss through the kidneys) starts to occur in dogs and cats when the serum glucose exceeds 180–200 mg/dL and 260–310 mg/dL, respectively. Hyperglycemia has also been linked to other deleterious consequences such as immunosuppression, increased inflammation, disruption of normal coagulation, and alterations of the endothelium.

Ketone levels

Ketones are produced as a consequence of fat store metabolism. While ketosis can occur with other disease states such as hepatic lipidosis, starvation, or errors of metabolism, the most common situation in veterinary patients in which measurement of ketones is important is in patients suspected or known to have diabetes mellitus. Diabetic ketoacidosis (DKA) is a life-threatening complication of diabetes mellitus marked by hyperglycemia with excessive ketone production and subsequent acidosis from the ketones. In DKA, a lack of insulin production and/or lack of insulin binding to its receptors on cells coupled with an increase in counter-regulatory hormones including glucagon, epinephrine, glucocorticoids, and growth hormone leads to an increase in glucose levels within the bloodstream. In addition, free fatty acid (FFA) breakdown increases in response to the counter-regulatory hormones in an attempt to create more glucose and provide more energy to the cells. The excessive amount of FFAs presented to the cells overwhelm their ability to oxidize these FFAs to acetyl coenzyme A to enter the TCA cycle and undergo aerobic metabolism to ATP. Instead, the excess FFAs are oxidized to ketone bodies that are released into the circulation.

There are three ketone bodies that are formed during this process: acetoacetate, 3-betahydroxybutyrate (3-HB), and acetone. Of these, acetoacetate is produced first from the oxidation of FFAs; it is then reduced in the mitochondria to yield 3-HB. Acetone is produced from the decarboxylation of acetoacetate. Acetone is produced in the smallest quantities and acetoacetate and 3-HB, *the two major ketone bodies in animals*, are normally present in equal proportions. However, in animals with DKA, 3-HB can be produced in amounts five to ten times those of acetoacetate. Once insulin therapy is initiated, the levels of 3-HB will decrease more rapidly than acetoacetate concentrations.

Lactate

There are two isoforms of lactate: L-lactate and D-lactate. L-Lactate is the isoform produced by mammals and is of the greatest significance in the small animal veterinary population. The production of excess L-lactate most commonly results from anaerobic metabolism secondary to poor oxygen delivery to tissues. L-Lactate therefore serves as a measurable biomarker for tissue hypoxia and hypoperfusion. However, because there is generally an excess of oxygen in the blood above basic tissue requirements, tissues are able to extract more oxygen from the blood in early states of hypoperfusion to maintain themselves. Cells will not switch to anaerobic metabolism (and produce lactate) until this excess oxygen is exhausted. Therefore, the appearance of lactate in the blood is considered 'late' versus the occurrence of hypoperfusion.

Normal lactate in adult canines and felines is considered to be less than 2.5 mmol/L. Lactate levels in neonates and younger animals have been documented to be considerably higher than those in adults. A study showed at the age of 4 days, the lactate ranged from 1.07–4.59 mmol/L in puppies, and between 10 and 28 days, the range was 0.80–4.60 mmol/L. This is thought to result from multiple factors including increased availability of lactate for use as an energy source for the brain in neonates and the small capacity and lack of complete development of normal clearance mechanisms at this age.

In normal adult dogs and cats, the breakdown of glucose via glycolysis produces pyruvate. In the presence of oxygen, pyruvate enters the TCA cycle and then undergoes oxidative phosphorylation, ultimately producing a total of 36 ATP molecules for energy utilization by cells. In the absence of oxygen, pyruvate is unable to enter the TCA cycle or undergo oxidative phosphorylation. As a result, it enters the Cori cycle for conversion to lactate. While this cycle prevents excessive buildup of pyruvate, it only yields two ATP molecules along with two lactate molecules (Fig. 1.1). While the liver is able to convert lactate back to pyruvate so that this energy reserve is not lost, it can only do so once oxygenation and perfusion are restored.

In contrast, D-lactate typically exists in only very tiny amounts in the body. It comes from three sources: bacteria (primarily in the colon), diet, and production in small quantities by the methylglyoxal pathway (an offshoot of glycolysis) prior to creation of pyruvate. Due to its tiny amounts and sources, D-lactate does not provide information about the patient's tissue oxygenation status, and is not measured by routine lactate analyzers. However, it can still cause a high-gap metabolic acidosis (see Chapter 5) if present in unusually large quantities, and has been rarely reported in small animals secondary to DKA, gastrointestinal (GI) disorders, or intoxications.

Typically, the majority of lactate produced by the body is cleared by the liver, although small amounts are metabolized by the kidneys and skeletal muscle. As the amount of lactate increases in the case of anaerobic metabolism, the ability of the liver to clear it is decreased. In addition, hepatic clearance itself is decreased by acidosis, hypoperfusion, and hypoxia.

1.2 How the Monitor Works

Physical examination

Tips for performing a good PE include establishing an organized approach, performing the PE in the same sequence each time, and always doing as complete a physical exam as the patient's status allows. By working in a methodical and organized fashion, such as examining the patient from the head to the tail or taking a body systems approach, and making every effort to perform the physical exam in the same sequence each time, the practitioner decreases the risk of missing key findings. It is also important to avoid focusing on only the obvious abnormality during the exam. As an example, in a patient that has been hit by a car that presents with an exposed bone associated with an open femoral fracture, it can be easy to fixate on the exposed bone and miss the heart rate of 200 beats per minute or the pale mucous membranes that support the patient is in shock. In a case such as this, failing to identify shock could delay initiation of lifesaving resuscitative therapy.

While it is important to practice doing physical exams in a repetitive sequential manner in an effort to prevent missing key findings, there are times when rearranging the sequence may be warranted. Such times might include situations where the patient's temperament will not allow a full or complete PE without chemical restraint or sedation, or emergent patients that require initiation of stabilization therapy prior to completing a full or complete physical exam. In cases such as this, it is acceptable to rearrange the sequence and begin stabilization measures or obtain appropriate sedation first. However, it is critical that once these initial concerns are met, the patient does receive a thorough and complete PE with evaluation of all body systems.

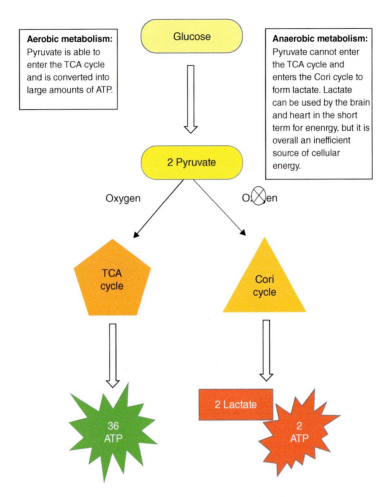

Fig. 1.1. Aerobic versus anaerobic metabolism. Pyruvate in the presence of oxygen is converted to acetyl coenzyme A and enters the tricarboxylic (TCA) cycle, resulting in the production of adenosine triphosphate (ATP) for cellular energy. Under anaerobic conditions, pyruvate is unable to enter the TCA cycle and instead enters the Cori cycle that ultimately produces lactate and minimal ATP for cellular energy.

The first step in a physical exam should be observation of the patient prior to making any physical contact. This includes noting such things as the patient's level of awareness, respiratory effort, posture, ability to ambulate, and looking for visible evidence of hemorrhage, wounds, and so on.

Next, a good physical exam includes basic vital signs: assessment of mentation, temperature, pulse (rate, quality), respiration (rate, quality), capillary refill time (CRT), and mucous membrane (MM) color. See Table 1.2 for normal reference ranges for canine and feline vital signs. Interestingly, very few of these variables and the currently accepted reference ranges associated with them have actually been scientifically studied or validated in veterinary medicine.

In addition to obtaining the basic vitals, a complete and thorough physical exam includes assessment of all body systems. See Table 1.3 for a list of body systems along with elements or techniques performed when assessing those systems. It is important to realize that the information obtained from a physical exam is only a piece of the puzzle; it should be considered along with data collected from other diagnostic testing as there is often a synergy between the two.

Table 1.2. Normal reference ranges for vital parameters in dogs and cats.

Vital parameter	Canine reference range	Feline reference range
Mentation	Appropriately responsive	Appropriately responsive
Temperature	100.0–102.5°F (37.38–39.17°C)	100.0–102.5°F (37.38–39.17°C)
Pulse	60–150 beats per minute	150–220 beats per minute
Respirations	12–24 breaths per minute	20–40 breaths per minute
Capillary refill time	<2 seconds	<2 seconds3
Mucous membrane color	Pink	Pink

Point-of-care blood testing

Packed cell volume/total protein

The PCV and TP is measured from a whole blood sample placed into a microhematocrit tube. The PCV represents the percent of total blood volume that is red blood cells (RBCs) as opposed to plasma. Total protein is the measurement of the plasma protein concentration in serum or plasma, expressed as g/dL (grams per deciliter). The protein is a reflection primarily of albumin and globulins. Besides the RBCs and plasma in the microhematocrit tube, there is also the presence of a buffy coat that appears between the red cells and the plasma after the tubes have been spun. The buffy coat contains white blood cells and platelets. The PCV/TP is relatively simple to perform and requires a minimal amount of fresh or anticoagulated whole blood, microhematocrit tubes and clay, a centrifuge capable of spinning microhematocrit tubes, a hematocrit reading card, and a refractometer. See Figs 1.2 and 1.3 for the equipment required to perform a PCV/TP and Table 1.4 for the normal reference ranges in dogs and cats.

Once a blood sample is obtained, it can be placed in heparinized or non-heparinized hematocrit tubes and spun at the recommended speed and for the recommended duration of time (usually 5 minutes or less) as per the manufacturer's guidelines for the centrifuge being utilized. Upon completion of spinning, and prior to reading the PCV and TP, the color of the plasma is assessed (see Section 1.3, Interpretation). Next, the PCV is determined utilizing the hematocrit reading card. If there is the presence of a visible buffy coat, the percentage of the buffy coat is also determined utilizing the hematocrit reading card. In order to measure the TP, the hematocrit tube is carefully broken at the level of the plasma and cellular sediment interface. The plasma is then evacuated from the tube onto the refractometer. The reading for the TP is taken from the scale labeled serum or plasma protein on the refractometer.

Blood glucose

The multitude of negative outcomes that can occur as a result of unregulated BG levels warrant diligent maintenance and monitoring BG. This monitoring can be accomplished by the use of handheld, transportable, point-of-care BG monitors. There are multiple commercially available units ranging from portable strip-based glucometers (Fig. 1.4) to cartridge-based systems (Fig. 1.5) and sensor card-based technology (Fig. 1.6). When using a cartridge-based system, the cartridge chosen determines the analytes measured. While there is a cartridge specifically to measure glucose, glucose values are included with other cartridges designed to measure parameters like electrolytes and blood gases. Table 1.5 provides a list of point-of-care BG monitors.

The methodology utilized by most handheld units (including strip-based and cartridge-based systems) to measure the glucose is based on a glucose oxidase reaction between the test strip or cartridge and the glucose in the blood. Glucose oxidase catalyzes an oxidation reaction that transforms glucose to gluconic acid and hydrogen peroxide. The amount of hydrogen peroxide produced is proportional to the amount of glucose in the blood. The change in the hydrogen peroxide concentration is measured based on the production of an electrical current that is sensed by an electrode in the glucose meter (this methodology is called enzymatic amperometry).

Ketone

Detection and measurement of ketones in urine or plasma is accomplished by utilizing reagent strips. These commercially available strips come in two forms: (i) the multi-stick that contains a test pad for ketones in addition to test pads for measurement of leukocytes, urobilinogen, pH, specific gravity, bilirubin, nitrites, protein, blood, and glucose (Fig. 1.7); and

Table 1.3. List of body systems along with elements and techniques utilized to evaluate each body system.

Body system	Examination[a]
Integument	Visual assessment of skin, being sure to part the hair and evaluate the ventral abdominal skin
Cardiovascular	Thoracic auscultation (heart sounds) Heart rate Rhythm Pulse quality/pulse rate Subjective assessment of vascular filling (jugular pulsations, lack of distention of vasculature while holding off a vessel)
Respiratory	Thoracic auscultation Audible upper airway sounds Posture/work of breathing Respiratory rate Respiratory pattern
Gastrointestinal	Abdominal palpation Rectal exam
Genitourinary	Visual ± palpation with sterile gloves
Musculoskeletal	Gait observation Range of motion and stability of joints, joint effusion Palpation of long bones
Neurologic	Gait observation Cranial nerves Peripheral reflexes Spinal palpation Assessment of mentation/awareness
Lymph nodes	Palpation and comparison of size bilaterally
Eyes	Visual survey Use of light source to evaluate pupillary responses Assessment of vision
Ears	Visual survey Smell Use of light source and cone to evaluate the ear canals and tympanic membrane
Oral cavity	Visual survey; often requires sedation/anesthesia for complete exam
Mucous membrane assessment	Moisture (hydration status) Color (pallor, cyanosis, icterus, hyperemia) Capillary refill time (prolonged, normal, brisk)
Body condition score	Typically compared to visual scale; may also include assessment of muscle mass

[a]More information about the various aspects of the exam are found in the accompanying text in Section 1.4.

(ii) the 'diastick' that contains only pads for glucose and ketones. Regardless of the exact reagent strip used, each test pad is a semi-quantitative test. When urine or plasma is placed on the test strip, if acetoacetate is present it will react with nitroprusside on the pad in an alkaline medium contained on the test pad. A positive reaction is indicated by a color change. The color change ranges from lavender (minimal ketone present) to a dark purple (large amount of ketone present). Unfortunately, the nitroprusside sticks do not detect 3-HB, the ketone present in greatest quantity in veterinary species. It is therefore possible to have false negative readings when the animal has ketonemia or ketonuria. While it is unlikely that the patient would have a negative reading if significant levels of ketones are present, the degree of color change may not accurately reflect the magnitude of ketones present.

In some settings, the reagent strips have been replaced by the use of point-of-care ketone meters (see Fig. 1.8). These meters are handheld, small,

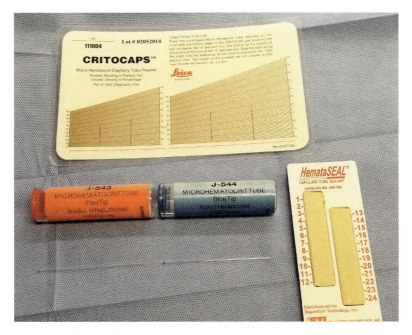

Fig. 1.2. Heparinized and non-heparinized microhematocrit tubes are demonstrated along with the clay used to seal one end of the tube and an example of the hematocrit reading card.

utilize minimal quantities of whole blood, and measure the ketone body 3-HB. Specifically, whole blood is placed within an electrochemical strip. Within that strip, hydroxybutyrate dehydrogenase oxidizes the 3-HB to acetoacetate while simultaneously reducing NAD$^+$ to NADH. The meter will then re-oxidize the NADH to NAD$^+$, generating a current detected and measured by the meter. The amount of current is directly proportional to the amount of NADH created (and hence the amount of 3-HB) in the blood sample. When operated properly, these units produce accurate results in a very short period of time and can be used serially to monitor response to therapy. Table 1.5 lists the various point-of-care meters available and indicates those that can also measure ketones. Normal ketone levels in heathy patients are reported as <0.32 mmol/L in dogs and 0.11 mmol/L in cats.

Lactate

The methodology utilized by most point-of-care testing units to measure L-lactate is enzymatic amperometry. Hydrogen peroxide produced by a reaction between L-lactate and lactate oxidase is oxidized and generates an electrical current that is proportional to the concentration of L-lactate in the sample. This method is utilized by all the handheld point-of-care units and by most blood gas analyzers to measure L-lactate.

Most commercially available units found in veterinary medicine are handheld. They are small, generally cost-effective, require very small amounts of blood, and require minimal maintenance or calibration. Most units use test strips or cartridges and the time to results is reliable and quick, usually seconds to minutes. For example, the i-STAT (Abbott Point-of-Care, Abbott Laboratories, Abbott Park, Illinois, USA; see Fig. 1.5) handheld instrument has a cartridge for measuring lactate. Figure 1.9 shows the Lactate Plus (Nova Biomedical, Waltham, Massachusetts, USA) that uses test strips. Table 1.6 provides a list of commercially available lactate meters.

1.3 Indications

Physical exam

The importance of the physical exam cannot be understated and it is an integral first step in evaluating ALL patients. A staged physical exam

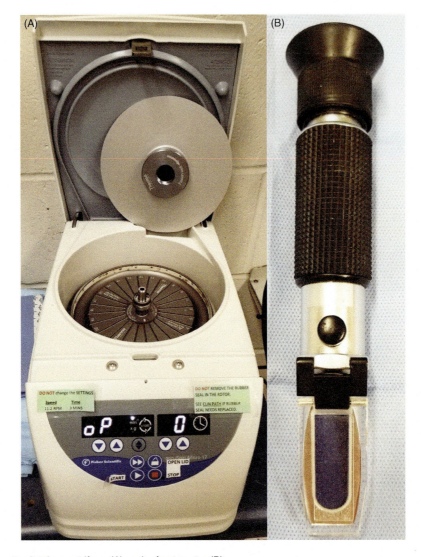

Fig. 1.3. Hematocrit tube centrifuge (A) and refractometer (B).

(e.g. focusing on assessment of the respiratory system in a respiratory distress patient while providing oxygen, reducing handling/mobility in a possible spinal fracture patient) should be considered depending on history and initial survey findings.

Point-of-care blood testing

Point-of-care testing is defined as testing at or near the site of the patient. It allows for efficient information collection about a patient's clinical status in order to make rapid therapeutic deci-

Table 1.4. Normal reference ranges for packed cell volume (PCV) and total protein (TP) for canines and felines.

Species	Normal PCV (%)	Normal TP (g/dL)
Canine	35–55	6.0–8.3
Feline	30–45	5.0–8.0

sions. Advantages associated with POCT include short turnaround time with rapid availability of patient data and a reduction in pre- and post-analytic errors due to rapidity of sampling and analysis. Since POCT instrumentation is generally

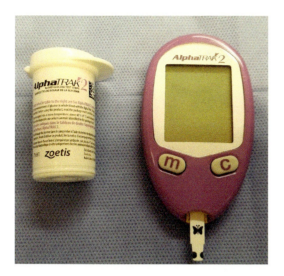

Fig. 1.4. The AlphaTRAK® 2 (Zoetis, Parsippany, New Jersey, USA) is a point-of-care glucometer developed specifically for veterinary species. It measures blood glucose in a whole blood sample where glucose is found both in the plasma and attached to the membrane of red blood cells. Because the distribution of glucose in these locations differs between species, the advantage of the AlphaTRAK® is that it is programmed with the normal distribution of glucose for both cats and dogs. Using a human glucometer will underestimate the blood glucose level because the distribution of glucose in humans is different.

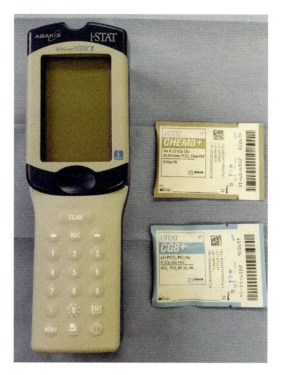

Fig. 1.5. The i-STAT (Abbott Laboratories, Abbott Park, Illinois, USA) handheld cartridge-based point-of-care instrument. Two of the available cartridges available for this system are pictured. Both of these cartridges include blood glucose readings.

self-contained, user friendly, easily transportable, and requires a relatively small volume of blood for multiple tests to be performed, it lends itself well to the emergent evaluation process. Some disadvantages of POCT include concerns regarding accuracy of results, quality control of the devices, and difficulty integrating patient data into the patient's medical record since these units are often self-contained and not networked into the electronic medical record. Over the years, POCT has advanced tremendously such that some of these concerns have been alleviated.

There are various instruments available to perform various types of testing but, as with every diagnostic test, any results from POCT should be interpreted in the context of the patient and its physical exam. In emergent patients, assessments of PCV/TP, BG ± lactate, and often some form of stat venous blood gas/electrolyte panel are commonly performed as part of data collection during initial stabilization.

1.4 Interpretation of Findings

Physical exam

Mentation

Changes in mental status can provide key information when assessing a patient. Determining if the patient is alert, responsive, aware, and appropriately engaged versus if the patient is nonresponsive, stuporous, obtunded, or comatose is often key when making initial recommendations for the need for immediate therapy. If there are changes in mentation, it is important to establish if the altered mental status is a result of primary neurologic disease versus being secondary to an 'extracranial' cause such as a toxin or poor perfusion from shock. If there is concern that the mentation changes are secondary, the focus should be identification and interventions to improve the underlying cause prior to reassessing the patient's mentation.

Alterations in mentation can be associated with or secondary to a wide variety of disease processes outside of the neurologic system including shock, trauma, infectious diseases, inflammatory diseases, electrolyte alterations, hypoglycemia, and many other causes. It is always valuable information to see if therapy improves mentation or not. For example, hypovolemic animals will have dull mentation as a result of decreased delivery of oxygen to the brain. If the patient is resuscitated appropriately, the mental status and responsiveness of the patient will improve. If the patient is not resuscitated and perfusion to the brain is not restored, the mental dullness could progress to stupor, obtundation, coma, and even death.

Temperature

Monitoring body temperature has been a foundation for assessing a patient's clinical status since the 1800s, and continues to be an important element of the PE. Monitoring body temperature in veterinary patients is usually done rectally; a rectal temperature is considered representative of the core body temperature. Multiple studies have investigated the accuracy of rectal temperature monitoring compared to the gold standard of core body temperature measurement: pulmonary artery thermometry. There is a strong correlation between rectal and pulmonary artery thermometry supporting the use of a rectal temperature to obtain a core body temperature.

See Table 1.2 for the normal rectal temperature of feline and canine species. Other forms of temperature monitoring (axillary, aural) are less accurate. In cats 22% of axillary temperatures and 49% of aural temperatures differed by more than ±0.9°F (±0.5°C) from rectal temperatures. In dogs, 98% of axillary temperatures and 56% of auricular temperatures differed from rectal temperatures by more than ±0.9°F (±0.5°C). While these methods may seem attractive in recalcitrant patients,

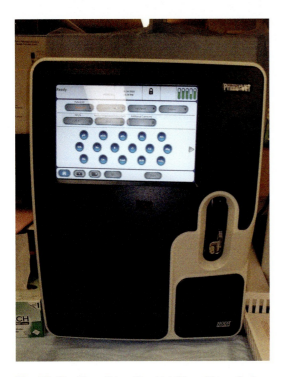

Fig. 1.6. The Nova Prime Plus Vet (Nova Biomedical, Waltham, Massachusetts, USA) unit. This is a sensor card-based instrument that can measure a variety of blood parameters including blood glucose.

Table 1.5. Commercially available point-of-care blood glucose and ketone meters.

Analyzer	BG/Ket	Range	Time to results (seconds)	Sample volume (μL)	Sample type	Strip/cartridge/sensor card
Nova Vet Meter[a]	BG	20–600 mg/dL	4	0.4	Whole blood	Strip
	Ket	0.1–8 mmol/L	10	0.8	Whole blood	Strip
Precision Xtra[b]	BG	20–500 mg/dL	5	0.7	Whole blood	Strip
	Ket	0.1–8 mmol/L	10	0.7	Whole blood	Strip
i-STATt[b]	BG	20–700 mg/dL	120	65–95	Whole blood	Cartridge
Nova Prime Plus Vet[a]	BG	15–500 mg/dL	60	135	Whole blood	Sensor card
AlphaTRAK® 2[c]	BG	20–750 mg/dL	5	0.3	Whole blood	Strip

[a]Nova Biomedical, Waltham, Massachusetts, USA; [b]Abbott Point of Care, Abbott Laboratories, Abbott Park, Illinois, USA; [c]Zoetis, Parsippany, New Jersey, USA.
BG, blood glucose; Ket, ketones.

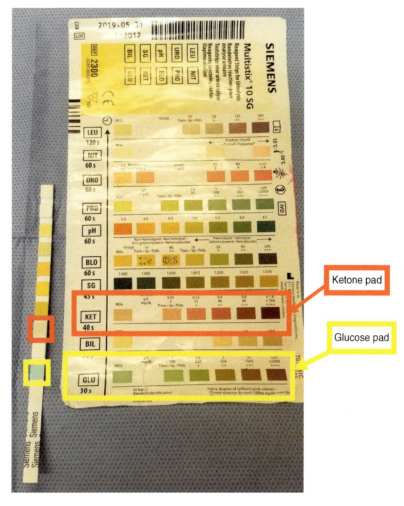

Fig. 1.7. A reagent strip test demonstrating the test pad for ketones and glucose among the other items for which the strip can test.

practitioners should be cautious in making clinical decisions based on these methods.

Obtaining a rectal temperature and determining if a patient is hypothermic or has a body temperature above normal can provide information related to a patient's clinical status, alert a clinician to changes in the animal's condition, and may lead to adjustments in the therapeutic plan. As an example: hypothermic patients could be so as a result of environmental exposure or as a result of shock, anesthesia, heart failure, or any other condition that might result in decreased cardiac output.

When an animal's body temperature is increased, the first decision point is to determine if the elevated temperature is due to hyperthermia (exogenous warming) or fever (increased body temperature as a result of alteration in the set point of the thermoregulatory center in the hypothalamus). Causes of true hyperthermia are usually associated with environmental changes leading to an inability to dissipate heat appropriately (e.g. being locked in a hot vehicle) or muscular activity such as in exercise or during generalized seizures. Hyperthermia commonly occurs in obese animals or those with airway disease such as laryngeal paralysis that cannot effectively pant and lose heat via evaporation. In contrast, fever can be a symptom of a wide variety of diseases whether infectious, inflammatory, immune-mediated, or neoplastic, and is not typically accompanied by any difficulties in dissipating heat.

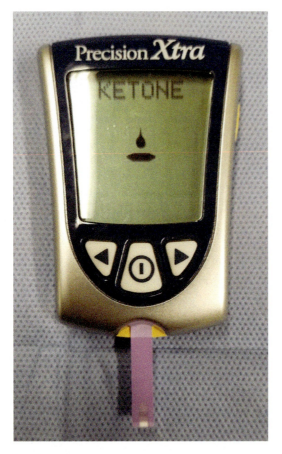

Fig. 1.8. An example of a commercially available ketone meter with test strip in place.

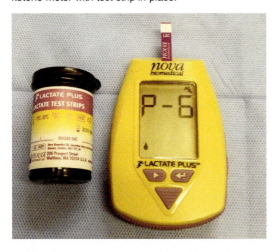

Fig. 1.9. Lactate Plus (Nova Biomedical, Waltham, Massachusetts, USA) monitor showing a test strip in place and ready for application of sample.

Heart rate/rhythm/pulse pressure

Heart rate, rhythm, and pulse quality can be evaluated via thoracic auscultation and palpation of the peripheral pulses simultaneously. During auscultation, heart sounds (murmurs, gallops, dull heart sounds) can be characterized as well as heart rate (i.e. beats per minute). It is important to simultaneously palpate the peripheral pulses during auscultation to allow further evaluation of the heart rate, heart rhythm, and pulse strength or intensity (i.e. pulse pressure). Arrhythmias are identified by palpable pulse deficits (absence of a peripheral pulse that coincides with auscultation of a heartbeat) or other abnormalities in rate or rhythm, especially compared to the audible heart rate/rhythm. Arrhythmias that are identified during this process should be further evaluated via electrocardiogram (ECG; see Chapter 3) to determine if anti-arrhythmic interventions are warranted.

During this process, the pulse pressure is assessed. Pulse pressure is the difference between systolic and diastolic arterial pressures and is responsible for the intensity of the palpated peripheral pulse. The pulse pressure is determined by stroke volume and aortic compliance (i.e. how stretchy the aorta is and how much it dilates in response to blood flow). Things to determine are if the strength of the pulse is normal, or if it is bounding, weak, thready, or absent. Typically, weak, thready, or absent pulses raise concern for hypovolemia or poor blood delivery to the site being palpated. Bounding/excessive pulse quality is most commonly caused by a decreased diastolic pressure and is associated with early vasodilatory states (e.g. systemic inflammation), severe anemia, or vascular anomalies such as patent ductus arteriosus.

Assessing the patient's cardiovascular status will help to determine that animal's stability. It is important to understand that some abnormalities such as extremes of heart rate (very fast or very slow) as well as poor to absent pulses warrant immediate therapy which could be lifesaving. Monitoring the patient's cardiovascular status via serial or sequential auscultation of the heart and palpation of pulses provides the opportunity to identify changes or trends that require adjustments to the patient's therapeutic protocol.

Respiratory rate/character

Thoracic auscultation allows for evaluation of lung sounds, respiratory rate, and effort. Reasons for alterations in a patient's respiratory parameters are

Table 1.6. Commercially available lactate meters.

Lactate analyzer	Mobility	Range (mmol/L)	Time to result (seconds)	Sample volume (µL)	Sample type	Strip/cartridge/sensor card
Stat Strip Lactate Connectivity[a]	Handheld	0.3–20	13	0.6	Whole blood	Strip
Lactate Scout 4[a]	Handheld	0.5–25	10	0.5	Whole blood	Strip
Lactate Plus[a]	Handheld	0.3–25	13	0.7	Whole blood	Strip
i-STAT[b]	Handheld	0.3–20	120	95	Whole blood	Cartridge
Nova Prime Plus Vet[a]	Transportable	0.4–20	60	130–135	Whole blood	Sensor card

[a]Nova Biomedical, Waltham, Massachusetts, USA; [b]Abbott Point of Care, Abbott Laboratories, Abbott Park, Illinois, USA.

often multifactorial and can involve one or more than one of the following: upper airway disease, pulmonary parenchymal disease, pleural space disease, thoracic wall injury, primary cardiovascular disease, pain, stress, or anemia. The respiratory rate is normally counted as breaths per minute (see Table 1.2 for normal rates in dogs and cats).

Assessing the quality of the respirations is also important and has the potential to provide information to help localize the problem to a specific location along the respiratory tract. Hearing crackles, wheezes, or rales (abnormal clicking, bubbling, or rattling sounds) within the lungs can be indicative of primary pulmonary parenchymal disease. Significant inspiratory stridor (sound produced as a result of disruption of airflow) in a patient could be indicative of laryngeal paralysis, upper airway obstruction as a result of a polyp or mass, or collapsing trachea to name a few examples. The presence of decreased lung sounds during auscultation might lead one to be concerned about the presence of pleural effusion or pneumothorax. In cases with severe respiratory distress, decreased lung sounds are an indication for immediate thoracocentesis to relieve the distress. If fluid is obtained and analyzed from thoracocentesis, it can be both a diagnostic and therapeutic intervention.

Capillary refill time

CRT is tested when a mucosal surface (usually the oral mucosa) is pressed until the color leaves and the tissue bed blanches. The time that it takes for the color (and therefore blood) to return to that tissue bed is called the CRT. It is generally considered to be prolonged when it takes >2 seconds for return of color. Reasons for prolongation include, but are not limited to, shock, dehydration, vasoconstriction, severe vasodilation, hypothermia, or any other condition that compromises circulation or delivery of blood to tissues or leads to poor vascular tone. CRTs can also be rapid (i.e. less than 1 second). This is most commonly seen in situations with supra-normal vascular tone such as compensatory shock (i.e. the smooth muscle in the vasculature is very taut allowing rapid return of blood to the tissue bed).

What actually constitutes a normal or abnormal CRT is a subject of debate. CRT in humans was first promoted in 1947 by Beecher as a way to assess a patient in shock. Initially, published parameters were considered 'normal' (no signs of shock), 'definite slowing' (slight to moderate shock), and 'very sluggish' ('severe' shock). In 1980, Champion and colleagues incorporated these ranges into the human 'Trauma Score' and in so doing set the normal CRT as less than 2 seconds despite a lack of scientific data to support this as being normal. Subsequently, studies related to CRT have determined that CRT actually varies with age and temperature (Schriger and Baraff, 1988) and that further research is needed to establish the true validity and usefulness of the CRT as an accurate measure of circulatory status.

To date no studies evaluating CRT and its use as a predictor of perfusion or circulatory status in veterinary medicine have been identified, and normal has continued to be the initially proposed <2 seconds. As such, the importance of the CRT is somewhat unclear. The authors propose that it is most important to serially examine the CRT and note changes rather than the actual documented CRT. Also, evaluating the CRT in the context of the remainder of the PE is more important than evaluating it on its own.

Mucous membrane color

Mucous membrane color is normally pink. Changes in MM color can be influenced by changes in tissue perfusion, vasomotor tone (venoconstriction or dilation), or the presence of deoxygenated hemoglobin or other pigments such as bilirubin (see Fig. 1.10). While assessing the color, it is important to be aware that the ability to assess the MM color is affected by gingival pigmentation, ambient lighting, and visual acuity, making assessment of MM color variable between operators.

Pale mucous membranes generally indicate vasoconstriction or anemia, both of which can have a variety of causes. Assessment for causes of shock based on other physical exam findings and measurement of PCV/TP should be prompted when pale MM are found. Determination of body temperature and glucose levels are also indicated as pallor also occurs in hypoglycemia and hypothermia. Yellow (icteric, jaundiced) MM may indicate pre-hepatic (hemolysis),

hepatic, or post-hepatic (biliary tree) abnormalities. Hyperemic/injected mucous membranes (also referred to as 'brick red') can occur in some patients as a result of septic conditions or endotoxemia, which cause vasodilation. The bright red color is caused by the presence of blood pooling in the dilated capillaries in the gingiva. Mucous membranes can also have a bluish color (i.e. cyanotic); this occurs as a result of the presence of excessive deoxygenated blood (see Chapter 4 for more information).

Point-of-care blood testing

Packed cell volume/total protein

Table 1.7 summarizes the information collected from evaluating the PCV/TP.

A decreased PCV could indicate anemia as a result of loss, destruction or lack of production of RBCs. An increased PCV could result from polycythemia or dehydration.

The presence of an increased TP is not pathognomonic for any particular disease process but could be indicative of such disorders as dehydration, inflammation, or even neoplasia. A decreased TP

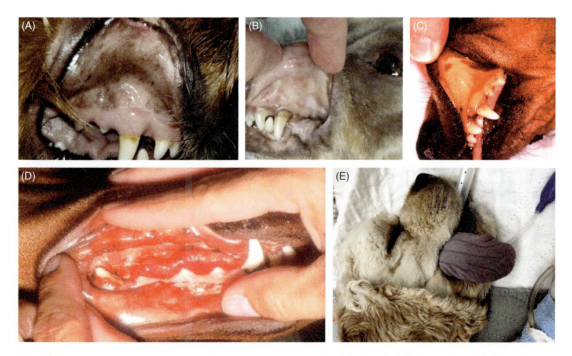

Fig. 1.10. A variety of appearances of mucous membranes color. (A) Normal mucous membrane color (pink); (B) pale mucous membrane color; (C) Icteric mucous membranes; (D) Brick red mucous membranes; (E) Cyanotic mucous membranes.

Table 1.7. Information collected when running a packed cell volume/total protein (PCV/TP).

PCV	Percentage of whole blood sample that is red blood cells Typically measured with hematocrit reading card	
Buffy coat	Percentage of whole blood sample that is buffy coat (platelets and white blood cells) Measured with hematocrit reading card	
Color of plasma	Color Clear to straw Yellow Red White	Interpretation of color Normal Bilirubinemia Hemolysis (pathologic or iatrogenic) Lipemia
Total protein	Protein concentration in the plasma Measure with refractometer	

could be indicative of inappropriate loss of protein (e.g. protein-losing nephropathy or protein-losing enteropathy), lack of production of protein (as with severe liver disease), iatrogenic dilution if following fluid therapy, or temporary downregulation of protein production as seen during inflammatory conditions (e.g. albumin is a negative acute phase protein and is not produced in normal quantities during severe systemic inflammatory conditions).

When measuring PCV/TP, it is important that both values are assessed and the information interpreted in concert with results of other data collected, and the clinical status of the patient. In situations where the patient has experienced acute whole blood loss resulting in hypovolemia, the PCV and TP would be expected to be decreased proportionally to one another. However, it should be remembered that the compensatory mechanisms for blood loss can also influence the values obtained when assessing PCV and TP.

In hypovolemic animals who have bleeding as a cause for their hypovolemia, compensation for low blood volume involves sympathetic nervous system stimulation and the release of catecholamines. Vascular contraction occurs in response to catecholamines, as does splenic contraction (primarily in dogs). Splenic contraction leads to release of RBCs without the proportionate release of protein. This can result in a measured PCV that is disproportionately increased compared to the TP of the blood. Thus, dogs with acute blood loss will often present with a 'normal' PCV (maintained by splenic contraction) but a low TP. If a clinician does not pay attention to this situation, ongoing blood loss can be overlooked especially during resuscitation from hypovolemia. It is important to monitor trends in the PCV and TP over time, especially when there has been blood loss and blood loss may be continuing (e.g. trauma cases).

For patients with 'non-blood loss' hypovolemia, who have largely lost fluid alone, hemoconcentration characterized by an elevated PCV/TP would be expected. In this situation, the number of RBCs in circulation remains the same but the plasma fluid content is decreased due to fluid loss from vomiting, diarrhea, effusing into cavities (e.g. pleural or abdominal effusions), or polyuria. However, if the fluid lost has a high protein content (septic abdominal effusions, hemorrhagic gastroenteritis), then the PCV may be elevated without a proportional increase in TP.

When conditions such as immune-mediated hemolytic anemia or primary bone marrow disease occur, both of these situations reduce red blood cell mass without a decrease in body fluid volume. Under these circumstances the PCV would be expected to be decreased while the TP would likely be normal.

In hypervolemic situations as seen with congestive heart failure or iatrogenic fluid overload, the PCV and TP can be proportionately decreased as a result of a dilutional effect. In this situation, more fluid in the blood vessels decreases the concentration of RBCs and TP equally. However, depending on the cause of the hypervolemia, this may not always be the case. For example, animals with liver failure often retain fluid but have disproportionately low TP due to lack of protein production by the failing liver. Or animals might display more severe decrease in their PCV versus the TP if they are anemic in addition to hypervolemic. Again, monitoring trends and taking the entire clinical picture of the animal into account is important when both interpreting the PCV/TP and evaluating changes in the animal's condition.

Blood glucose

A variety of diseases and situations can lead to hypoglycemia and hyperglycemia. See Table 1.8 for the most common causes of each condition as well as associated clinical signs.

Anorexia is unlikely to be a cause of hypoglycemia in an adult animal unless they are severely cachectic, so hypoglycemia should prompt further investigation beyond mild-to-moderate anorexia. In contrast, in juveniles, especially toy breeds, poorly developed liver function can cause these patients to become hypoglycemic within hours of decreased food intake.

Animals that initially present with normal BG can become hypoglycemic quickly in the face of progressive disease. Serial monitoring of BG in patients with underlying conditions such as sepsis or hepatic failure is therefore recommended, and rechecking BG in any patient who has had an acute change in hemodynamic or neurological status that cannot be easily explained by other causes is warranted.

Ketones

As indicated previously, the presence of ketones is most important in diabetic animals in whom there is concern for DKA. Early identification and therapeutic intervention in cases of DKA increases the chances for a positive outcome and provides information to the owner as to the degree of intervention and cost their pet may require. Therefore, having the capability to identify the presence of ketones is critical to success not only to make an early diagnosis, but also to make repeated assessments to monitor response to therapy.

Diabetic patients with low to trace ketones, no acidosis, and who are still eating and drinking can often be managed as outpatients with adjustments to insulin and treatment of underlying disease conditions (e.g. urinary tract infection, pancreatitis) that may have led to the development of ketosis. Patients with significant ketone levels causing acidosis often require more extensive supportive care that is best provided in a hospital environment.

Healthy dogs generally have 3-HB levels <0.32 mmol/L. A 3-HB level cutoff above 3.8 mmol/L has been suggested by Duarte *et al.* (2002) as having the best predictive value for diagnosis of DKA in dogs. In cats, a normal reference limit of <0.11 mmol/L has been reported, with all cats with DKA in a study by Weingart (2012) having 3-HB concentrations >3.8 mmol/L. However, cats with other disease processes such as hepatic lipidosis can also have elevated ketone levels, which have been reported to be as high as 2.78 in one study by Gorman *et al.* (2016). Therefore, while severe elevations in ketones are almost always associated with DKA, mild-to-moderate

Table 1.8. Clinical signs and causes of hypoglycemia and hyperglycemia.

	Hypoglycemia	Hyperglycemia
Clinical signs	Abnormal behavior Mental dullness Weakness Hypersalivation Tremors Seizures Death	Increased thirst Increased urination Weight loss Polyphagia Dehydration Alterations in mental status Coma
Common underlying causes	Sepsis Juvenile and toy breeds Insulinoma Paraneoplastic Hypoadrenocorticism Insulin overdose Toxins: (Xylitol, ethylene glycol) Hepatic insufficiency Spurious (sample storage) Severe starvation Glycogen storage diseases	Diabetes mellitus Pheochromocytoma Hyperadrenocorticism Iatrogenic dextrose administration Administration of dextrose containing fluids Drugs: glucocorticoids Parenteral nutrition Stress hyperglycemia/excessive catecholamines

elevations may be associated with other concurrent comorbidities such as lipidosis and interpreted accordingly.

Lactate

Lactic acidosis is an increase in blood lactate that results in an acidemia. Hyperlactatemia is classified as type A or type B. Type A hyperlactatemia occurs as a consequence of decreased delivery of oxygen to tissues. Type B hyperlactatemia is divided into three categories related to the cause. See Table 1.9 for classifications of hyperlactatemia and their causes.

The use of lactate clinically as an indicator of severity of disease and response to therapy has been evaluated. Its use as an adjunct diagnostic indicator when assessing cavitary effusions has also been investigated. Table 1.10 lists a variety of disease entities where lactate has been evaluated as a biomarker for severity of disease or prognosis and includes recommendations as to how to use lactate for monitoring. Key points to remember when including lactate as a diagnostic tool are: (i) a single isolated reading is of little diagnostic or prognostic value; (ii) serial values or trends should be monitored; and (iii) lactate values are only one piece of the global picture and should be reviewed in combination with other diagnostic results and physical exam findings.

1.5 Pitfalls of the Point-of-care Meters

Blood glucose

As simple as the use of point-of-care glucose meters is, there are some pitfalls to be aware of with this instrumentation. It is important to ensure the instrument as well as any necessary disposables are stored and handled properly. Make sure all strips and cartridges are in date and strips are kept in a sealed container. Proper

Table 1.9. The classifications of lactic acidosis and potential causes of each.

Classification	Pathophysiology	Disease examples
Type A	Systemic hypoperfusion	Shock Sepsis SIRS
	Local hypoperfusion	Arterial thromboembolism Burns Organ torsion
	Impaired hemoglobin carrying capacity for oxygen	Carboxyhemoglobinemia Methemoglobinemia
	Severe anemia	Hemoglobin <5 g/dL (PCV <15%)
	Severe hypoxemia	PaO_2 <30 mmHg
	Increased oxygen demand	Exercise Seizures Shivering Trembling/tremors
Type B1	Diseases associated with decreased lactate clearance	Severe liver failure Neoplasia Sepsis Diabetes mellitus Thiamine deficiency Kidney Injury
Type B2	Drugs and toxins that impair oxidative phosphorylation	Propylene glycol Prednisone
Type B3	Metabolic defects leading to abnormal mitochondrial function	Insufficient pyruvate hydrogenase Mitochondrial myopathies

SIRS, systemic inflammatory response syndrome; PCV, packed cell volume; PaO_2, arterial partial pressure of oxygen.

Table 1.10. Diseases where lactate has been reported as a biomarker for either severity of disease or prognosis. Recommendations and points to consider regarding its use for each disease are also included.

Disease entity	Points to consider
Shock and resuscitation	Serial measurements useful to guide resuscitation and predict mortality in critically ill patients
	Useful to gage efficacy of fluid therapy, cardiovascular supportive measures, and blood administration
	Use with caution when treating later stages of sepsis as elevation in lactate can result from adaptive responses and not poor perfusion
Septic peritonitis	Failure to normalize within 6 hours of admission associated with nonsurvival
Babesiosis	Lactate concentration higher than 2.5 mmol/L at 8, 16, and 24 hours following admission associated with higher mortality
	Increase in lactate or failure to decrease by more than 50% within 8–16 hours associated with higher mortality
Immune-mediated hemolytic anemia	Initial lactate not associated with outcome
	Persistently increased lactate within 6 hours of admission despite therapy associated with increased mortality
Gastric dilation and volvulus	Decreased lactate following fluid resuscitation and decompression good predictor of survival
Traumatic brain injury	Serial lactate measurements to guide resuscitation may be helpful
Cavitary effusions	*Peritoneal fluid*
	A blood to effusion lactate difference of >2.5 mmol/L can help differentiate septic effusions from other types
	Lactate concentration in effusion used in conjunction with cytology can help differentiate neoplastic and septic effusions from other types
	Pericardial fluid
	Lactate not useful to differentiate neoplastic from non-neoplastic effusions
	Synovial fluid
	Septic effusions had higher synovial fluid lactate concentrations than blood lactate levels
	Use of synovial fluid lactate in conjunction with cytology could be useful diagnosis or increasing suspicion of septic arthritis

sample handling is also crucial; collection of samples in the proper tube and in an appropriate volume is important for valid results. Since glucose is labile, it is important to assess BG immediately after blood collection. Allowing blood samples to sit prior to testing without separating the red cells from the plasma will result in falsely decreased glucose readings as the RBCs continue to metabolize glucose present in the sample.

There is inherent error in the manufacturing and accuracy from glucose strip to glucose strip within a manufactured lot and even from manufactured lot to lot. However, strips are theoretically required to be within ±15 mg/dL of each other for BG readings below 100 mg/dL and ±15% of each other for readings above 100 mg/dL. Also, glucose meters need to be used at normal room temperatures. If used at temperature extremes, changes in the speed of red blood cell metabolism and alterations of enzymatic reactions can cause artificially high or low glucose measurements. Ideally, cellular phones are kept at least 50 m away from glucose meters as the electromagnetic radiation has been shown to change glucose measurements by up to 10 mg/dL.

In addition, patient factors such as red blood cell concentration, acid–base status, and oxygenation level can alter BG readings. Acid–base abnormalities will alter the distribution of glucose between plasma and RBCs, thus rendering the pre-programmed calibration in units like the AlphaTRAK (Zoetis, Parsippany, New Jersey, United States) incorrect. Point-of-care units measure BG in whole blood rather than plasma, so hemoconcentration will allow less non-RBC–bound glucose interaction with the sensors in the test strip, artifactually lowering BG. Anemia will have the opposite effect, artifactually raising BG due to less RBCs to bind it. Oxygen supplementation can interfere with glucose oxidase in the test strips, taking electrons from the enzyme and decreasing the ability of the enzyme to convert glucose to gluconic acid and hydrogen peroxide. Therefore, high levels of oxygen in the blood (as might be seen under general anesthesia) can falsely lower the BG reading.

Certain drugs can also interfere with BG assessment when glucose is measured on point-of-care units. Ascorbic acid, acetaminophen, dopamine, and mannitol can all interfere with BG readings by affecting glucose oxidase's conversion of glucose or by being broken down by the glucose oxidase and therefore being misinterpreted as glucose. Thus, drug therapy can falsely increase or decreased BG readings depending on the situation. If patients are receiving these drugs, it is better to verify any glucose reading obtained from a point-of-care instrument against a glucose result done on a standard laboratory analyzer.

Ketones

When dealing with ketone strips, the same concerns for manufacturing and storage as indicated above for glucose strips are true. There is much less research into this area versus glucose strips, however. Hematocrit changes can also alter ketone results. Low hematocrits can falsely increase ketone levels; some meters have proprietary built-in corrections for hematocrit levels, but to the author's knowledge these have not been validated in veterinary species. Ketone testing is similar to glucose testing in that substances such as vitamin C can interfere with the enzymatic conversion of ketones to nitroprusside because it alters the alkaline environment needed for that conversion. The degree of change of ketones in response to vitamin C is still under investigation in humans. Vitamin C is likely not important in most animal patients.

As previously discussed, when using colorimetric reagent urine ketone test pads with either urine or serum, they do not detect 3-HB. This can lead to a decreased estimation of severity or even potentially a false negative reading in a patient with ketosis.

Lactate

The most common situations affecting lactate levels are not related to the lactate meter itself, but rather to pre-analytical variables. The first obstacle is that there is no standardization between lactate values meaning that lactate meters cannot be compared to a single standard reference and as such cannot be compared to each other. Also, delays in testing lactate will falsely increase the lactate level because red blood cell metabolism in the sample will continue to increase lactate levels.

The other large consideration with lactate testing is how sample collection can impact the lactate levels. Specifically, lactate levels can be falsely increased when obtaining the blood sample. This occurs when a blood vessel is held off for long periods, or, in the case with animals, there is significant restraint required to obtain the sample. In the former example, holding off blood flow from an area can decrease oxygen delivery to those local tissues, leading to anaerobic metabolism and lactate production. Similarly, more significant restraint can either lead to increased lactate production from a similar effect or possibly secondary to increased muscle activity related to the restraint. Sampling from an ischemic limb (e.g. in a cat with an aortic thromboembolism affecting blood flow to its rear legs) can falsely increase lactate levels due to the anaerobic metabolism naturally taking place in ischemic tissue that lacks blood flow. This 'artifact' is sometimes used diagnostically; if lactate in one limb is significantly higher than peripheral blood, it would raise concern for decreased regional perfusion to that limb (e.g. possible thrombosis).

Whole blood samples have a lower lactate level than plasma samples. This is because the RBCs will sequester some of the circulating lactate, thus falsely lowering the lactate levels. Similarly, lactate levels in venous blood will naturally be higher than levels in arterial blood due to diffusion of lactate from metabolizing cells into the venous blood.

1.6 Case Studies

Case study 1: Diabetic ketoacidosis

Jazzy, a 10-year-old female spayed Cocker Spaniel presented to the emergency service with a 2-week history of increased drinking and urination along with a decreased appetite. In the week just prior to presentation, she began having intermittent episodes of vomiting that increased in frequency leading up to presentation. On the day of presentation she was noted to be very lethargic and depressed and she urinated where she was lying in the house. Jazzy had previously been a healthy dog with the exception of obesity and ear infections.

At presentation Jazzy was able to stand and walk but was very lethargic. Although she seemed dull she was appropriately responsive. Her temperature was 99.5°F (37.5°C), heart rate 120 beats per minute, respiratory rate 30 breaths per minute, CRT >2 seconds, and MM color pink. See Box 1.1 for the remaining results of the PE for Jazzy.

Box 1.1. Jazzy: Physical exam by body system.

- Integument: increased skin tent
- Cardiovascular:
  - Thoracic auscultation: grade II/VI left sided systolic murmur
  - Rate: within normal limits
  - Rhythm: within normal limits
  - Pulse quality/pulse pressure: strong and synchronous pulses, normal quality
- Respiratory:
  - Thoracic auscultation: normal lung sounds
  - Rate: 30 breaths per minute
  - Pattern: eupneic breathing pattern, no increased effort noted
- Gastrointestinal:
  - Abdominal palpation: mild pain elicited upon palpation of the cranial and mid abdomen
  - Rectal exam: within normal limits, normal stool present
- Genitourinary: within normal limits
- Musculoskeletal:
  - Ambulation: normal (reluctant to move)
  - Range of motion: within normal limits
- Neurologic:
  - Cranial nerves: within normal limits
  - Reflexes: within normal limits
- Lymph nodes: submandibular lymph nodes slightly enlarged, all other peripheral lymph nodes within normal limits
- Eyes: within normal limits
- Ears: moderate amount of brown exudate present in both ears
- Oral cavity: moderate dental tartar present
- Body Condition Score (scale 1–9): 8.0/9.0

Blood and urine samples were obtained for both point-of-care and laboratory testing. Point-of-care tests completed included: PCV = 40%, TS = 9.6 g/dL (serum slightly yellow). BG was 624 g/dL and the urine dipstick was negative for ketones but 4+ positive for glucose. Blood ketones on a meter was positive (4.0 mmol/dL).

Based the information gathered from the history, PE, and point-of-care testing, Jazzy's initial diagnosis was DKA with abdominal pain due to suspected pancreatitis.

An i-STAT Chem8 was also performed and revealed: Na 130 mmol/L (norma139–150 mmol/L), potassium 3.3 mmol/L (normal 3.4–4.9 mmol/L), chloride 91 mmol/L (normal 106–127 mmol/L), ionized calcium 1.04 mmol/L (normal 1.12–1.40 mmol/L), TCO_2 15 mmol/L (normal 17–25 mmol/L), blood urea nitrogen 65 mg/dL (normal 10–26 mg/dL), creatinine 1.4 mg/dL (normal 0.5–1.3 mg/dL), glucose 614 mg/dL (normal 60–115 mg/dL), hematocrit 37% (normal 35–50%), anion gap 2825 mmol/L (normal 8–25 mmol/L), and hemoglobin 12.6 g/dL (normal 12–17 g/dL). All of these abnormalities were consistent with the DKA diagnosis.

Additional diagnostic testing included submission of blood for a complete blood count, chemistry profile, and a pancreatic lipase level. Urine was submitted for a complete urinalysis and urine culture. Thoracic and abdominal radiographs were also performed with full diagnostic abdominal ultrasound planned for the following day.

Initial therapy for Jazzy included a 20 mL/kg bolus of isotonic crystalloid fluids, followed by a rate of isotonic crystalloid fluid that would provide maintenance fluids plus correction of a 7% deficit over 12 hours. The fluids were supplemented with potassium after the initial bolus since she was found to be hypokalemic. She was started on maropitant, pantoprazole, and a fentanyl constant rate infusion (CRI) for her abdominal pain. An insulin CRI was initiated.

Results of the additional diagnostics revealed that the initial diagnoses made based on the PE and POCT were correct: Jazzy had DKA with severe concurrent pancreatitis. Monitoring for Jazzy included vital signs every 4 hours in the first 24 hours, then every 6 hours. Full physical exam was performed a minimum of twice a day for the first few days. Body weight was measured twice daily. Her BG was monitored every 2 hours for the first 4 days then every 4 hours (the rate of the insulin CRI was adjusted based upon the measured BG). Blood ketones were checked a minimum of once every 24 hours. Other bloodwork including electrolytes, blood urea nitrogen, and creatinine were monitored every 4 hours in the first 24 hours then twice daily thereafter. Adjustments were made to her fluid type and fluid additives (primarily potassium, phosphorus, and dextrose) based on the results of the various bloodwork results. Physical exam findings dictated her fluid rate.

She remained in hospital for a total of 12 days but she was successfully discharged after treatment of both conditions.

Case study 2: Hit by car

Duke, a 9-year-old male neutered Standard Poodle (24 kg) presented to the emergency department 45 minutes after being hit by a car. Prior to the accident, Duke had previously been a healthy dog.

Upon presentation Duke was laterally recumbent and unable to stand. His vital signs were as follows: mentation dull but responsive, temperature 100.0°F (37.78°C), pulse rate 190–200 beats per minute, respiratory rate 50 breaths per minute, MM color pale, and CRT >3 seconds.

Box 1.2. Duke: Physical exam by body system.

- Integument: multiple abrasions and open wounds on the left rear leg, wound on right rear leg with open wound and visible fracture, abrasions of ventral abdomen
- Cardiovascular:
    - Thoracic auscultation: no murmur ausculted
    - Rate: tachycardia
    - Rhythm: sinus tachycardia
    - Pulse quality/pulse pressure: weak and thread pulses, synchronous
- Respiratory:
    - Thoracic auscultation: harsh lung sounds ventrally, dull lung sounds in the dorsal lung fields
    - Rate: 50 breaths per minute
    - Pattern: tachypnea with mild increased respiratory effort
- Gastrointestinal:
    - Abdominal palpation: soft nonpainful abdomen
    - Rectal exam: small amount of blood noted on glove, normal stool present
- Genitourinary: normal
- Musculoskeletal:
    - Ambulation: unable to stand at presentation
    - Range of motion: normal range of motion and palpation of both forelimbs, left rear limb has normal range of motion, right rear limb has open tibial fracture with bone protruding through the skin

Continued

> **Box 1.2. Continued.**
>
> - Neurologic:
>   - Cranial nerves: within normal limits
>   - Reflexes: forelimbs and left rear limb within normal limits right rear limb not assessed initially
> - Lymph nodes: within normal limits
> - Eyes: within normal limits
> - Ears: within normal limits
> - Oral cavity: blood coming from mouth, small wound on tongue
> - Body Condition Score (scale 1–9): 4/9

Point-of-care testing for Duke included: PCV = 45%, TS = 6.0 g/dL, BG 110 g/dL, lactate 5.4 mmol/L.

Diagnoses based on PE and POCT: Duke's diagnoses were shock, possible pneumothorax, and an open right tibial fracture.

Duke was diagnosed with shock based on his tachycardia, dull mentation, weak pulses, pale MM with delayed CRT, and tachypnea. Intravenous crystalloid and colloid therapy was initiated (see Table 1.11 to see the trends in Duke's response to therapy).

Due to concerns for pneumothorax based on his PE and auscultation, a thoracocentesis was performed and 1000 mL of air was removed from the right pleural space. Duke's breathing significantly improved after fluid therapy and thoracocentesis.

Duke was given flow by oxygen and further testing such as blood pressure, ECG monitoring, pulse oximetry, and an abdominal FAST scan (see Chapters 2, 3, 4, and 7 for more details regarding these monitoring modalities) to further characterize his condition. Blood was collected for laboratory testing.

Continued monitoring for Duke included checking his vital signs, repeat assessment of his mentation status, PCV/TP, and lactate. He was also monitored with continuous pulse oximetry, intermittent blood pressure readings, and ECG monitoring. His wounds were cleaned and covered during the stabilization period. See below for details regarding the trends in his status/POC testing and the therapies administered during this initial stabilization period.

Note that initially (time 0–55 minutes), Duke's clinical condition and lactate values seemed to indicate a positive response to therapy. He was more alert, seemed to recover from his shock, and showed a decline in the lactate values. However, at ~95 minutes after presentation, his PCV/TP showed continued declined along with an increase in the lactate. At the same time, Duke seemed to be quieter than previously and PE revealed an increase in the size of his abdomen, all of which implied a hemoabdomen. The presence of the hemoabdomen was confirmed by an abdominal FAST scan and sampling of the intra-abdominal fluid. He was resuscitated with a bolus of colloid fluids and an abdominal compression wrap was applied to tamponade the bleeding.

Attention should be paid to the decrease in the PCV and TP, particularly the disproportionate decrease between the two values. This is an indication of ongoing blood loss (loss of blood and proteins with a concurrent splenic contraction which blunted the drop in PCV), and, in Duke's case, was consistent with development of a hemoabdomen. The abdominal compression wrap was placed tightly for two hours (with observation that Duke could easily breathe with the wrap). When his clinical condition and PCV/TP seemed to stabilize, the abdominal compression was loosened gradually over 2 hours and completely removed 8 hours after presentation.

Duke was stable enough to go to surgery for fracture repair 48 hours after presentation. He was discharged from the hospital on day 6. Six weeks after discharge, Duke's fracture was healed and he was doing well.

Bibliography

American College of Surgeons (2008) *ATLS, Advanced Trauma Life Support Program for Doctors*. American College of Surgeons, Chicago, Illinois, USA, pp. 58.

Astrup, P., Jorgensen, K., Siggaard-Anserson, O., et al. (1960) Acid-base metabolism: new approach. *Lancet* 1, 1035.

Astrup P. (1961) New approach to acid-base metabolism. *Clinical Chemistry* 7, 1.

Table 1.11. Trends in Duke's response to therapy.

Time (minutes)	Heart rate (bpm)	PCV/TP (% / g/dL)	Lactate (mmol/L)	Assessment	Therapy
0	190–200	45/6.0	5.4	Lateral recumbency, dull mentation	Isotonic crystalloid bolus 22 mL/kg
20	180	–	–	Lateral recumbency, dull mentation	Isotonic crystalloid bolus 22 mL/kg
35	168	–	–	Sternal recumbency, quiet but responsive	Colloid bolus 5 mL/kg Fentanyl bolus 3 µg/kg
55	150	38/4.5	2.7	Sternal recumbency, alert and responsive	Continue isotonic crystalloid 120 mL/kg/day Fentanyl CRI for pain (3 µg/kg/h)
70	140	–	–	Sternal recumbency, alert and responsive, Exhibiting pain	Continue isotonic crystalloid 120 mL/kg/day Fentanyl CRI for pain
95	165	34/3.0	3.5	Sternal recumbency, but quieter than previous, abdomen noted to be distended	Repeat abdominal fast scan confirmed hemoabdomen, **apply abdominal compression wrap**, continue isotonic crystalloid 120 mL/kg/day, fentanyl CRI, colloid bolus 2.5µmL/kg
120	155	–	–	Sternal recumbency, continues to be quiet but responsive, abdomen no change	Isotonic crystalloid 120 mL/kg/day, **maintain abdominal wrap**, fentanyl CRI Antibiotics started (open fracture)
140	146	34/3.0	3.0	Sternal recumbency, quiet but responsive, abdomen no change	Isotonic crystalloid 120 mL/kg/day, **maintain abdominal wrap**, fentanyl CRI
160	138	30/3.0	2.5	Sternal recumbency, quiet but responsive, abdomen no change	Isotonic crystalloid rate decreased to 90 mL/kg/day, **maintain abdominal wrap**, fentanyl CRI
215	135	–	–	Sternal recumbency, but will change positions, more alert responsive, engaged, abdomen no change	Isotonic crystalloid rate decreased to 90 mL/kg/day, **loosen abdominal wrap**, fentanyl CRI
270	130	32/2.8	2.2	Sternal recumbency, but will change positions, more alert responsive, engaged, abdomen no change	Fluid rate decreased to 90 mL/kg/day, fentanyl CRI, **maintain loosened abdominal wrap**

CRI, constant-rate infusion.

Badgett, R.G., Lucey, C.R., Mulrow, C.D. (1997) Can the clinical examination diagnose left-sided heart failure in adults? *Journal of the American Medical Association* 277, 1712–1719.

Bakovic, D., Eterovic, D., Saratlija-Novaković, Z., et al. (2005) Effect of human splenic contraction on variation in circulation blood cell counts. *Clinical and Experimental Pharmacology and Physiology* 32, 944–951.

Bakovic, D., Pivac, N., Maslov, P.Z., et al. (2013) Spleen volume changes during adrenergic stimulation with low doses of epinephrine. *Journal Physiology and Pharmacology* 64, 649–655.

Chakko, S., Woska, D., Martinez, H., et al. (1991) Clinical, radiographs, and hemodynamic correlations in chronic congestive heart failure: Conflicting results may lead to inappropriate care. *American Journal of Medicine* 90, 353–359.

Champion, H.R., Sacco, W.J., Carnazzo, A.J., et al. (1981) Trauma score. *Critical Care Medicine* 9, 672–676.

Cichocki, B., Dugat, D., Payton, M. (2017) Agreement of axillary and auricular temperature with rectal temperature in systemically healthy dogs undergoing surgery. *Journal of the American Animal Hospital Association* 53, 291–296.

Chong, S.K., Reineke, E.L. (2016) Point-of Care Glucose and ketone monitoring. *Topics in Companion Animal Medicine* 31, 18–26.

Clark, B.W., Derakhshan, A., Desai, S.V. (2018) Diagnostic errors and the bedside clinical examination. *Medical Clinics of North America* 102, 453–464.

Conti-Patara, A., de Araujo Caldeira, J., de Mattos-Junior, E., et al. (2012) Changes in tissue perfusion parameters in dogs with severe sepsis/septic shock in response to goal-directed hemodynamic optimization at admission to ICU and the relation to outcome. *Journal of Veterinary Emergency and Critical Care* 22, 409–418.

DeLaforcade, A., Silverstein, D.C. (2014) Shock. In: Silverstein, D., Hopper, K. (eds) *Small Animal Critical Care Medicine*, 2nd edn. Elsevier, Ontario, Canada, pp. 26–28.

Dhatariya, K. (2016) Blood ketones: measurement, interpretation, limitations, and utility in the management of diabetic ketoacidosis. *The Review of Diabetic Studies* 13, 217–225.

DiMauro, F.M, Schoeffler, G.L. (2016) Point of care measurement of lactate. *Topics in Companion Animal Medicine* 31, 35–43.

Duarte, R., Simoes, D.M., Franchini, M.L., et al. (2002) Accuracy of serum beta-hydroxybutyrate measurements for the diagnosis of diabetic ketoacidosis in 116 dogs. *Journal of Veterinary Internal Medicine* 16, 411–417.

Erbach, M., Freckmann, G., Hinzmann, R., et al. (2016) Interferences and limitations in blood glucose self-testing: an overview of current knowledge. *Journal of Diabetes Science and Technology* 10, 1161–1168.

Gorman, L., Sharkey, L.C., Armstrong, P.J., et al. (2016) Serum beta hydroxybutyrate concentrations in cats with chronic kidney disease, hyperthyroidism, or hepatic lipidosis. *Journal of Veterinary Internal Medicine* 30, 611–616.

Guerci, B., Benichou, M., Floriot, M., et al. (2003) Accuracy of an electrochemical sensor for measuring capillary blood ketones by fingerstick samples during metabolic deterioration after continuous subcutaneous insulin infusion interruption in Type 1 diabetic patients. *Diabetes Care* 26, 1137–1141.

Hackett, T.B. (2014) Physical examination and daily assessment of the critically ill patient. In: Silverstein, D., Hopper, K. (eds) *Small Animal Critical Care Medicine*, 2nd ed.. Elsevier, Ontario, Canada, pp. 6–10.

Hart, S., Drevets, K., Alford, M., et al. (2013) A method-comparison study regarding the validity and reliability of the Lactate Plus analyzer. (2013) *British Medical Journal Open* 3, e001899.

Henderson, D.W., Schlesinger, D.P. (2010) Use of a point-of-care beta-hydroxybutyrate sensor for detection of ketonemia in dogs. *Canadian Veterinary Journal* 51, 1000–1002.

Hill, R.D., Smith, R.B. III. (1990) Examination of the extremities: Pulses, bruits, and phlebitis. In: Walker, H.K., Hall, W.D., Hurst, J.W. (eds) *Clinical Methods: The History, Physical, and Laboratory Examinations*, 3rd edn. Butterworths, Boston, Massachusetts, USA, Chapter 30.

Hopper, K., Silverstein, D., Bateman, S. (2012) Shock syndromes. In: Dibartola, S.P. (ed.) *Fluid, Electrolyte, and Acid Base Disorders in Small Animal Practice*, 4th ed. Elsevier, St. Louis, Missouri, USA, pp. 557–576.

Koenig, A. (2014) Hypoglycemia. In: Silverstein, D., Hopper, K. (eds) *Small Animal Critical Care Medicine*, 2nd ed. Elsevier, Ontario, Canada, pp. 352–356.

Lunn, K.F., Johnson, A.S., James, K.M. (2012) Fluid therapy. In: Little, S.E. (ed.) *The Cat: Clinical Medicine and Management*. Elsevier, Ontario, Canada, pp. 52–89.

Mathews, K.A. Monitoring fluid theraphy and complications of fluid theraphy. In: Dibartola, S.p. (ed.) *Fluid, Electrolyte, and Acid Base Disorders in Small Animal Practice*, 4th ed. Elsevier, St. Louis, Missouri, USA, pp. 386–399.

Maurer, C., Wagner, J.Y., Schmid, R.M., Saugel, B. (2017) Assessment of volume status and fluid responsiveness in the emergency department: a systematic approach. *Medizinische Klinik – Intensivemedizin und Notfallmedizin* 112, 326–333.

McMichael, M.A., Lees, G.E., Hennessey, J., et al. (2005) Serial plasma lactate concentrations in 68 puppies aged 4 to 80 days. *Journal of Veterinary Emergency and Critical Care*, 15,17–21.

Miller, J.B. (2014) Hyperthermia and fever. In: Silverstein, D., Hopper, K. (eds) *Small Animal Critical Care Medicine*, 2nd edn. Elsevier, Ontario, Canada, pp. 55–59.

Nguyen, H.B., Rivers, E.P., Knoblich, B.P., et al. (2004) Early lactate clearance is associated with improved outcome in severe sepsis and septic shock. *Critical Care Medicine* 32, 1637–1642.

NOVA Stat profile prime instructions for use manual. Available at: https://physiology.case.edu/media/eq_manuals/eq_manual_STAT_Profile_Prime_Instructions_for_Use_Manual.pdf (accessed 20 August 2019).

Rosenstein, P.G., Hughes, D. (2014) Hyperlactatemia. In: Silverstein, D., Hopper, K., (eds) *Small Animal Critical Care Medicine*, 2nd edn. Elsevier, Ontario, Canada, pp. 300–305.

Saugel, B., Ringmaier, S., Holzapfel, K., et al. (2011) Physical examination, central venous pressure, and chest radiography for the prediction of transpulmonary thermodilution–derived hemodynamic parameters in critically ill patients: A prospective trial. *Journal of Critical Care* 26, 402–410.

Schriger, D.L., Baraff, L. (1988) Defining normal capillary refill: variation with age, sex, and temperature. *Annals of Emergency Medicine* 17, 932–935.

Smith, V.A., Lamb, V., McBrearty, A.R. (2015) Comparison of axillary, tympanic membrane and rectal temperature measurements in cats. *Journal of Feline Medicine and Surgery* 17, 1028–1034.

Southward, E.S., Mann, F.A., Dodam, J. (2005) A comparison of auricular, rectal and pulmonary artery thermometry in dogs with anesthesia induced hypothermia. *Journal of Veterinary Emergency and Critical Care* 16, 172–175.

Wadell, L.S., Brown, A.J. (2014) Hemodynamic monitoring. In: Silverstein, D., Hopper, K. (eds) *Small Animal Critical Care Medicine*, 2nd edn. Elsevier, Ontario, Canada, pp. 957–961.

Weingart, C., Lotz, F., Kohn, B. (2012) Measurements of β-hydroxybutyrate in cats with nonketotic diabetes mellitus, diabetic ketosis, and diabetic ketoacidosis. *Journal of Veterinary Diagnostic Investigation* 24, 295–300.

Zaman, J.A. (2017) The enduring value of the physical examination. *Medical Clinics of North America* 102, 417–423.

Zollo, A.M., Ayoob, A.L., Prittie, J.E. (2019) Utility of admission lactate concentration, lactate variables, and shock index in outcome assessment in dogs diagnosed with shock. *Journal of Veterinary Emergency and Critical Care* 29, 1–9.

2 Blood Pressure Monitoring

Daniel S. Foy*

College of Veterinary Medicine, Midwestern University, Glendale, Arizona, USA

2.1 Basic Physiology and Anatomy

When discussing and evaluating blood pressure, the reference is almost always to systemic blood pressure. However, the two sides of the heart (more specifically the two ventricles) each create their own pressure; the right ventricle generates the pulmonary blood pressure, while the left ventricle generates the systemic (arterial) blood pressure (Fig. 2.1). The pulmonary circulation is a lower pressure system with systolic pressures normally ~25 mmHg. The systemic circulation is a far higher pressure system with the systolic pressures normally ~120 mmHg. This chapter will focus on the systemic blood pressure generated by the left ventricle.

Systemic blood pressure is first generated by the contraction of the left ventricle. Isovolumetric contraction increases pressure within the left ventricle until the pressure exceeds the resting (diastolic) pressure in the aorta. At that point, blood is ejected from the left ventricle into the aorta; the maximal pressure in the aorta achieved during the contraction phase of the left ventricle is called the *systolic pressure*. As the contraction phase of the left ventricle ends, the aortic pressure begins to drop and the aortic valves close, preventing retrograde flow of blood back into the left ventricle. The lowest aortic pressure achieved during the left ventricular relaxation phase is the *diastolic pressure*. The difference between the systolic pressure and diastolic pressure is the pressure that may be felt when palpating pulses and is termed the *pulse pressure*.

A pressure tracing can be created which illustrates the pressure in the aorta throughout the entire contraction and relaxation cycle of the left ventricle (Fig. 2.2). The area under this curve is the *mean arterial pressure* (MAP). The wide base and relatively narrow peak of this curve illustrates the MAP is almost always closer to the diastolic pressure than the systolic pressure.

Many factors are incorporated into the MAP, which is physiologically defined by the following equation:

$$MAP = cardiac\ output \times systemic\ vascular\ resistance$$

There are individually many components that can affect cardiac output. Cardiac output is defined as stroke volume (amount of blood ejected by the left ventricle per beat) multiplied by the heart rate (contractions per minute). Therefore, any factor that increases the *heart rate* (providing all other variables remain constant) will increase MAP, and any factor that increases the *stroke volume* (providing all other variables remain constant) will increase MAP, and vice versa. Heart rate and stroke volume are both affected by variables ranging from blood volume to neurohormonal factors affecting the return of blood to the heart and/or the passage of blood out of the heart into the vessels (Fig. 2.3).

Regulation of mean arterial pressure: Stroke volume

As the blood volume is increased in the body, the veins will generally increase the volume of blood within their walls. In most physiologic states, as the volume of blood in the veins increases, the pressure within the vena cava returning blood to the heart increases. The volume of returned blood will affect the degree of ventricular myocardial distension prior to contraction (i.e. increased return of blood causes increased ventricular distension). It is this myocardial distension which defines the *preload*. Therefore in most instances, as the blood volume increases, the return of blood to the right side of the heart increases and myocardial distension (i.e. preload) increases.

---

* Corresponding author: dfoy1@midwestern.edu

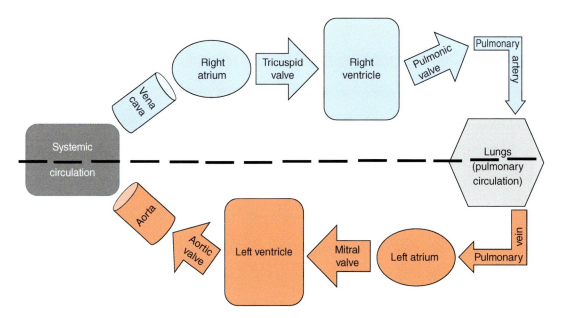

Fig. 2.1. A diagrammatic representation of blood flow through both the systemic and pulmonary circulatory systems. With the exception of the pulmonary artery and pulmonary vein, the dotted black line separates the venous blood flow (top) from the arterial blood flow (bottom). Oxygenated blood is represented by the red shaded symbols while deoxygenated blood is represented by the blue shaded symbols. Deoxygenated blood originating in the systemic circulation returns to the right-hand side of the heart via the venous circulation. Eventually all venous blood empties into the vena cava – the large vein that returns blood to the right atrium. This blood equates to the venous return. In a normal setting, the blood comprising the venous return passes through the tricuspid valve into the right ventricle. Right ventricular contraction then generates a pulmonary systolic pressure of ~25 mmHg and propels blood through the pulmonary artery into the pulmonary circulation where carbon dioxide is offloaded to the alveoli and the blood is oxygenated. This oxygenated blood leaves the lungs through the pulmonary veins and returns to the left atrium. The left atrial blood volume then travels past the mitral valve into the left ventricle where it is pumped past the aortic valve and into the aorta and the systemic arteries, delivering oxygen to the tissues. The pressure generated by left ventricular contraction creates the systemic arterial systolic pressure, which is typically ~120 mmHg.

Generally speaking, the same amount of blood pumped out by the right ventricle into the pulmonary circulation will return to the left side of the heart and be pumped into the aorta by the left ventricle. Thus, presuming normal myocardial function, increasing preload on the right-hand side of the heart leads to increasing stroke volume on the left-hand side of the heart. In other words, as long as the heart can pump the amount of blood it receives, the increasing venous return to the heart will lead to an increasing stroke volume. An increased stroke volume in a normal physiologic setting will lead to an increased blood pressure.

In addition to preload, stroke volume is also determined by inotropy (or contractility). Increasing inotropy means that as the preload increases (causing filling and stretching of the ventricular muscle), the ventricle will contract harder and more completely, ejecting more blood into the aorta. Increasing inotropy leads to increasing stroke volume and an increase in MAP (again, presuming no changes occur in other variables). Inotropy is under neurohormonal control and regulated by the autonomic nervous system. Sympathetic nerves and hormones (such as epinephrine and norepinephrine) increase inotropy and can increase blood pressure.

Regulation of mean arterial pressure: Heart rate

Heart rate is also under neurohormonal control and will increase with sympathetic nervous system stimulation. The sympathetic nervous system can increase blood pressure by increasing heart rate

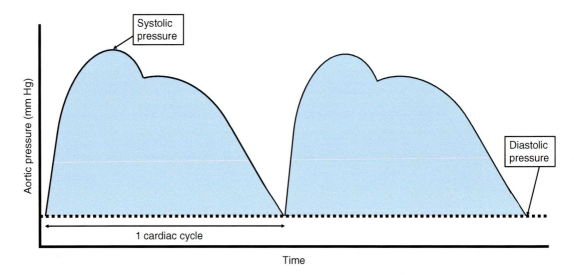

Fig. 2.2. A diagrammatic representation of the aortic pressure tracing over two left ventricular contraction cycles. The pressure in the left ventricle increases as the left ventricle contracts until the pressure in the left ventricle exceeds the diastolic aortic pressure and the aortic valve opens. Blood rapidly flows into the aorta, causing a rapid increase in aortic pressure until it reaches its peak pressure (also known as the systolic pressure). As the blood leaves the aorta and the left ventricle relaxes, the pressure in the aorta gradually declines back to baseline (diastolic pressure). The mean arterial pressure is represented by the shaded area under the curve – due to the wider base and narrower peak, the mean arterial pressure lies closer to the diastolic pressure than the systolic pressure.

and, therefore, cardiac output. In addition to the effects on heart rate and inotropy, the sympathetic nervous system also plays a major role in vascular tone and systemic vascular resistance (SVR). Increasing SVR will serve to increase blood pressure. Resistance of an individual vessel is inversely related to its radius; Poiseuille's equation explains that resistance is related to the radius raised to the fourth power. If the radius doubles, then the resistance will decrease by a factor of 16, and if the radius is halved, then the resistance increases by a factor of 16. Vascular tone is maintained by the smooth muscle surrounding the vessel. This muscle layer can relax (or dilate) to increase blood flow downstream of the vessel or can constrict to limit downstream blood flow; small changes in vessel diameter will have large changes in resistance and blood flow to tissues.

Regulation of mean arterial pressure: Systemic vascular resistance

The systemic arterial network includes large, medium and small arteries and arterioles, all of which have a smooth muscular layer that allows for maintenance of vascular tone. The small arteries and arterioles are the component of the network most responsible for SVR and the distribution of vascular tone. Beyond this network, capillaries, venules, and veins all exist but they are low-resistance vessels with little to no muscular tone, meaning that the vast majority of the aortic systolic pressure has dissipated by the time the blood reaches this part of the circulation. The systolic blood pressure decreases by approximately 50–70% as it travels through the small arteries and arterioles. This leads to a blood pressure at the arterial side of the capillaries that has dropped to 25–30 mmHg from the starting pressure of approximately 120 mmHg in the aorta.

A multitude of factors are involved in establishing a vessel's vascular tone. Extrinsic factors originate outside of the tissue in which the blood vessel is located. These factors include hormones such as angiotensin II and sympathetic nervous system stimulation, which tend to cause a more global change in vascular tone and therefore, SVR. Intrinsic factors arise from the vessel itself or local tissues and have a greater role regulating local blood flow; such factors include histamine, arachidonic acid metabolites, and oxygen tension.

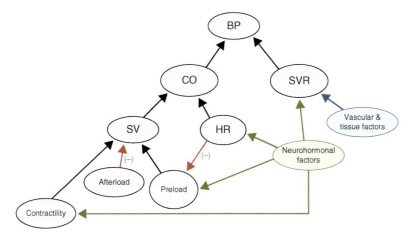

Fig. 2.3. A diagrammatic representation of the various factors affecting the cardiac output (CO) and systemic blood pressure (BP). The cardiac output represents the blood ejected out of the left ventricle into the systemic circulation over time. One of the determinants of the arterial blood pressure is the volume of blood that leaves the heart (CO). The other determinant of the blood pressure is the vascular tone or systemic vascular resistance (SVR). As the SVR increases, the blood pressure increases and as the SVR decreases, the vessels dilate and the blood pressure decreases. The cardiac output is in turn made up of the stroke volume (SV) and the heart rate (HR). The SV is the blood volume that leaves the left ventricle and enters the aorta during a ventricular contraction while the HR is the number of ventricular contractions over time. The SV increases as more blood is returned to the ventricle (the preload increases). The SV is also increased when the heart contracts more vigorously (has increased contractility) and when the afterload (pressure that the heart is pumping against) is lower (shown in the diagram by a minus (−) sign). Typically, as the heart rate increases, the CO increases. However, as shown in the diagram by the minus sign (−), if the heart rate increases too much, the ventricle does not have adequate time to relax and it will not fill completely (i.e. a decreased preload), leading to a decreased SV and decreased CO. Neurohormonal factors can have a wide array of effects on CO and BP. For example, systemic nervous system stimulation may improve SVR, increase HR, and increase contractility. In addition, the renin–angiotensin–aldosterone system may lead to improved SVR and improved water retention, which leads to increased preload. Local tissue factors (such as hypoxia or increased activity) can have regional effects on SVR.

Regulation of mean arterial pressure: Blood volume

Extrinsic factors not only play a role in the maintenance of vascular tone, but also in the regulation of blood volume. The renin–angiotensin–aldosterone system (RAAS) is involved in blood pressure regulation through control of both vascular tone and blood volume. The first component of the system (renin) is stored in the juxtaglomerular cells in the kidney, which are associated with the renal afferent arteriole. A drop in the renal afferent arteriole pressure leads to the release of renin. The juxtaglomerular cells can also release renin in response to sympathetic nervous system stimulation. Furthermore, cells (called the macula densa) within the distal renal tubules sense sodium and chloride concentration; a decrease in distal tubule sodium concentration also leads to renin release.

Once released into the bloodstream, renin acts on circulating angiotensinogen and cleaves angiotensinogen to angiotensin I. Angiotensin converting enzyme (ACE) lies predominantly in the pulmonary endothelium and further cleaves angiotensin I to angiotensin II. The formation of angiotensin II is critical to the clinical effects of the RAAS as angiotensin II acts as a potent vasoconstrictor (increasing SVR and blood pressure). At the same time, angiotensin II is involved in controlling blood volume. It stimulates sodium reabsorption within the kidney, increases aldosterone release from the adrenal cortex, and stimulates release of antidiuretic hormone (ADH, vasopressin) from the pituitary gland. Aldosterone also leads to sodium reabsorption largely in the distal tubule and collecting ducts of the kidney. As water generally follows sodium, reabsorption of sodium by any mechanism will lead to retention of water and, subsequently, an increase in blood volume. In addition to the RAAS system, ADH release also contributes to water reabsorption in the renal collecting ducts as well as vasoconstriction, and helps maintain an appropriate blood volume and pressure (Fig. 2.4). The RAAS is a common site of pharmacologic intervention in patients with hypertension (see Section 2.4, Interpretation of the Findings).

Regulation of mean arterial pressure: Local regulation of vascular tone

In addition to the various factors controlling systemic vascular tone and blood volume, the circulatory system has the ability to regulate vascular tone within individual tissues in order to deliver a relatively constant flow of blood to organs over a wide range of arterial pressures. This 'autoregulation' causes arterial blood vessels in a particular organ or tissue bed to dilate when exposed to lower perfusion pressure. The resulting arterial dilation improves blood flow to that tissue bed. Conversely, if the perfusion pressure should increase, the arterial vasculature will constrict to 'block' increased blood flow to tissues and help maintain more constant organ perfusion.

The ability of an organ to autoregulate blood flow varies. For example, the renal, cerebral, and coronary circulatory beds exhibit excellent autoregulation while the skeletal muscle circulatory bed shows only moderate autoregulation and the cutaneous circulatory bed offers almost no autoregulation.

Measuring the blood pressure

The diastolic pressure measured within the vessels is relatively constant when measured in the aorta extending distally to the larger peripheral arteries. In contrast, the systolic pressure and MAP increase over this same range in healthy patients. Again, the pulse pressure (which is appreciated clinically during physical examination), is the difference between the systolic and diastolic pressures.

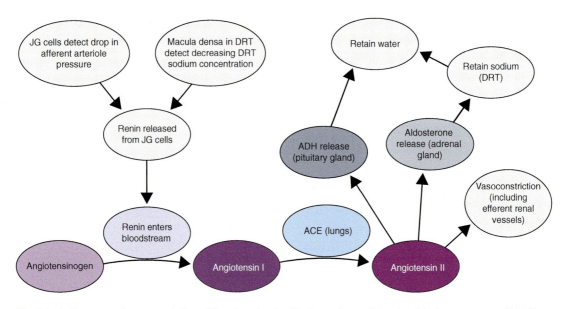

Fig. 2.4. A diagrammatic representation of the steps involved in the renin–angiotensin–aldosterone system (RAAS). The juxtaglomerular (JG) cells in the kidney detect a drop in the afferent arteriole pressure. In addition, the macula densa within the distal renal tubules (DRT) can sense a decrease in urine sodium concentration. Either change leads to the JG cells releasing renin. In the bloodstream, renin cleaves circulating angiotensinogen to angiotensin I. Angiotensin I is converted to angiotensin II by angiotensin converting enzyme (ACE), which lies predominantly in the pulmonary endothelium. Angiotensin II has multiple effects which can improve blood pressure: (i) vasoconstriction leading to increased systemic vascular resistance; (ii) release of aldosterone from the adrenal gland which leads to sodium and subsequent water retention in the DRT; and (iii) release of antidiuretic hormone (ADH) which leads directly to water retention. Water retention leads to increased circulating volume and improved cardiac output.

An approximate calculation for MAP has been written as:

$$\text{MAP} = \text{diastolic pressure} + \left(\frac{1}{3} \times \text{pulse pressure}\right)$$

A healthy aorta is relatively compliant and wall distension along with reflective waves maintains a lower pulse pressure in the aorta. Although the primary role of the aorta and large arteries is to act as a conduit for blood delivery to the tissues, a secondary role is to dampen the pressure changes that occur in the cardiac cycle. Approximately 10% of the energy produced during left ventricular contraction is directed toward distension of the aortic walls. During diastole, the distended arterial walls recoil and reflect energy back into the aorta and this energy continues to squeeze blood forward even while the heart is not contracting. This in turn helps ensure forward blood flow throughout both systole and diastole. The more compliant or distensible a vessel wall, the greater the wall recoil and return of energy to the vessel during diastole. Therefore, a more distensible vessel will have a diastolic pressure closer to the systolic pressure and a lower pulse pressure.

As blood travels away from the heart, the arterial walls become less compliant (increasingly stiff), which leads to an increasing systolic pressure as the stiffer arterial walls can no longer distend as easily with the pressure wave. As mentioned above, since the diastolic pressure does not exhibit as large a change as blood travels peripherally, the increasing systolic pressure leads to an increasing pulse pressure in the peripheral vessels versus the aorta. Visually this leads to a taller and narrower peripheral arterial pressure waveform versus the wider and less tall aortic pressure waveform shown in Fig. 2.2. Therefore, the *peripheral* non-invasive blood pressure measurements that are routinely obtained may overestimate the *aortic* systolic and pulse pressures. However, the MAP measured in the aorta versus the MAP in a peripheral vessel should be similar since the *area under the curve* remains the same despite the alterations in the waveform as the systolic pressure and pulse pressures increase (Fig. 2.5). The consistent MAP pressure is more important from a cardiac cycle perspective (compared to changes in systolic and diastolic pressure) as tissue perfusion is more aligned with the MAP than the systolic pressure.

Normal blood pressure readings for dogs and cats are listed in Table 2.1; however, as discussed later,

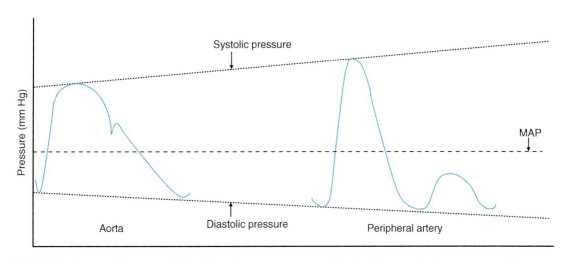

Fig. 2.5. A diagrammatic representation of how the pressure wave varies from the aorta to the peripheral arteries (where non-invasive blood pressure monitoring typically occurs). As the walls of the aorta are more compliant, these walls distend during systole and then recoil during diastole. This property causes some of the energy created during systole to be stored and then released by the walls of the aorta during diastole and has the effect of dampening the pressure changes in the aorta. The peripheral artery walls are less compliant and do not absorb as much of the systolic pressure. This leads to taller and more narrow pressure profiles in the peripheral arteries. However, since mean arterial pressure (MAP) is the area under the curve, this value remains relatively constant as blood travels from the aorta to the peripheral arteries.

Table 2.1. Normal blood pressure values in dogs and cats.

	Systolic blood pressure	Mean arterial pressure	Diastolic pressure
Dogs	90–140 mmHg	60–100 mmHg	50–80 mmHg
Cats	80–140 mmHg	60–100 mmHg	55–75 mmHg

many additional variables may interfere with precise non-invasive blood pressure monitoring. From this table, one may deduce that a normal or strong pulse pressure is 40–60 mmHg (i.e. the difference between the systolic and diastolic pressures).

2.2 How the Blood Pressure Monitor Works

Direct arterial blood pressure measurement

The gold standard method of measuring arterial blood pressure is via an arterial catheter, typically placed in a hindlimb dorsopedal artery. Although less commonly placed, femoral artery, auricular artery, or coccygeal artery catheterization may also be performed. The arterial catheter is in turn connected to a transducer via a continuous column of saline (i.e. direct arterial blood pressure measurement). The transducer converts the pressure to an electrical signal which is displayed on a monitor that amplifies the signal and filters the noise.

There are several important advantages to direct arterial blood pressure monitoring: (i) providing beat-to-beat monitoring; (ii) production of accurate readings at low pressures; and (iii) avoiding repeated cuff inflations. However, there are several disadvantages including discomfort and skill level required for placing the arterial catheter, risk of thrombosis in the arterial system due to catheter placement, and the challenge in maintaining a functional arterial catheter in an ambulatory cat or dog. Although direct blood pressure monitoring may be used with some frequency in anesthetized patients, anecdotal impressions suggest that maintaining function and patency of these catheters for >24 hours post-anesthesia is difficult.

For these reasons, in a clinical setting, indirect blood pressure monitoring is performed more frequently, especially in non-anesthetized patients. Indirect blood pressure monitoring is performed using either Doppler flow detection or oscillometry (see below for more details).

Indirect blood pressure measurement
Doppler

The Doppler flow detection unit (ultrasonic method) employs a probe containing two piezoelectric quartz crystals (Fig. 2.6). One crystal serves as the transmitter and emits a constant ultrasound wave at a set frequency (2–10 MHz). The second crystal functions as a continuous receiver. The Doppler unit probe has a concave surface which is placed against the skin surface (any fur must be shaved prior to placing the probe) and positioned over a peripheral artery parallel to the direction of arterial blood flow.

The ultrasound signal is emitted from the transmitting crystal and waves reflect back from moving red blood cells within the artery and are detected by the receiving crystal. These reflected waves have a different wavelength dependent on the velocities of the moving red blood cells. If the red blood cells are moving toward the probe, the sound wave frequency is increased and if the red blood cells are moving away from the probe, the sound wave frequency is decreased. The change in wavelength is

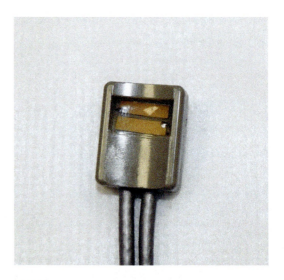

Fig. 2.6. A close-up photograph of the piezoelectric quartz crystals in the Doppler ultrasonic unit. One of these crystals serves as a transmitter and emits an ultrasound wave at a frequency of 2–10 MHz. The second crystal serves as a receiver.

termed the Doppler effect or Doppler shift; the difference in sound wave frequencies are converted to equivalent electrical impulses by the receiving piezoelectric crystal and are appreciated as a characteristic 'whoosh' noise with the pulsatile arterial flow. It is essential that the transmitter is placed over a blood vessel as movement (such as red blood cells) within the vessels is necessary to detect the Doppler shift. In this way, the change in frequency is amplified and audible to the person obtaining the pressure.

A cuff connected to a sphygmomanometer is required to obtain a Doppler blood pressure reading (Fig. 2.7). The circumference of the limb should be measured at the intended cuff placement site with a soft measuring tape and width of the selected cuff should be 30–40% of the limb circumference. The cuff is placed proximally relative to the peripheral artery where the Doppler probe will be located. When the cuff is subsequently inflated to a pressure greater than that within the artery, blood flow will be prevented. This effect will be clinically appreciated through a loss of the 'whoosh' sound.

Doppler blood pressure readings are typically obtained over the distal aspect of the limbs at the level of either the tarsus or carpus, or from the tail. Rather than a preference for one site over another, it is more important to be consistent in measurements and use the same site at each measurement period. In the forelimb, the medial palmar artery is appreciated just proximal to the metacarpal pad. The cuff should ideally be placed halfway along the antebrachium between the elbow and carpus (Fig. 2.8A). If using the hindlimb, the dorsal pedal artery can be detected just distal to the tarsus on the dorsomedial aspect of the metatarsus and the medial plantar superficial artery proximal to the metatarsal pad. Dependent on the artery used, the cuff on a hindlimb may be placed between the stifle and hock (Fig. 2.8B) or just distal to the tarsus when monitoring the dorsal pedal artery or the medial plantar superficial artery, respectively. When measuring blood pressure from the coccygeal artery on the tail, the cuff is placed at the tail base and the artery is identified along the ventral midline of the tail just distal to the cuff site.

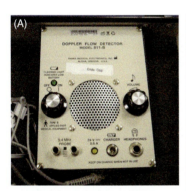
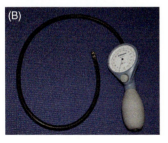
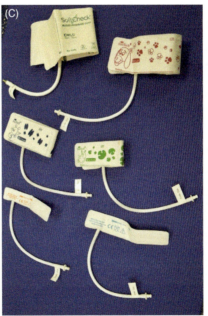
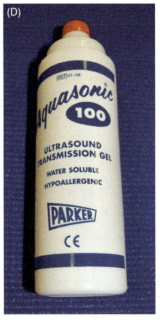

Fig. 2.7. The components (excluding the piezoelectric quartz crystals) used in obtaining a Doppler blood pressure. (A) The Doppler ultrasonic unit which processes the signal received from the piezoelectric quartz and emits sound. (B) A sphygmomanometer which is attached to the cuffs. The sphygmomanometer is utilized to inflate the cuff and the needle reflects the pressure (in mmHg) within the cuff. (C) An array of different sizes of cuffs used in both indirect blood pressure monitoring techniques. (D) The ultrasound gel which must be placed on the probe to permit transmission and reception of the ultrasound waves.

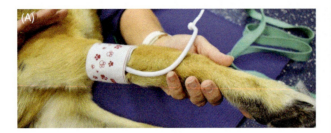
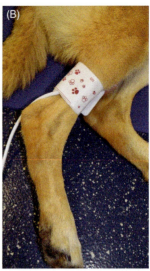

Fig. 2.8. The placement of cuffs when performing indirect blood pressure monitoring (similar location is used for both Doppler blood pressure measurement and oscillometric blood pressure monitoring). (A) The cuff is placed between the elbow and carpus when utilizing the forelimb's medial palmar artery for blood pressure monitoring. (B) The cuff is placed between the stifle and hock when utilizing the hindlimb's dorsal pedal artery for blood pressure monitoring.

The cuff should be placed snugly on the limb and secured with a hook and loop fastener on the cuff (Fig. 2.8). Occasionally, white medical tape can be used to augment the hook and loop fastener to prevent the cuff from opening up during cuff inflation. If tape is used, it should be placed loosely so as to not alter the pressure reading of the cuff during inflation. Prior to inflation, the cuff should be placed tightly enough that a finger cannot be inserted between the cuff and the patient's limb or tail.

The fur at the intended arterial detection site is clipped and ultrasound gel is placed on the Doppler transducer. Ultrasound gel is critical as air between the probe and the skin will not clearly conduct sound (Fig. 2.9). Once the 'whoosh' audible signal is noted, the transducer is held gently over the artery. It should be noted that excessive pressure should not be used to hold the transducer over the site as it may affect the blood flow and generation of an audible signal. The sphygmomanometer is then used to inflate the cuff until the audible sound is no longer heard. The cuff is inflated 20–30 mmHg beyond the point at which the sound is no longer audible and then the pressure is slowly released. The pressure at which the 'whoosh' sound is again heard represents the systolic blood pressure.

A change in the sound or a second sound may be noted as the pressure drops. This is theoretically

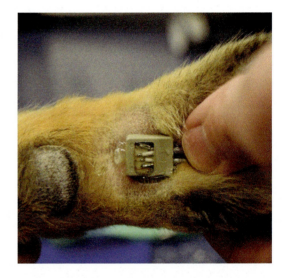

Fig. 2.9. The clipped fur proximal to the metacarpal pad. Ultrasound gel is placed on the probe and the probe is then placed against the skin and the position adjusted until an audible 'whoosh' is heard (this sound confirms the probe is detecting arterial blood flow).

representative of the diastolic pressure; however, the measurement of diastolic pressure is inconsistent and unreliable. Therefore, when using the Doppler in veterinary medicine, only the systolic pressure is documented. The initial Doppler measurement should be discarded as the patient may be acclimating to the environment or the sensation of the inflated cuff. As long as the measurements are reasonably consistent (i.e. within 10% of each other) and appear to have plateaued, between five and seven measurements should be recorded and averaged. If the measurements continue to drop or increase with subsequent readings, measurements should continue until a plateau is reached. In some situations (e.g. patient temperament), obtaining five to seven readings may not be feasible. As long as the obtained readings are relatively consistent, fewer than five to seven measurements may be acceptable.

Oscillometry

Oscillometry is the second method used for indirect blood pressure monitoring. The oscillometric unit (Fig. 2.10) is connected to a blood pressure cuff; the size of the cuff is selected in the same way as outlined above in the Doppler ultrasonic method (see Fig. 2.8). The oscillometric unit inflates the cuff to a pressure greater than the arterial blood flow; at that point, no arterial blood flow passes distal to the cuff and no wall oscillations are present. The unit then gradually deflates the cuff at a rate of 3–4 mmHg per second until arterial pulsations are detected. Once arterial blood flow returns, a slight increase in the blood volume of the limb occurs and the movement of blood past the cuff and through a partially compressed artery creates a detectable arterial wall vibration. The oscillometric unit detects these small arterial wall vibrations and the variation in the vibrations allows for assessment of the MAP, systolic, and diastolic blood pressures. The units commonly used in veterinary medicine measure heart rate and MAP and calculate the systolic and diastolic pressures.

The first pressure at which small oscillations are detected corresponds to the systolic arterial pressure. As the cuff is slowly deflated and the pressure decreases, greater pulsatile flow occurs, which leads to greater oscillations in the arterial wall. The peak amplitude of the oscillations is considered the MAP. Finally, as the cuff pressure is reduced sufficiently, blood flows normally through the artery, the arterial wall vibrations will no longer be detectable and this reading is considered the diastolic pressure. Although some units used in people do measure all three pressures, the units currently available in the veterinary marketplace use the data collected at different pressures to determine the MAP. Proprietary algorithms are then used to analyze the data and calculate the systolic and diastolic pressures. Based on the pulsatile flow and changes in cuff pressure, the oscillometric unit will also measure a heart rate. Specifically, the machine interprets each vibration or oscillation of the vessel wall as originating from the heart, and therefore, can determine a heart rate.

If the detected signal of arterial wall vibration is insufficient or inconsistent or the algorithm cannot convert the collected data into a calculated systolic or diastolic pressure, the unit will re-cycle and repeat the attempt to measure the patient's blood pressure. Dependent on the pulse palpation and numbers calculated for the systolic and diastolic pressures, the operator may determine if the readings are reliable. For example, if the palpable pulse pressure in a patient (e.g. physical palpation of a patient's femoral pulse) is subtle but a large difference is noted between the systolic and diastolic pressures reported by the oscillometric unit (i.e. reported systolic minus diastolic value is a large number), the operator may interpret the findings of the oscillometric unit as poor or potentially

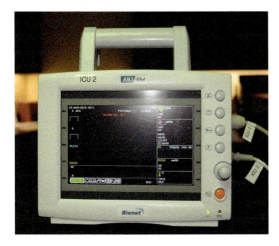

Fig. 2.10. An example of an oscillometric blood pressure unit. This unit is attached to a cuff and inflates the cuff to a pressure necessary to occlude arterial flow. The unit will gradually deflate the cuff (at a rate of 3–4 mmHg per second). As the cuff deflates, arterial wall vibrations are detected and the intensity and change in arterial wall vibrations allows the unit to measure the mean arterial pressure. Once the MAP is calculated, a proprietary algorithm is used to calculate the systolic and diastolic pressure.

inaccurate since large differences in the systolic and diastolic pressures should yield an easy-to-detect femoral pulse.

As mentioned above, the oscillometric unit should always report the heart rate at the time the pressure was measured based on the number of oscillations of the blood vessel detected per minute. It is important for the operator to ensure that the heart rate reported at the time of the blood pressure reading is accurate and representative of the patient's true heart rate. If a discrepancy is noted, the blood pressure measurement should be discarded since the unit was not able to accurately distinguish the blood vessel wall oscillations over time.

Similar to pressures measured using the Doppler flow method, the first oscillometric measurement should be discarded and the next five to seven measurements recorded and averaged to determine the patient's blood pressure. The oscillometric units require less technical skill than the Doppler ultrasonic equipment and have an advantage that they may be programmed to cycle at pre-determined intervals to obtain oscillometric readings over time.

Regardless of the indirect technique used, many studies have illustrated that indirect blood pressure monitoring is inconsistent and may not be representative of direct blood pressure readings. In an effort to reduce variability within a given patient, measurements should always be obtained consistently. The patient's position (recumbency), limb used for measurement, cuff size, and disposition should all be recorded to ensure repeatability. In addition, the indirect blood pressure monitoring modality used and environment (e.g. with owner, location/room used) should also be documented.

2.3 Indications

Which veterinary patients warrant a blood pressure measurement is not always easily determined and there are many factors that contribute to this debate. In addition, as discussed later, a blood pressure measurement that is consistently representative of the arterial blood pressure is not easily and predictably obtained.

Hypertension

When a clinician is concerned about hypertension, it is important to remember that some patients develop high sympathetic tone simply from traveling to or entering the hospital, and therefore will tend to have a higher blood pressure reading in the hospital environment than in their home environment. Furthermore, hypertension appears to be a relatively rare phenomenon in the healthy dog or cat. In the healthy pet population with a low incidence of disease, measuring a high blood pressure may be more likely to be a false positive measurement than truly represent hypertension. As a result, it is not recommended that healthy cats and dogs automatically have their blood pressure measurement obtained at every appointment.

There may be a reasonable argument to measure blood pressure in a patient periodically (e.g. 2–3 years old, 4–6 years old, and 7–9 years old) to establish a baseline of what may be normal in that patient in the event changes occur which do warrant blood pressure measurement. Age-related increases in blood pressure have been documented in people and a small (<3 mmHg/year) increase in blood pressure has been variably reported in dogs. The relationship between age and blood pressure in cats is not clear based on the current literature.

In contrast, there are several organs that are more susceptible to damage in patients suffering from hypertension, especially if prolonged. This damage is often referred to as target organ damage (TOD). When an animal exhibits signs of TOD during an exam, it warrants blood pressure evaluation. Target organs include the eyes, central nervous system (CNS), heart, and kidneys. The most common effect of hypertension on the eyes is retinal detachment. However, hypertension may also manifest as additional changes in the eye including retinal hemorrhage, retinal blood vessel tortuosity, retinal edema, hyphema, and retinal degeneration. Central nervous system changes may be referred to as hypertensive encephalopathy and can range from lethargy to seizures, altered mentation, and vestibular changes. Hemorrhage and infarction in the CNS have also been reported. Central nervous system changes are more likely to occur after an acute increase in blood pressure. Cardiac changes in response to chronic hypertension include murmurs, gallop rhythms, and left ventricular hypertrophy. Chronic hypertension also consistently increases the degree of proteinuria or albuminuria in experimental settings and may contribute to renal damage.

In addition, there are numerous diseases (see Table 2.2) that have been shown to have an association with hypertension. Dogs or cats with these diseases (or highly suspected of having these diseases) should

Table 2.2. Conditions known to be associated with secondary hypertension in dogs and cats.

Associated conditions	Examples
Kidney disease	Chronic kidney disease Acute kidney injury Glomerular disease
Endocrinopathy	Diabetes mellitus Hyperadrenocorticism (dogs) Hyperthyroidism (cats)
Neoplasia	Primary hyperaldosteronism Pheochromocytoma
Drugs	Glucocorticoids Mineralocorticoids Phenylpropanolamine Toceranib phosphate Erythropoiesis-stimulating agents Ephedrine/pseudoephedrine
Miscellaneous	Obesity Brachycephalic airway disease (dogs)

also have a blood pressure measurement performed. Furthermore, some drugs (e.g. phenylpropanolamine) are known to cause hypertension. Patients receiving such drugs should have their blood pressure routinely monitored before starting and while taking the medication. Dogs or cats receiving medication aimed at lowering blood pressure should also have their blood pressure monitored after starting therapy.

Hypotension

Hypotension usually occurs in more critically ill animals. Patients suffering from various forms of shock are at risk for hypotension and warrant blood pressure monitoring. Major presentations of shock include hypovolemic shock (e.g. marked blood loss either through external hemorrhage or internal/cavitary hemorrhage), distributive shock (e.g. anaphylaxis with diffuse vasodilation), obstructive shock (e.g. gastric dilatation-volvulus placing pressure on the vena cava and occluding the venous blood supply), cardiogenic shock (e.g. dilated cardiomyopathy leading to markedly reduced forward blood flow from the left ventricle), and septic shock. Animals with obstructive or distributive shock have a diminished venous return to the heart, which in turn leads to a decreased stroke volume and blood pressure (Fig. 2.3). Animals with cardiogenic shock experience decreased forward flow from the left ventricle and also have a decreased stroke volume/blood pressure (Fig. 2.3), while patients in hypovolemic shock have a decreased circulating blood volume which, when sufficiently diminished, leads to a decreased venous return to the heart (preload) and a subsequent drop in stroke volume and blood pressure (Fig. 2.3). Animals suffering from septic shock frequently exhibit multiple forms of shock as their illness likely leads to some measure of hypovolemia while the systemic inflammatory response may easily have a depressive effect on both cardiac function (inotropy) and maintenance of vascular tone.

Anesthesia can also be associated with hypotension for numerous reasons, necessitating blood pressure monitoring. Many anesthetic drugs cause cardiopulmonary depression (decreased heart rate or inotropy) or affect vasomotor tone leading to decreased SVR (Fig. 2.3). Positive pressure ventilation during anesthesia may lead to decreased venous return to the heart by compressing the vena cava or other components of the venous system, in turn decreasing preload and negatively affecting stroke volume (Fig. 2.3). Hypoxemia during anesthesia can deplete energy reserves and lead to peripheral vasodilation as individual tissues make efforts to preserve oxygen delivery. At a local level, such responses to tissue hypoxia are advantageous; however, if tissue hypoxia is more global, widespread peripheral vasodilation can contribute to hypotension. Moreover, hypercapnia occurring under anesthesia causes global smooth muscle relaxation as a direct effect of carbon dioxide on the smooth muscle of the vasculature. For many of these reasons, mild hypotension is frequently noted even in healthy animals undergoing anesthesia, and unhealthy animals are even more likely to display hypotension.

2.4 Interpretation of the Findings

A blood pressure measurement may be interpreted as either elevated (hypertension), normal, or low (hypotension).

Hypertension

When considering the potentially hypertensive patient, a reading <140 mmHg is generally considered to be normal. The vast majority (>80%) of hypertensive veterinary patients develop hypertension secondary to another disease process (see Table 2.2). Therefore, if a patient is assessed as hypertensive, further evaluation to deduce the underlying condition should be pursued and, if warranted, appropriate therapy for that condition should be implemented. The classification of the degree of hypertension is based on the risk of TOD and is outlined in Table 2.3.

Dogs and cats measuring in the range of pre-hypertension are not usually treated with antihypertensive medications. However, monitoring the patient's blood pressure more frequently (e.g. every 6 months) may be warranted to ensure the animal does not develop true hypertension.

If the patient is diagnosed with hypertension or severe hypertension, anti-hypertensive therapy is indicated. Efforts should be directed at diagnosing and treating any underlying disease while anti-hypertensive therapy is initiated. The goal for antihypertensive therapy in most cases is a gradual reduction in blood pressure over the course of several days with repeated blood pressure evaluation performed 7–10 days later. This slower adjustment is preferable because autoregulatory vascular function within the target organs, especially within the brain and kidneys, may have become relatively well-adapted to chronic hypertension. When that has occurred, sudden normalization or decrease in blood pressure may potentially lead to hypoperfusion within those organs. Therefore, treatment is initially started at the lower end of the dose range with a gradual increase in dose or frequency as indicated by the patient's clinical response.

Occasionally dogs suffer from a disease process that mandates specific therapy for hypertension (e.g. aldosterone secreting tumor requiring aldosterone blockade). However, in most cases, dogs are initially treated with drugs which inhibit RAAS (see Fig. 2.4). Angiotensin converting enzyme inhibitors (ACEi) are currently most widely used in veterinary medicine, but alternative options include angiotensin receptor blockers (ARB) and aldosterone receptor blockers. Both ACEi and ARB serve to block angiotensin II production. Common ACEi include both enalapril and benazepril, while the most studied ARB in veterinary medicine is currently telmisartan. Aldosterone blockage (e.g. spironolactone) can have antihypertensive effects by reducing blood volume. The effect is typically mild and this class of drugs is infrequently used in the treatment of hypertension.

One effect of angiotensin II is efferent arteriole constriction in the kidney glomerulus; therefore, angiotensin II blockade via ACEi or ARB induces efferent arteriolar dilation. This can have the effect of decreasing glomerular filtration rate (GFR). Therefore, care should be taken before starting either of these medications in dehydrated patients which may already have a decreased GFR. Whenever ACEi or ARB are prescribed, renal values should be monitored.

In addition, blockade of the RAAS, and specifically the aldosterone regulation of sodium and potassium, can lead to hyperkalemia; electrolytes must be periodically monitored in patients receiving ACEi or ARB, and require repeated monitoring as the drug dose is increased. Although hyponatremia is a theoretical concern, the degree of aldosterone blockade is usually insufficient to cause drastic changes in sodium; water movement with sodium typically maintains normal sodium levels.

In cases of severe hypertension, multimodal therapy is likely indicated and is achieved through a combination of RAAS inhibition and calcium channel blockade. Calcium channel blockers (CCB) function by preventing calcium entry into excitable cells. As calcium is critical to smooth muscle contraction, CCB cause smooth muscle dilation; this mechanism leads to a decrease in SVR and (presuming the cardiac output stays constant) a decrease in blood pressure (Fig. 2.3). Dogs should not receive CCB treatment as their lone treatment for hypertension as CCB have the effect of afferent arteriole dilation within the kidney glomerulus. This can blunt the protective effects of autoregulation in the kidney and subject the glomerulus to a greater degree of hypertension and potential damage. In some cases, CCB

Table 2.3. Categories of hypertension in dogs and cats.

	Pre-hypertensive (low risk of TOD)	Hypertensive (moderate risk of TOD)	Severely hypertensive (high risk of TOD)
Systolic blood pressure (mmHg)	140–159	160–179	≥180

TOD, target organ damage.

can also reduce GFR and lead to renal damage. Combination therapy appears safer for the kidneys as RAAS inhibitors preferentially dilate the efferent glomerular arteriole and the joined effect of both afferent and efferent glomerular arteriole dilation will ideally spare the glomerulus exposure to increased hydrostatic pressures. Even so, any patient receiving CCB even with RAAS inhibition should have renal values monitored. Amlodipine is the most commonly prescribed CCB used to treat hypertension in dogs and cats.

Cats receiving CCB therapy alone have not been shown to suffer the same ill effects on the glomerulus that have been documented in dogs. Therefore, the first-line treatment of hypertensive cats is generally amlodipine. Telmisartan (ARB) has been shown to be efficacious as single-agent therapy in hypertensive cats, although the efficacy has not been studied in severely hypertensive cats. In cats, ACEi are not recommended as first-line therapy as the reduction in systolic blood pressure is usually minimal (~10 mmHg) with those drugs.

The reader is referred to the Further Reading section for more detail on dosing and specific monitoring regiments for dogs and cats being treated for hypertension.

Rarely, a hypertensive crisis may become evident in a patient leading to acute severe TOD. Some potential causes for a hypertensive crisis include sudden catecholamine release from a tumor (e.g. pheochromocytoma), drug or toxin exposure (e.g. methylxanthines, phenylpropanolamine), or glomerulonephritis. Retinal detachment or acute central neurologic effects may be related to severe and/or acute hypertension. In such cases, 24-hour care is often necessary to control and monitor the hypertension using parenteral treatment titrated to affect. Precise recommendations for therapy do not exist at this time, but considerations include fenoldopam, labetolol, hydralazine, nitroprusside, and phentolamine. Please see the Further Reading section for more detail on parenteral treatment of hypertensive crises.

Hypotension

Decreased blood pressure, or hypotension, is the other extreme of blood pressure measurement. Hypotension is commonly appreciated during the evaluation of patients with varying causes of shock or in critically ill patients. Due to the potential effects of anesthetic medications on either myocardial function or maintenance of vascular tone as detailed in Section 2.3, documentation of hypotension in anesthetized patients is also quite common; anesthetic hypotension has been documented in >25% cats and dogs in various studies.

The body's autoregulation of the cardiovascular system suggests that a relatively constant delivery of blood to the organs exists with a MAP between roughly 60–160 mmHg in awake otherwise healthy animals. However, in disease or anesthetic states, the body's normal autoregulatory processes may not be fully maintained. Hypertensive cases typically focus on the systolic blood pressure to assess the risk of TOD (dependent on degree of blood pressure elevation or rate of change in blood pressure elevation). However, as the perfusion pressure is more closely related to the MAP than the systolic blood pressure, in hypotensive patients there may be a greater focus on the MAP than the systolic blood pressure. Although MAP is more associated with perfusion pressure, assessment of the MAP in a small and/or hypotensive patient may not be easily achieved, so degrees of hypotension are still often described in terms of the systolic blood pressure. The degree of hypotension may be classified as outlined in Table 2.4.

If hypotension is convincingly documented, steps should be pursued immediately to correct this condition as it can lead to death. The initial step, with rare exceptions (e.g. conditions marked by poor cardiac contractility such as dilated cardiomyopathy), is additional fluid support. Usually the first fluid administered is an intravenous crystalloid delivered as a fluid bolus. Multiple crystalloid boluses are often performed if the patient fails to show an appreciable or acceptable response. Colloid bolus(es) may subsequently be administered to a persistently hypotensive patient. Please see the Further Reading section for more detail related to fluid therapy in hypotensive patients.

Laboratory and routine examination and monitoring are also critical in the hypotensive patient to

Table 2.4. Categories of hypotension in dogs and cats.

	Mild hypotension	Moderate hypotension	Severe hypotension
Systolic blood pressure (mmHg)	80–90	60–80	<60

look for additional abnormalities that caused or contributed to the hypotension (or that might result from the hypotension). For example, electrolyte derangements (e.g. hypokalemia, hyponatremia) or hypoglycemia may also contribute to hypotension; a patient may not demonstrate an appropriate response to fluid therapy until those abnormalities are corrected. Marked hypokalemia (<3.0 mEq/L) leads to neuromuscular weakness and decreased smooth muscle function. Hyponatremia (≥5.0 mEq/L below the lower limit of the reference range) can be associated either with volume depletion with concurrent sodium loss or water retention associated with ADH release (diluting the sodium concentration). Therefore, in the former setting, hyponatremia may result in a decreased circulatory volume, contributing to hypotension. Hypoglycemia will interfere with appropriate smooth muscle function and potentially cause peripheral arterial vasodilation and a subsequent drop in blood pressure. Tachyarrhythmias or bradyarrhythmias found during an examination can both lead to hypotension that will not easily respond to intravenous fluid infusion (see Chapter 3). Also, profoundly hypothermic or hypoxemic dogs or cats will likely only show minimal blood pressure response to fluid support. Decreased cardiovascular function may begin to occur as the core body temperature drops to <97°F (36.1°C); vasomotor tone similarly cannot be maintained at low body temperatures.

Some patients remain hypotensive despite appropriate resuscitative fluid therapy and correction of laboratory abnormalities. In these cases, additional sympathetic support is recommended to improve cardiac inotropy and peripheral vasoconstriction. Norepinephrine and vasopressin are often the initial medications utilized to improve vascular tone and may be titrated to effect as a constant rate infusion. Some patients may have a greater need for positive inotropy and, in those cases, a dobutamine constant rate infusion should be considered. Please see the Further Reading section for more information on the use of positive inotropes and vasopressive drugs in dogs and cats.

2.5 Pitfalls of the Monitor

One of the greatest challenges with blood pressure monitoring in companion animals is obtaining measurements that the reader can be confident represent the true blood pressure. Currently, no indirect monitoring blood pressure device has met the human standards of validation in conscious dogs or cats. Therefore, results must always be critically evaluated and interpreted with caution and no blood pressure measurement should be accepted without also assessing the patient. Additional factors including the patient's presentation or condition, examination findings (e.g. capillary refill time, heart rate, pulse quality), and perfusion indices (e.g. lactate – see Chapter 1) should be considered as a component of indirect blood pressure monitoring assessment.

Machine/operator factors

Steps must also be taken to improve the reliability of the acquired measurements; the more trustworthy the monitoring, the more useful the readings may be for clinical decision making. For example, it is important to reduce the effect of situational hypertension on the measured blood pressure. Situational hypertension occurs when a dog or cat is especially anxious or excited, leading to falsely elevated blood pressure measurements. To attempt to reduce situational hypertension, patients should be allowed to acclimate to a quiet area for at least 5–10 minutes prior to taking any blood pressure measurements. All readings should be obtained with the owner present and ideally involved in restraint of the animal. The first blood pressure measurement should be discarded and the average of the subsequent five to seven readings should be calculated to represent the patient's blood pressure. When collecting the representative measurements, readings should only be accepted if they are reasonably consistent; readings with substantial variation (>10%) should also be discarded. If the readings continue to decrease, measurements should be repeated until a plateau is reached and then five to seven measurements should be obtained.

Patient movement can also affect the results (or ability to obtain an accurate measurement) in both Doppler and oscillometric units. Movement during Doppler blood pressure measurement can alter the probe placement over the peripheral artery leading to either a loss of signal or artifactual noise; this makes proper assessment of the 'whoosh' noise difficult to impossible. Motion during oscillometric readings can cause artifactual signals, making accurate detection of the arterial wall vibration difficult or inconsistent.

Changing conditions or personnel may also create inconsistency in blood pressure monitoring. It is important to be as consistent as possible when measuring serial blood pressures. The patient's position (e.g. left lateral recumbency), limb utilized for the measurement (e.g. right forelimb), and cuff size should be accurately recorded. In addition, the environment, patient's disposition or attitude, and indirect monitoring device should all be documented. The staff obtaining the measurements is also important as positioning of the patient, cuff location, and cuff tightness may vary between personnel. Subsequent checks should take pains to recreate a similar environment and condition each time a blood pressure is measured to reduce variability.

Frequent mistakes include the choice of cuff size, patient positioning, and the type of indirect monitoring equipment used. Cuff size is important as using too large a cuff will generally result in falsely low blood pressure readings. Conversely, using a cuff that is too small will result in falsely increased blood pressure measurements. Cuffs that are too small transmit pressure inefficiently to the underlying tissues, meaning a greater pressure than appropriate is necessary to occlude the arterial blood flow. The opposite is the case when too large a cuff is selected for the patient.

Blood pressure measurement (i.e. the location of the cuff) should occur at the level of the right atrium which is generally estimated by the location of the thoracic inlet in lateral recumbency or the point of the shoulder in sternal recumbency. Patients having a blood pressure measured while in a sternal or standing position often have significant vertical distance between the cuff site (usually on a limb) and the right atrium. This leads to false elevation of the blood pressure due to the weight of the blood column between the right atrium and the cuff site. If a blood column exists between the cuff site and the right atrium, the measured blood pressure includes both the actual blood pressure (generated by left ventricular contraction) and the weight of the vertical blood column which exerts force on the cuff.

An adjustment for the cuff distance (in centimeters; cm) below the right atrium may be incorporated to adjust the blood pressure and appropriately decrease the measured blood pressure. The cuff distance below the right atrium (measured in cm) can be subtracted from the measured blood pressure (in centimeters of water; cmH_2O). The measured blood pressure (in mmHg) can be converted to cmH_2O by multiplying it by a conversion factor of 1.36. However, this approach to blood pressure measurement is not advisable as it is difficult to accurately measure the distance between the cuff and the right atrium. Furthermore, precise positioning will likely be difficult to recreate for subsequent monitoring leading to poor repeatability of the measurement between time points.

All oscillometric measurements must be interpreted carefully. The unit provides systolic and diastolic pressures as well as MAP. When evaluating the results, the clinician must consider the quality of the pulse pressure on physical examination. The palpated pulse may be interpreted as strong, fair, poor, or absent, dependent on the situation. When the oscillometric unit displays the systolic and diastolic pressures, a calculated pulse pressure can be determined from the measurements (see Equation 2.2). On occasion the machine may provide either very wide/large or very narrow/small pulse pressures, and this data should be compared carefully with the clinician's impression of the pulse pressure noted during examination. As mentioned previously, a normal or strong pulse pressure is approximately 40-60 mmHg. If the subjective assessment of the pulse strength is inconsistent with the calculated pulse pressure, the result displayed on the oscillometric unit should be interpreted cautiously.

Likely attributable to difficulty sensing and assessing the arterial wall oscillations, cats and small dogs (<10 kg) should not have their blood pressure measured with oscillometric equipment as this tool tends to underestimate blood pressure. There is also some controversy as to the interpretation of Doppler blood pressure readings in small dogs and cats. Some sources state that Doppler blood pressure readings in these animals (especially in hypotensive patients) may be more representative of MAP than systolic blood pressure. However, there is no consistent research data to support this claim.

Patient factors

Patients with peripheral limb disease affecting the vasculature or interstitium may have unreliable readings by either indirect method. Any state of shock may create pulses with a lower pulse pressure, leading to a greater degree of difficulty in pulse detection and measurement. Furthermore, states of obstructive shock (such as gastric dilatation and volvulus) can compromise blood flow to the caudal aspect of the body and make blood pressure measurements on the tail or hindlimb very difficult to obtain. The presence of peripheral edema necessitates a greater pressure in the cuff to occlude arterial flow and subsequently will tend to overestimate systolic blood pressure.

Any condition causing peripheral vasoconstriction can compromise blood pressure readings. Detectable pulsatile flow is a prerequisite for indirect blood pressure monitoring. The foundation of the Doppler blood pressure reading is the reflection of ultrasonic sound waves off moving red blood cells. Without this detectable motion, the 'whoosh' associated with the unit cannot be obtained and the reading is not possible. The oscillometric unit also requires arterial pulsatile flow to generate the arterial wall oscillations; if these oscillations are absent or below the limits of detection, this measurement is also not possible. Patients with advanced shock are likely to have significant peripheral vasoconstriction as blood flow is directed to more critical organs. Hypothermic patients (e.g. secondary to shock, secondary to anesthesia, environmental exposure) will also experience peripheral vasoconstriction in an effort to minimize further heat loss. Some drugs (e.g. α-2 agonists) induce peripheral vasoconstriction and may cause inconsistent indirect blood pressure readings.

In some situations, indirect blood pressure measurement is simply not the ideal option for the patient. As mentioned above, no indirect device has met the human standards of validation for blood pressure measurement in dogs or cats and no indirect device continuously displays blood pressures. Patients at risk or suffering from either marked hypertension or hypotension or with rapidly changing blood pressures are more likely to benefit from direct blood pressure monitoring.

There are several examples of situations where patients should ideally have direct blood pressure monitoring. One example are those suffering from a hypertensive crisis and undergoing therapy, who may require accurate, minute-to-minute monitoring to evaluate both the degree of hypertension and the response to therapy. Also, as discussed previously, many patients with moderate-to-marked hypotension are also likely to suffer from peripheral vasoconstriction, further complicating accurate indirect blood pressure monitoring. Direct blood pressure monitoring enables more accurate initial assessment and evaluation of the patient's response to fluid and vasopressor therapy. A final example are animals which may be normotensive or only mildly hypotensive or hypertensive prior to anesthesia but are at risk for developing marked blood pressure changes during the surgical/anesthetic procedure (e.g. adrenal gland surgery, biliary surgery, thoracic/pleural space surgery, septic abdomen surgery). These patients should ideally be monitored via direct blood pressure measurements throughout anesthesia and for 24 hours post-anesthesia to allow for more rapid reaction to changes in blood pressure.

2.6 Case Studies

Case study 1: Hypertension

A 9-year old neutered male Labrador retriever is presented for acute onset of blindness. Vital signs are normal and the physical examination is unremarkable aside from a bilaterally absent menace response. The fundic evaluation reveals bilaterally detached retinas. Following that finding, blood pressure readings are obtained and the result of the Doppler unit measurement is 200 mmHg averaged over five readings. The readings are consistent with minimal variation and the patient is calm at the time of the measurements. The blood pressure is double-checked with an oscillometric unit and the reading is a systolic pressure of 205 mmHg, a MAP of 155 mmHg, and a diastolic pressure of 130 mmHg. The dog is diagnosed with severe systemic hypertension with evidence of TOD (the blindness).

Severe hypertension is unlikely to be effectively controlled with ACEi or ARBs alone, but dogs should not receive a CCB (e.g. amlodipine) without some measure of efferent arteriole dilation. Therefore, multimodal therapy is indicated in this patient. Options for starting medical therapy include ACEi (either benazepril or enalapril) at a 0.5 mg/kg dose likely administered twice daily combined with a CCB (likely amlodipine) at a 0.1–0.2 mg/kg dose administered once daily. An ACEi may be administered once or twice daily, but given the degree of hypertension, twice daily therapy would appear more appropriate in this dog. Another initial option would be the use of an ARB (e.g. telmisartan) at a 1 mg/kg dose administered once daily combined with amlodipine.

A common recommendation for blood pressure monitoring is to re-check the patient's blood pressure 7 days after institution or adjustment of therapy. Given this dog's severe hypertension and TOD, a blood pressure re-check is indicated within 1–2 days, and, if the patient's hypertension is not satisfactorily controlled, the dose of medication may be increased or a third medication may be considered. If the starting regimen is an ACEi combined with a CCB, then an ARB may be a reasonable third option. Alternatively, hydralazine (direct vasodilator) may be a more potent third option at a starting dose of 0.5 mg/kg twice daily.

In addition to the management of the dog's hypertension, further diagnostics are indicated to look for an underlying cause of the hypertension (Table 2.2). Considered diagnostics should include a minimum database (complete blood count, chemistry with electrolytes, and a urinalysis, potentially with the urine protein-to-creatinine (UPC) ratio also calculated). Imaging is frequently necessary and thoracic radiographs along with abdominal radiographs or abdominal ultrasound are options. CNS imaging (either through computed tomography or magnetic resonance imaging) may be indicated in patients with evidence of CNS TOD, but neither appear indicated as this patient was not noted to have other neurologic deficits.

In this dog's case, significant proteinuria was documented with a UPC ratio of 20.0 (reference: <0.5). The albumin was slightly low (2.2 g/dL); however, the renal values were normal. Thoracic radiographs were normal and an abdominal ultrasound was normal outside of diffusely hyperechoic renal cortices. Additional testing was performed after proteinuria was documented but a heartworm test, rickettsial polymerase chain reaction and antibody titer testing, aerobic urine culture, and a low-dose dexamethasone suppression test were all negative. The dog was presumed to have primary glomerular proteinuria and secondary hypertension. The dog was initially treated with benazepril at a 0.5 mg/kg dose administered twice daily and amlodipine at a 0.1 mg/kg dose administered once daily. In addition, the dog was switched to a commercial diet aimed at improved renal health. The systolic blood pressure remained elevated at 175 mmHg when checked after 7 days of therapy. At that time the amlodipine dose was increased to 0.2 mg/kg dose administered once daily. The blood pressure had decreased to a prehypertensive level with a systolic pressured measured at 150 mmHg after 7 days of the increased amlodipine dose. At that point, the UPC ratio had decreased to 11.2. A renal biopsy was recommended but declined by the owner and therapy continued unchanged.

Case study 2: Hypotension

A 5-year old spayed female Golden Retriever is presented for evaluation after three days of vomiting and anorexia with progressive weakness and lethargy over the last 12 hours. Abnormal vital signs include pyrexia (40.2°C) and tachycardia (180 beats/min). Physical examination abnormalities include pale pink mucous membranes, delayed capillary refill time (2 seconds), bilaterally weak but synchronous femoral pulses, and diffuse abdominal discomfort noted during palpation. Blood pressure readings are consistent and hypotensive using both the Doppler ultrasonic method (78 mmHg) and oscillometric machine (systolic pressure 75 mmHg, MAP 50 mmHg, diastolic pressure 40 mmHg). The dog's blood pressure readings are consistent with moderate hypotension and the physical examination findings are consistent with a patient who may be hypotensive (evidence of decompensatory shock with weak pulses, tachycardia, pallor and lethargy).

Treatment of hypotension typically addresses fluid deficits prior to pharmacologic intervention. A peripheral intravenous catheter was placed expeditiously and blood was collected from the catheter to perform a complete blood count, chemistry profile, and possibly a lactate measurement. Once the intravenous catheter was placed, replacement crystalloid fluids (Normosol-R) was administered as a bolus. This dog was given a quarter of her 90 mL/kg shock fluid bolus (~22 mL/kg) over 10–15 minutes. Due to only a partial improvement in the monitored parameters (heart rate reduced to 160 beats/min and Doppler blood pressure increased to only 85 mmHg), the same ~22 mL/kg bolus was repeated. After another only marginal improvement (heart rate reduced to 150 beats/min and Doppler blood pressure increased to only 90 mmHg), a 5 mL/kg colloid bolus (e.g. hydroxyethyl starch) was administered over 10–15 minutes. A more substantial improvement was noted after the colloid bolus (heart rate reduced to 130 beats/min, capillary refill time improved to 1–2 seconds, and Doppler blood pressure increased to 110 mmHg).

While performing the necessary fluid boluses, a rapid abdominal ultrasound scan revealed free fluid. Sampling of the fluid revealed a marked inflammatory response with both degenerate and non-degenerate neutrophils. Many of the neutrophils contained rod bacteria, and the diagnosis of septic peritonitis was confirmed in this patient. A full abdominal ultrasound was later performed that confirmed a small intestinal foreign body; intestinal perforation secondary to the foreign body was highly suspected at that time and emergency surgery was indicated for the patient.

Regardless of the dog's response to the intravenous fluids administered after presentation, she is at a high risk of further hypotension once under anesthesia (many commonly used inhalant drugs have vasodilatory effects) and her cardiovascular status is likely to be further compromised. In order to provide the greatest chance of a successful anesthetic experience and diminish secondary organ damage, it is essential that efforts are directed toward maintaining appropriate blood pressure both throughout anesthesia and in the hours following surgery. Important considerations prior to anesthesia include ensuring the patient is volume replete and placement of an arterial catheter for direct blood pressure monitoring.

Continuous rate infusion (CRI) of multiple pharmacologic agents may be necessary and potential drugs can be prepared prior to surgery to improve response time under anesthesia. Consideration is given to sympathomimetics for their vasopressor effects; these drugs have short half-lives (only 2–3 minutes) and need to be administered as a CRI. In this case, norepinephrine was infused at 0.1 µg/kg/min (epinephrine infused at 0.01–0.03 µg/kg/min is another consideration). Additional vasopressor support was necessary and was provided by the use of vasopressin at a rate of 0.002 IU/kg/min. A concern with vasopressors is that the vasoconstriction (and increase in SVR) may increase blood pressure readings, but this change may not be associated with an increase in cardiac output and perfusion. Therefore, these drugs should be used for as short a period as possible. Positive inotropic therapy may be combined with the aforementioned vasopressor therapy; dobutamine improves cardiac output through β-1 receptor stimulation. In this case, dobutamine was infused at a rate of 3 µg/kg/min. Sympathomimetic drugs have the potential to cause cardiac arrhythmias and electrocardiographic monitoring should be available during such infusions. Following anesthesia, continued care must be directed at blood pressure monitoring, maintenance of appropriate fluid balance, and pharmacologic intervention.

Further Reading

Acierno, M.J., Labato, M.A. (2005) Hypertension in renal disease: diagnosis and treatment. *Clinical Techniques in Small Animal Practice* 20, 23–30.

Acierno, M.J., Brown, S., Coleman, A.E., Jepson, R.E., Papich, M., et al. (2018) ACVIM consensus statement: guidelines for the identification evaluation, and management of systemic hypertension in dogs and cats. *Journal of Veterinary Internal Medicine* 32, 1803–1822.

Berger, A. (2001) Oscillatory blood pressure monitoring devices. *British Medical Journal* 323, 919.

Bodey, A.R., Michell, A.R. (1996) Epidemiological study of blood pressure in domestic dogs. *Journal of Small Animal Practice* 37, 116–125.

Crowe, D.T., Spreng, D.E. (1995) Doppler assessment of blood flow and pressure in surgical and critical care patients. In: Bonagura, J.D. (ed.) *Kirk's Current Veterinary Therapy XII*. W.B. Saunders, Philadelphia, Pennsylvania, USA, pp. 113–119.

Duke-Novakovski, T. (2017) Basics of monitoring equipment. *The Canadian Veterinary Journal* 58, 1200–1208.

Duke-Novakovski, T., Carr, A. (2015) Perioperative blood pressure control and management. *Veterinary Clinics of North America: Small Animal Practice* 45, 965–981.

Jepson, R. (2011) Feline systemic hypertension: classification and pathogenesis. *Journal of Feline Medicine and Surgery* 13, 25–34.

Joles, J.A. (1998) Obesity in dogs: effects on renal function, blood pressure, and renal disease. *Veterinary Quarterly* 20, 117–120.

Klabunde, R.E. (2016) Cardiovascular physiology concepts. Available at: www.cvphysiology.com (accessed 21 July 2019).

Mazzaferro, E.M. (2009) Arterial catheterization. In: Silverstein, D.C., Hopper, K. (eds) *Small Animal Critical Care Medicine*. Saunders, St. Louis, Missouri, USA, pp. 206–208.

Remillard, R.L., Ross, J.N., Eddy, J.B. (1991) Variance of indirect blood pressure measurements and prevalence of hypertension in clinically normal dogs. *American Journal of Veterinary Research* 52, 561–565.

Rondeau, D.A., Mackalonis, M.E., Hess, R.S. (2013) Effect of body position on indirect measurement of systolic arterial blood pressure in dogs. *Journal of the American Veterinary Medical Association* 242, 1523–1527.

Simmons, J.P., Wohl, J.S. (2009) Hypotension. In: Silverstein, D.C., Hopper, K. (eds) *Small Animal Critical Care Medicine*. Saunders, St. Louis, Missouri, USA, pp. 27–30.

Stepien, R.L. (2011) Feline systemic hypertension: diagnosis and management. *Journal of Feline Medicine and Surgery* 13, 35–43.

Vincent, J. (2008) Understanding cardiac output. *Critical Care* 12, 174–176.

Whittemore, J.C., Nystrom, M.R., Mawby, D.I. (2017) Effects of various factors on Doppler ultrasonographic measurements of radial and coccygeal arterial blood pressure in privately owned, conscious cats. *Journal of the American Veterinary Medical Association* 250, 763–769.

3 Electrocardiography

JESSICA L. WARD*

Iowa State University, Ames, Iowa, USA

3.1 Physiology: How Does Normal Cardiac Conduction Occur?

Before cardiac myocytes can contract (and thus before the heart can beat), myocytes must first receive electrical signals that cause cellular depolarization. The goal of an electrocardiogram (ECG) is to depict these electrical events involved in cardiac conduction. Waves of depolarization and repolarization are sensed using metal electrodes placed around the body, and electrical activity is represented as deflections on graph paper. In order to understand ECGs, one must first understand how electricity normally moves through the heart (see Fig. 3.1).

Normal cardiac conduction begins with depolarization of the *sinoatrial (SA) node*, a small group of cells located high in the right atrium that has the fastest rate of spontaneous diastolic depolarization of any cardiac tissue. In other words, the SA node 'fires' fastest; therefore, in normal animals, the SA node sets the pace of the heart. From the SA node, the wave of depolarization travels cell-to-cell throughout the atria, creating the *P wave* on ECG (see Table 3.1 and Fig. 3.2). The impulse also travels along specialized interatrial tracts to the *atrioventricular (AV) node*, located low in the right atrium near the tricuspid valve and interventricular septum. Impulse conduction slows in the AV node during the *PR interval* (also called the PQ interval), giving time for active atrial contraction to occur before the ventricles depolarize. AV nodal delay allows extra blood from atrial contraction (the 'atrial kick') to augment passive ventricular filling, thus increasing stroke volume. In the normal heart, the AV node is the *only* pathway by which electrical stimulation can travel from the atria to the ventricles; the top and bottom of the heart are electrically 'insulated' from one another (no electrical conduction tissue present) at all locations other than the AV node. From the AV node, the wave of depolarization crosses from atria to ventricles through the *bundle of His*, and splits into left and right *bundle branches* that subdivide further before terminating as *Purkinje fibers* (see Fig. 3.1). Depolarization of ventricular myocytes follows as the *QRS complex*, normally the tallest and most distinctive waveform on the ECG. The specialized ventricular conduction pathway (His bundle, bundle branches, and Purkinje fibers) quickly spreads the electrical impulse throughout the ventricles, allowing rapid ventricular depolarization and synchronous ventricular contraction. This pathway allows the normal QRS complex to be relatively narrow (approximately the same width as the P wave), despite representing electrical activity for a much larger mass of tissue (ventricles versus atria). If the specialized conduction pathway cannot be utilized for some reason, the ventricles must depolarize cell-to-cell, resulting in QRS complexes that are wide and bizarre. After ventricular depolarization has completed, ventricular repolarization follows, represented by the T wave on ECG.

Knowing how normal cardiac conduction is depicted on an ECG allows identification of abnormal electrical activity within the heart. If P waves are absent, then the atria did not depolarize. If a P wave is present with no QRS complex following, then electrical conduction was 'blocked' at the level of the AV node. If QRS complexes are wide and bizarre, then the ventricles depolarized cell-by-cell rather than using the specialized ventricular conduction pathway; this can occur if the impulse originated within the ventricles (as with ventricular premature complexes) or if delay occurred within the specialized conduction system (as with bundle branch block).

The rate of SA node depolarization, as well as the rate of AV nodal conduction, are regulated by

---

*Corresponding author: jward@iastate.edu

the autonomic nervous system. Stimuli that increase sympathetic nervous system (SNS) activity (causing increased β1-adrenergic stimulation to the heart) will increase the rate of SA node depolarization and AV nodal conduction (see Table 3.2). In contrast, stimuli that increase parasympathetic nervous system (PNS) activity (causing increased vagal stimulation to the heart) will decrease the rate of SA node depolarization and AV nodal conduction (see Table 3.2). The two arms of the autonomic nervous system thus have a major influence on heart rate and occurrence of certain ECG abnormalities discussed in this chapter.

3.2 The Monitor: How Does an ECG Machine Work?

The ideal way to measure cardiac conduction is to place catheters inside the heart that can measure electrical activation at each point within the heart. Obviously, this is not practical in most settings. Instead, metal *electrodes* are placed on the outside of the body to measure electric potentials moving between them. The pattern of electric potentials measured on the body surface can be used to infer how electricity is moving through the heart. For example, if electricity is measured moving from an electrode placed on the right forelimb to an electrode on the left forelimb, then one can infer that the electricity moved from right to left within the heart.

An ECG *lead* is created by placing two electrodes on opposite 'sides' of the heart in some configuration (for example, on the right and left forelimbs, or on the left forelimb and left hindlimb). The ECG machine arbitrarily labels one electrode in the pair as the 'positive' electrode and one as the 'negative' electrode. When the ECG detects electricity moving *towards the positive electrode*, the machine creates a *positive deflection* on the screen or paper for that lead. When the ECG detects electricity moving away from the positive electrode (*towards the negative electrode*), the machine creates a *negative deflection* on the screen or paper for that lead. Finally, if electricity is moving exactly perpendicular to the two electrodes, no deflection is recorded for that lead (termed *isoelectric*).

Having multiple leads allows the ECG to 'look' at electricity moving through the heart from different angles. The most common electrode and lead configuration involves three electrodes

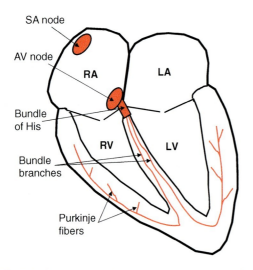

Fig. 3.1. Schematic depiction of the cardiac conduction system. See text for details. RA, right atrium; RV, right ventricle; LA, left atrium; LV, left ventricle; SA, sinoatrial; AV, atrioventricular.

Table 3.1. Events in cardiac conduction as depicted on an ECG.

Depolarization of this structure	Causes this waveform on an ECG
Sinoatrial node	Before P wave
Atria	P wave
Atrioventricular node	PR interval
His bundle / bundle branches	PR interval
Ventricles	QRS complex Q = first negative deflection R = first positive deflection S = first negative deflection after R wave
Ventricular repolarization	T wave

placed on the right forelimb, left forelimb, and left hindlimb. Sometimes a fourth 'grounding' electrode is placed on the right hindlimb to reduce electrical interference. In this configuration, the limbs act as volume conductors of electricity, so placing the electrodes as distal as feasible generally improves the recording. By convention in the United States, colored electrodes are placed as follows: white electrode on the right forelimb; black electrode on the left forelimb; red electrode on the left hindlimb; and the optional green 'grounding' electrode on the right hindlimb. When using standard right lateral positioning for recording ECGs, a number of mnemonic devices can be used to recall proper color configuration; these include 'white on right, smoke above fire' (black cranial to red), and 'snow (white) and grass (green) are on the ground; Christmas (red and green) comes at the end of the year (caudal end of the animal)' (Fig. 3.3). Tips for electrode placement and reducing artifact are listed in Box 3.1.

Relationships between pairs of these electrodes are then used to generate the three *bipolar leads*. *Lead I* represents electricity moving from the right forelimb electrode (white) to the left forelimb electrode (black). *Lead II* represents electricity moving from the right forelimb electrode (white) to the left hindlimb electrode (red). *Lead III* represents electricity moving from the left forelimb (black) to the left hindlimb (red). These three bipolar leads are often represented as an equilateral triangle showing electrical potential moving in three different directions, each separated by an angle of 60 degrees (see Fig. 3.3). Advanced ECG machines are also capable of comparing electric potential from one of these three electrodes to an *average* of the other two electrodes, generating *augmented unipolar leads* (aVR, aVL, and aVF). Addition of augmented unipolar leads to bipolar leads allows evaluation of electrical potential at 30-degree intervals around the entire heart.

Although evaluation of multiple leads can be useful to calculate the exact overall vector of ventricular depolarization for a patient (termed the *mean electrical axis*), in practice, most clinically relevant information can be obtained from a single-lead tracing. Most ECG monitors used in emergency settings or for anesthetic monitoring display only one lead at a time. *Lead II is most commonly chosen for single-lead evaluation because it evaluates electricity along a path that*

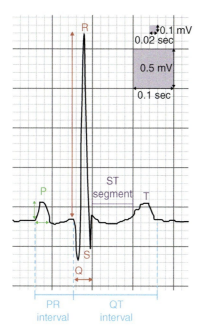

Fig. 3.2. Labeling portions of the ECG waveform. The following example ECG is recorded at a paper speed of 25 mm/s with calibration 1 cm = 1 mV. Image courtesy of Dr. Melissa Tropf.

Table 3.2. Common causes of sympathetic and parasympathetic activation that can influence rate of depolarization of the SA and AV nodes.

Causes of SNS activation (increased 'sympathetic tone')	Causes of PNS activation (increased 'vagal tone')
Pain	Drugs/toxins (opioids, digoxin, general anesthesia)
Anxiety/excitement/exercise	Ocular disease
Hypovolemia (or any cause of circulatory shock)	Central nervous system disease
Congestive heart failure	Respiratory disease
Drugs/toxins (methylxanthines, ketamine, methamphetamines, anticholinergics)	Gastrointestinal disease

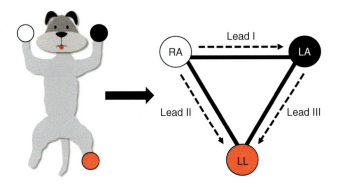

Fig. 3.3. Electrode placement and directionality for three bipolar leads (lead I, II, III). RA, right atrium; LA, left atrium, LL, left hind limb.

Box 3.1. Tips for performing a high-quality ECG.

Patient positioning: lateral recumbency preferred; right lateral recumbency is the standard for ECG complex measurements

Electrode placement: clip or attach metal electrodes to skin folds on the appropriate limbs, as distally as feasible (based on skin tautness)

Electrical contact: apply isopropyl alcohol or conductive paste to the electrode–skin interface (avoid alcohol if defibrillation may be required)

Reducing artifact: avoid crossing/touching wires; avoid contact between electrodes and other metal; avoid nearby electronic devices; reduce patient trembling/panting/purring

---

most closely approximates normal ventricular conduction. Recall that in a normal heart, the ventricles depolarizes *cranial to caudal* and *right to left*. This occurs because the wave of ventricular depolarization comes from the AV node in the right atrium, and terminates with individual myocyte depolarization within the more massive left ventricle. Among bipolar leads, lead II (right forelimb to left hindlimb) most closely approximates this path. QRS complexes should normally be positively deflected in lead II. Negatively deflected QRS complexes in lead II are abnormal in cats and dogs, and suggest abnormal ventricular myocyte mass (e.g. right ventricular hypertrophy) or abnormal ventricular conduction (e.g. ventricular origin of QRS complexes or bundle branch block). Evaluation of lead II is sufficient to diagnose *heart rate* and *heart rhythm*, which are the most critical components of ECG analysis in the emergency setting.

Recall that ECGs are simply lines on graph paper that show electrical potential (on the Y-axis) plotted over time (on the X-axis) for a given lead (direction between two electrodes). Once an ECG tracing is generated, the operator can manipulate several aspects of how the ECG appears visually, based on how electrical signals are translated into linear deflections. All ECGs are printed on graph paper standardized such that one small box measures 1 mm in length and height (and therefore one large box measures 5 mm); but the operator can control how these measures of *length (mm)* are translated into either *electrical potential (mV)* on the Y-axis or *time (s)* on the X-axis. First, the operator can adjust the ECG *calibration* or *amplitude*, meaning how tall the Y-axis deflections will be for a given amount of electrical potential. Using 'standard' ECG calibration, detection of 1 mV of electrical potential results in a deflection that is 1 cm 'high' on the graph paper (1 cm = 1 mV). However, for patients with very small QRS complexes (especially cats), it may be useful to change calibration such that 1 mV of electrical potential results in a deflection that is 2 cm 'high' (2 cm = 1 mV), or vice versa for patients with very large QRS complexes (0.5 cm = 1 mV).

Second, operators can adjust *paper speed*, meaning how quickly time passes along the X-axis.

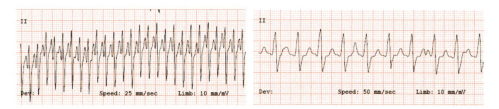

Fig. 3.4. Relationship between length (mm) and time (s) on the graph paper used for ECGs. One 'small box' always measures 1 mm in length, while one 'large box' always measures 5 mm. 'Slower' paper speed (25 mm/s) makes ECG complexes appear narrower, since more heartbeats occur within a given length of paper. 'Faster' paper speed (50 mm/s) makes ECG complexes appear wider, since fewer heartbeats occur within the same length of paper. The figure shows two ECGs taken from the same patient at the same time, shown at 25 mm/s and 50 mm/s.

Changing paper speed will change how complexes appear on an ECG: 'faster' paper speed will make complexes appear wider (think of the paper being 'pulled out' of the machine more quickly while deflections are being recorded), while 'slower' paper speed will make complexes appear narrower (Fig. 3.4). The most commonly used paper speed for patient monitoring and rhythm diagnosis is 25 mm/s, while the standard paper speed for measuring ECG complexes is 50 mm/s. At a paper speed of 25 mm/s, each small box represents 0.04 s (40 ms), and each large box represents 0.2 s (200 ms). At a paper speed of 50 mm/s, each small box represents 0.02 s (20 ms), and each large box represents 0.1 s (100 ms).

A recent advancement in heart rate and rhythm monitoring in veterinary patients is the existence of smartphone applications to analyze and record ECG tracing (e.g. Alivecor, Kardia Mobile). A small rectangular device consisting of two metal electrodes is placed directly over the chest wall (using alcohol ± coupling gel) oriented with one electrode on either side of the heart. An ECG tracing is transmitted wirelessly to a nearby smartphone. The tracing can be viewed in real time or recorded/downloaded as a PDF file that can subsequently be emailed to veterinarians or other caregivers. Because of the electrode configuration, smartphone ECGs project only a single 'base–apex' lead (rather than the bipolar leads I–III). These tracings cannot be used to calculate mean electrical axis or perform P-QRS-T complex measurements, but smartphone ECG apps have shown good agreement with traditional ECGs for calculation of heart rate and determination of heart rhythm. Similar to other ECG systems, the smartphone user interface allows manipulation of paper speed and calibration.

3.3 Indications: What Can an ECG Monitor Tell You?

ECGs depict how electricity moves through the heart. This provides a number of different pieces of information that differ in clinical relevance and whether the ECG is the 'best' tool to obtain that information. Potential uses of ECGs are outlined in Table 3.3. Fundamentally, ECGs are most useful for *calculation of heart rate* and *determination of heart rhythm*, both of which provide critically important clinical information in the triage assessment of emergent veterinary patients. ECG assessment of heart rate and rhythm can prompt emergency treatment and intervention, and no other diagnostic tests perform better than an ECG for these purposes. Additional information provided by ECGs includes mean electrical axis (overall vector of ventricular depolarization) and presence of conduction disturbances (such as bundle branch block). Although intraventricular conduction abnormalities can be clinically useful (e.g. they can suggest presence of underlying heart disease), they are rarely relevant in an emergency setting and do not require directed treatment. Historically, ECG complex measurements (e.g. P wave or QRS complex amplitude) were commonly used as a screening tool for cardiac chamber enlargement. However, ECGs are relatively insensitive indicators of cardiac chamber size. Echocardiography is a vastly superior modality for assessment of cardiac structure and function, and is now widely available. For these reasons, *ECG analysis in an emergency patient should focus on assessment of heart rate and rhythm*.

There are a number of indications for ECG monitoring in the emergency setting. An ECG is certainly indicated for any patient with an arrhyth-

Table 3.3. Applications of electrocardiography in cardiovascular assessment of veterinary patients.

What information can an ECG tell you?	How good / reliable is the ECG at telling you this?	How many ECG leads do you need?	How difficult is it to use an ECG to get this?	How useful is this information clinically?
Heart rate	****	Lead II only	Easy	****
Heart rhythm / Arrhythmias	****	Lead II only	Medium	****
Conduction disturbances	****	Lead II required, others helpful	Medium	**
Mean electrical axis	***	At least two orthogonal leads, ideally six	Hard	*
Chamber enlargement	*	Lead II only	Hard	*

The number of asterisks represent a subjective assessment of reliability or clinical utility, with (*) representing the least reliable or useful, and (****) representing the most reliable or useful.

mia (including tachycardia or bradycardia) ausculted on triage examination. Continuous ECG monitoring is useful for patients with trauma and/or hemodynamic instability (shock) to assess response to treatment (fluid resuscitation, blood products, analgesics, etc.). ECGs should also be performed to monitor cardiovascular stability in heavily sedated or anesthetized patients, since these drugs can have cardiodepressant actions. In critically ill or anesthetized patients, heart rate trends act as a surrogate for autonomic nervous system activity; an increase in heart rate can signal increased SNS stimulation that may indicate hypotension, pain, or inadequate anesthetic plane (see Table 3.2).

3.4 Interpretation of the Findings: How to Analyze an ECG

The first step to analyzing an ECG is *calculation of heart rate*. There are two general methods of heart rate calculation: average heart rate and instantaneous heart rate (see Table 3.4 and Fig. 3.5). *Average heart rate* represents the mean heart rate over a defined period of time (generally 3 or 6 seconds is chosen as a representative sample); this method is typically preferred for clinical assessment. *Instantaneous heart rate* represents the heart rate between two QRS complexes only; this method can be useful for transient tachyarrhythmias (e.g. instantaneous rate between two VPCs) or bradyarrhythmias (e.g. instantaneous rate during a period of sinus arrest). If heart rhythm is regular (i.e. if R–R intervals are all the same), then heart rate calculated by the two methods will be identical; if the heart rhythm is irregular (R–R intervals vary), then the heart rate calculated by the two methods may differ.

The 'ballpoint pen method' has been described as a shortcut to calculating average heart rate on an ECG. A standard ballpoint pen (with cap on) is approximately 15 cm (150 mm) long; therefore, the length of the pen represents approximately 6 seconds of ECG recording at a paper speed of 25 mm/s. Heart rate (at 25 mm/s) can thus be estimated as the number of QRS complexes occurring within the length of a pen multiplied by 10 ('pen times ten').

The next step in ECG analysis is *determination of cardiac rhythm*. Rhythm analysis requires first *labeling individual waveforms* to identify P, QRS, and T waves. For some ECGs these distinctions are easy, while other cases are less obvious (see Fig. 3.6). Remember that every heart beat (ventricular contraction) *must* be preceded by a QRS complex (ventricular depolarization). Every time the ventricle depolarizes (QRS), it *must* repolarize (T wave); however, depending on the lead and size of the patient, T waves may not always be visible. Depending on the rhythm, P waves may or may not be present. Therefore, it is typically easiest to start by identifying QRS complexes, since these are the waveforms most consistently present. Usually (but not always), QRS complexes are the largest (highest amplitude) waveform identified on the ECG. When visible, T waves always occur after QRS complexes at a consistent Q–T intervals. In sinus

Table 3.4. Instructions for calculating average and instantaneous heart rate at different paper speeds.

Paper speed (mm/s)	Average heart rate	Instantaneous heart rate
@ 25 mm/s	Mark off 15 LARGE boxes (3 seconds) Count # of QRS complexes Multiply by 20 = beats/minute	Count # of SMALL boxes between single R–R interval 1500/(# small boxes) = beats/minute
@ 50 mm/s	Mark off 30 LARGE boxes (3 seconds) Count # of QRS complexes Multiply by 20 = beats/minute	Count # of SMALL boxes between single R–R interval 3000/(# small boxes) = beats/minute

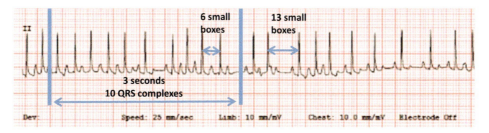

Fig. 3.5. Example calculation of average and instantaneous heart rate. In this ECG recorded at 25 mm/s, the average heart rate is equal to the number of QRS complexes occurring in 3 seconds (15 large boxes) multiplied by 20: 10 × 20 = 200 beats per minute (bpm). Instantaneous heart rate is equal to the number 1500 divided by the number of small boxes between two consecutive QRS complexes, and ranges from a minimum of 1500/13 (115 bpm) to 1500/6 (250 bpm). The average heart rate for this irregular rhythm is between the maximum and minimum instantaneous heart rates.

rhythm, P waves preced QRS complexes at consistent P–R intervals.

Once waveforms are identified and labeled, the next step in ECG analysis involves *asking a series of questions about the relationships between these waveforms* (see Table 3.5). Answers to these questions will lead to a clear rhythm diagnosis in the majority of cases.

3.5 Pitfalls of Electrocardiography: When Can the Machine Lead You Astray?

ECG machines can sometimes provide false or misleading information. ECG *artifacts* are defined as deflections on the graph paper caused by a source other than actual electrical conduction activity within the heart. Common causes of ECG artifact include patient motion (panting, trembling, or cat purring), extraneous metal touching leads (such as the operator's watch), or interference from nearby electronic devices. Cellular telephones have been reported to cause electrical interference if held within 7.5 cm (3 inches) of the ECG electrodes, but not at longer distances.

ECG waveforms can also be misleading if electrodes are placed on the incorrect limbs, or if the machine amplitude or paper speed settings are inappropriate. Inappropriate amplitude settings can cause complexes to appear either too small (e.g. P waves may not be visible) or too large (e.g. the top and bottom of QRS complexes are 'cut off' from the monitor view, causing waveforms to appear square or rectangular). Unconventional paper speed settings can cause complexes to appear too wide or too narrow.

Most ECG machines have an automated function to calculate heart rate, and most will display this machine-generated heart rate. *Operators should never rely solely on an automated heart rate assessment*, because ECG monitors are not calibrated to sense dog and cat QRS complexes and thus often calculate improperly. Based on the lead and amplitude settings, ECG monitors may either fail to sense small QRS complexes (leading to an underestimation of heart rate) or oversense large P or T waves (leading to an overestimation of heart rate). For this reason, heart rate and ECG findings should be confirmed and correlated with the cardiovascular physical examination, including auscultation of heart rate and palpation of femoral pulses (see Chapter 1).

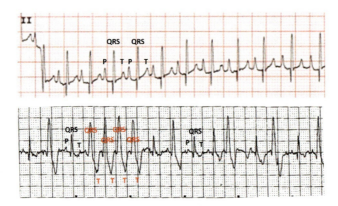

Fig. 3.6. Examples of labeling P, QRS, and T waves on ECGs. In the first example, QRS complexes are easily identified as the tallest waveforms; P waves precede the QRS at consistent P–R intervals, and T waves follow the QRS at consistent Q–T intervals. The rhythm diagnosis is sinus tachycardia. In the second example, there are two different ECG complex morphologies, each of which requires identification of waveform elements. For the normal sinus complexes (labeled in black), P–QRS–T waveforms are all present at consistent intervals. For the ventricular premature complexes (labeled in red), QRS complexes are identified as the initial large positive deflections. For abnormal depolarizations (wide bizarre QRS complexes), the T waves are the large deflections of the opposite polarity (negative deflections) following the QRS complexes.

Most ECG pitfalls can be avoided by use of appropriate electrical coupling medium (isopropyl alcohol), connecting electrodes to the appropriate limb, adjusting paper speed and calibration settings, and minimizing electrical interference and patient motion. When considering possible ECG artifact of any kind, the operator should auscult the patient's heart and palpate femoral pulses to confirm whether ECG findings match the patient's actual heart rate and rhythm.

3.6 Common Cardiac Rhythms in Veterinary Medicine

Sinus rhythms

Sinus rhythm is characterized electrocardiographically by the presence of normal P–QRS–T morphology for each beat with consistent P–R, Q–T, and R–R intervals. Sinus rhythm implies that cardiac depolarization utilized the 'normal' conduction pathway as shown in Fig. 3.1: the impulse began in the SA node, was conducted through the atria to the AV node, and traversed the AV node before depolarizing the ventricles. Sinus rhythm is the normal expected rhythm in dogs and cats. *Sinus arrhythmia* is a variant of sinus rhythm that is also normal in dogs. It is defined electrocardiographically as a sinus rhythm with greater than 10% variation in R–R interval between beats (Fig. 3.7). Sinus arrhythmia is mediated by variations in PNS activation (vagal tone) of the SA node. This rhythm is often associated with the cyclical alterations in vagal tone associated with breathing (*respiratory sinus arrhythmia*), but can also occur independently of breathing pattern. Presence of a sinus arrhythmia suggests relatively high vagal tone (see Table 3.2), which can help to rule out significant hemodynamic instability (shock, congestive heart failure, etc.).

Sinus bradycardia is defined as a sinus rhythm occurring at a rate below the expected heart rate for that patient and context (typically <60 bpm for an awake dog or <140 bpm for an awake cat). Sinus bradycardia is caused by a decreased firing rate of the SA node, and is typically a manifestation of either increased vagal tone (see Table 3.2) or drug administration (especially sedatives such as opioids or α-2 agonists). In contrast, *sinus tachycardia* reflects accelerated normal automaticity of the SA node (Fig. 3.8). Sinus tachycardia generally occurs secondary to stimuli that increase SNS activity, such as pain, anxiety, or hypovolemia (see Table 3.2). Less common causes include drugs or toxins (chocolate, β-adrenergic agonists, or anticholinergics such as atropine). Heart rate in sinus tachycardia rarely exceeds 240–250 bpm in the dog or 260–280 bpm in the cat. Onset and termination of sinus tachycardia typically occur as gradual increase or decrease in rate ('warm-up' or 'cool-down'), rather than abrupt start or end of tachycardia.

Table 3.5. Questions to guide analysis of ECG waveforms in determinig rhythm diagnosis.

Question	Options	What does this mean?	Examples with rhythm diagnosis
How many rhythms are present?	One rhythm only	Calculate single HR and rhythm diagnosis	Supraventricular tachycardia
	>1 rhythm	Calculate HR and describe rhythm diagnosis for each rhythm separately	Supraventricular tachycardia with conversion to normal sinus rhythm
Are the R-R intervals regular or irregular?	Regular	Multiple differential diagnoses possible	Supraventricular tachycardia
	Irregular with pattern (regularly irregular)	Consistent with sinus arrhythmia	Sinus arrhythmia
	Irregular with no pattern (irregularly irregular)	Suggests atrial fibrillation	Atrial fibrillation

Continued

Electrocardiography

Table 3.5. Continued.

Question	Options	What does this mean?	Examples with rhythm diagnosis
How are P waves and QRS complexes related?	One P wave precedes every QRS complex at consistent P-R interval	Sinus rhythm (electrical impulse originated in SA node and conducted through AV node)	Sinus tachycardia
	>1 P wave precedes QRS complexes (at least sometimes)	2nd or 3rd degree AV block	High-grade 2nd degree AV block (4:1 P:QRS ratio)
	P waves are present but not consistently related to QRS complexes	AV dissociation; suggests either ventricular ectopy or 3rd degree AV block	Ventricular tachycardia
	No P waves present	Suggests atrial fibrillation or atrial standstill	Atrial standstill
Do QRS-T waveforms look normal or abnormal?	QRS–T waveforms normal	Past the AV node, electrical impulse was conducted using specialized conduction system (His bundle, bundle branches, Purkinje system)	Normal sinus rhythm with single supraventricular premature complexes

Table 3.5. Continued.

Question	Options	What does this mean?	Examples with rhythm diagnosis
	QRS–T waveforms abnormal	Abnormal electrical impulse origin (ventricular origin), abnormal ventricular conduction (bundle branch block), or abnormal ventricular mass/volume (enlargement or hypertrophy)	Normal sinus rhythm with frequent ventricular premature complexes (single VPCs and short paroxysm of ventricular tachycardia)
			Normal sinus rhythm with left bundle branch block
			Sinus arrhythmia with right axis deviation (secondary to right ventricular hypertrophy)
When do abnormal QRS complexes occur?	Early (before next expected sinus beat)	Suggests ventricular premature complexes	Normal sinus rhythm with ventricular premature complexes (single VPC and ventricular couplet)
	Late (after a long pause)	Suggests ventricular escape complexes	3rd degree AV block with ventricular escape rhythm
	At approximately the same time as the next expected sinus beat	Suggests accelerated idioventricular rhythm	Accelerated idioventricular rhythm

Electrocardiography

Because variants of sinus rhythm (sinus arrhythmia, sinus bradycardia, sinus tachycardia) almost always occur as a physiologic response to changes in autonomic tone, these 'arrhythmias' rarely require directed treatment. Rather, the underlying cause of sinus tachycardia or bradycardia (see Table 3.2) should be identified and treated if needed. Persistent sinus tachycardia that occurs secondary to drug toxicity or autonomic imbalance is typically treated with a β-blocker (such as oral atenolol or IV short-acting esmolol; see Table 3.6) to directly counteract SNS overstimulation and slow sinus rate. Persistent sinus bradycardia causing hypotension (e.g. during general anesthesia) can be treated with an anticholinergic (atropine, glycopyrrolate; see Table 3.6).

Common tachyarrhythmias in small animals

Ventricular tachyarrhythmias

A ventricular ectopic complex is recognized electrocardiographically by (i) wide, bizarre QRS morphology compared to normal sinus complexes; (ii) the presence of a large T wave of opposite polarity; and (iii) the absence of a preceding P wave. Ventricular ectopy can be caused by abnormal automaticity (ectopic activity) in ventricular myocytes or re-entrant loops of electrical activity within the ventricles. A number of terms are used to designate how frequently ventricular ectopic beats occur. A single ventricular ectopic beat that occurs before the next expected sinus beat is called a single (or isolated) *ventricular premature complex*. Two VPCs in a row is called a ventricular *couplet*; three VPCs in a row is called a ventricular *triplet*; and more than three VPCs in succession is termed *ventricular tachycardia (VT)* (see Fig. 3.9). Periods of VT alternating with sinus rhythm are often called 'runs' or 'paroxysms' of VT. Ventricular ectopy (the umbrella term for these arrhythmias) can occur in patients with structural heart disease (and is particularly common in dogs with dilated cardiomyopathy or arrhythmogenic right ventricular cardiomyopathy) or cardiac trauma. However, ventricular ectopy can

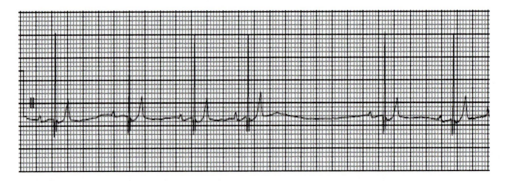

Fig. 3.7. Lead II ECG (25 mm/s, 10 mm/mV) showing sinus arrhythmia / sinus bradycardia. The heart rate is approximately 60 bpm. The rhythm is irregular, with greater than 10% variation in R–R interval between beats. Normal P–QRS–T complexes are identifiable for each beat.

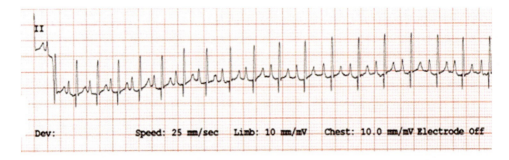

Fig. 3.8. Lead II ECG (25 mm/s, 10 mm/mV) showing sinus tachycardia. The heart rate is approximately 180 bpm. The rhythm is regular, and normal P–QRS–T complexes are identifiable for each beat.

Table 3.6. Anti-arrhythmic drugs commonly used in small animal emergency practice. Medications are grouped by their Vaughn–Williams classification (Class I-IV), based on cellular mechanism of action.

Drug	General indications	Dose (dog)	Dose (cat)
Class I: Na⁺ channel blockers; decrease rate of myocardial depolarization			
Lidocaine	Emergency treatment of VT	IV: initial slow bolus of 2 mg/kg; can repeat up to cumulative dose of 8 mg/kg (over ≥10 min) CRI: 25–80 µg/kg/min	(Generally avoid) IV: initial slow bolus of 0.2 mg/kg CRI: 10–40 µg/kg/min
Mexiletine	Long-term oral treatment of VT/VPCs	PO: 5–8 mg/kg q8h	–
Procainamide	Emergency treatment of VT (if unresponsive to lidocaine)	IV: initial slow bolus of 4 mg/kg; can repeat up to cumulative dose of 16 mg/kg CRI: 10–50 µg/kg/min	IV: initial slow bolus of 1-2 mg/kg; can repeat up to cumulative dose of 10 mg/kg CRI: 10–20 µg/kg/min
Class II: β-blockers; decrease SNS activation			
Atenolol	Long-term oral treatment of SNS-mediated VT/VPCs or SVT/SVPCs; heart rate reduction in AF	PO: 0.25–1.0 mg/kg q12h (start low and up titrate)	PO: 6.25 mg/cat q12h
Esmolol	In-hospital treatment of persistent sinus tachycardia (usually secondary to toxicity)	IV: initial bolus of 50–100 µg/kg over 5 min CRI: 25–50 µg/kg/min	IV: initial bolus of 50–100 µg/kg over 5 min CRI: 25–50 µg/kg/min
Class III: K⁺ channel blockers; prolong repolarization			
Sotalol	Long-term oral treatment of ventricular or supraventricular arrhythmias	PO: 2–3 mg/kg q12h	PO: 10–20 mg/cat (2–4 mg/kg) q12h
Amiodarone	Emergency treatment of ventricular tachycardia (if unresponsive to lidocaine); long-term oral treatment of VT/VPCs or SVT/SVPCs	PO: loading protocol of 15 mg/kg q12h for 7 days, then 15 mg/kg q24h, then 7.5 mg/kg q24hr IV (aqueous formulation only): 3–5 mg/kg slow IV over 15 min CRI: 0.05 mg/kg/min	IV (aqueous formulation only): 2.5 mg/kg slow bolus over 15 min
Class IV: Ca²⁺ channel blockers; decrease SA node rate and AV node conduction			
Diltiazem	Emergency treatment of SVT; long-term oral treatment of SVT/SVPCs; heart rate reduction in AF	IV: 0.05–0.2 mg/kg over 2–5 min; can repeat if needed up to 0.5 mg/kg CRI: 2–5 µg/kg/min PO (regular formulation): 0.5–1.5 mg/kg q8h (start low and up titrate) PO (sustained-release formulation, Diltiazem ER): 3–6 mg/kg q12h	IV: 0.05–0.2 mg/kg over 2–5 min; can repeat if needed up to 0.5 mg/kg PO (regular formulation): 7.5 mg/cat q8h PO (sustained-release formulation, Diltiazem ER): 30 mg/cat q12h PO (sustained-release formulation, Cardizem-CD): 10 mg/kg q24h
Positive chronotropes (drugs that increase heart rate)			
Atropine	Hemodynamically relevant bradyarrhythmias; response test for vagal influence	IV/IM/SQ: 0.02–0.04 mg/kg Atropine response test: 0.04 mg/kg SQ	IV/IM/SQ: 0.02–0.04 mg/kg Atropine response test: 0.04 mg/kg SQ

Continued

Table 3.6. Continued.

Drug	General indications	Dose (dog)	Dose (cat)
Glycopyrrolate	Hemodynamically relevant bradyarrhythmias	IV/IM/SQ: 0.01–0.02 mg/kg	IV/IM/SQ: 0.01–0.02 mg/kg
Theophylline	Long-term treatment of SSS; bronchodilation	PO: 10 mg/kg q12h	PO: 10 mg/kg q12h
Propantheline	Long-term treatment of SSS	PO: 0.25–0.5 mg/kg q8-12h	–
Hyoscyamine	Long-term treatment of SSS	P: 0.003–0.006 mg/kg q8h	–
Other anti-arrhythmic medications			
Magnesium chloride (or sulfate)	Adjunct treatment of VT/VPCs	IV: 0.3 mEq/kg over 15 min	IV: 0.3 mEq/kg over 15 min
Digoxin	Heart rate reduction in AF (especially if concurrent CHF)	IV: loading protocol of 2.5 µg/kg slow bolus repeated hourly × 4 hours (total 10 µg/kg) PO: 3–5 µg/kg q12h	PO: 5 µg/kg q48h

AF, Atrial fibrillation; CHF, congestive heart failure; CRI, continuous rate infusion; IM, intramuscular; IV, intravenous; PO, by mouth; SQ, subcutaneous; SNS, sympathetic nervous system; SSS, sick sinus syndrome; SVPC, supraventricular premature complex; SVT, supraventricular tachycardia; VPC, ventricular premature complex; VT, ventricular tachycardia.

also occur in patients with noncardiac diseases, including electrolyte derangements (hypokalemia, hypomagnesemia), splenic disease, gastric dilatation-volvulus, and sepsis. Another variant of ventricular ectopy is called *accelerated idioventricular rhythm (AIVR)*. AIVR, sometimes oxymoronically called 'slow VT,' refers to a ventricular rhythm that occurs at heart rates close to the sinus rate of the patient (e.g. <140 bpm in the dog). AIVR most commonly occurs in patients with *noncardiac* causes of ventricular ectopy (see above) or in patients under general anesthesia/sedation. Because the heart rate in AIVR is similar to the sinus rate for that patient, AIVR does not lead to hemodynamic compromise and generally does not require treatment.

Isolated VPCs are typically easy to recognize because QRS morphology differs from the surrounding sinus beats; however, sustained VT may be more difficult to identify without normal sinus beats present for comparison. VT is perfectly regular (identical R-R intervals) unless there are multiple ventricular foci involved, in which case QRS morphology also varies between beats (polymorphic VT; see Fig. 3.10). Because the ectopic beats originate within the ventricles, the presence of VT does not affect the firing of the SA node; the atria and ventricles are controlled by two independent 'pacemakers' (termed *AV dissociation*). Therefore, P waves of normal morphology may be noted intermittently between ventricular QRS complexes, with no consistent temporal relationship to QRS complexes (see arrows in Fig. 3.9). Most P waves are not visible because they occur simultaneously with QRS complexes and are thus 'hidden' on the ECG. VT is often most often seen as an intermittent rhythm; that is, the patient has an underlying normal sinus rhythm with frequent VPCs and paroxysms of VT. If a sinus beat and VPC occur at the same time, wave fronts from both stimuli may cause the ventricle may depolarize from both 'above and below' simultaneously, leading to an abnormal QRS complex that is a morphologic hybrid of the patient's ventricular and sinus complexes. Such complexes are called *fusion beats* and can be helpful in confirming the diagnosis of VT.

Ventricular ectopy warrants treatment if the ventricular arrhythmias lead to hemodynamic compromise (hypotension) or place the patient at risk for sudden cardiac death. The first-line emergency treatment for VT in dogs is intravenous lidocaine; adjunctive treatments if lidocaine is unsuccessful include procainamide or amiodarone (see Table 3.6). In cats, lidocaine is generally avoided or used at much lower doses due to adverse effects. Hypokalemia and hypomagnesemia should also be corrected if present. Long-

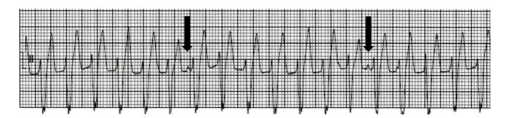

Fig. 3.9. Lead II ECG (25 mm/s, 10 mm/mV) showing ventricular tachycardia. The heart rate is approximately 180 bpm. The rhythm is regular. QRS complexes are wide and bizarre, negatively deflected in lead II, with large positive T-waves. Occasional P-waves are seen (see arrows) but are not temporally related to QRS complexes.

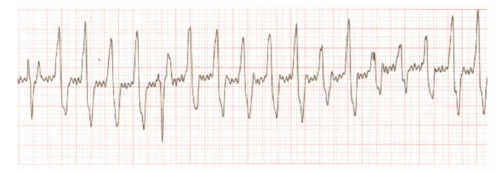

Fig. 3.10. Lead II ECG (25 mm/s, 10 mm/mV) showing polymorphic ventricular tachycardia. The heart rate is approximately 160 bpm. All QRS complexes are wide and bizarre, but are of different morphology, with some positively and some negatively deflected in lead II. All QRS complexes have large T waves of opposite polarity to the QRS complex. There is a large amount of baseline artifact due to patient motion and panting (may be mistaken for flutter/fibrillation waves). Because ectopic beats originate from multiple foci within the ventricles, the rhythm is not perfectly regular.

term management of ventricular arrhythmias most commonly involves oral sotalol (combined potassium-channel blocker and weak nonselective β-blocker) and/or mexiletine (sodium-channel blocker; see Table 3.6).

Supraventricular tachyarrhythmias

Supraventricular ectopy is caused either by abnormal automaticity (ectopic activity) in atrial cells or re-entrant loops of electrical activity involving the atria. Supraventricular ectopy most commonly occurs in patients with structural heart disease and severe left atrial enlargement. These arrhythmias can also be seen as an isolated phenomenon in dogs (particularly Labrador Retrievers) with abnormal 'accessory pathways' of conduction tissue linking the atria and ventricles, allowing cardiac depolarization to return to the atria via a re-entrant loop that bypasses the AV node ('bypass tracts'; see Fig. 3.11). Occasionally, supraventricular ectopy can be caused by drug toxicity, trauma, and severe systemic diseases. From a practical perspective, *supraventricular* and *atrial* ectopy are synonymous terms; technically 'supraventricular' is more anatomically correct since it includes ectopic beats originating from the region of the AV node itself.

Supraventricular ectopic QRS complexes appear the same as sinus complexes for that patient, since the abnormal impulse or circuit still conducts through the AV node, and ventricular depolarization past the AV node proceeds as normal. Normal P waves are not present for these beats since the impulse for atrial depolarization does not originate in the SA node. Abnormal atrial depolarization waveforms (P′ waves) can occur before, during, or after the QRS complex and may be positive, negative, or isoelectric depending on where the ectopic activity or re-entrant circuit are located within the atrium. A single supraventricular ectopic beat that occurs before the next expected sinus beat is called a single (or isolated) *supraventricular premature complex* (SVPC). As with ventricular ectopy, the terms *couplet* and *triplet* can be used to describe two or three SVPCs in a row, respectively; more than three VPCs in succession is termed *supraventricular tachycardia* (SVT) (see Fig. 3.12); and periods of SVT alternating with sinus rhythm are often called 'runs' or 'paroxysms' of SVT. SVT is perfectly regular (identical R–R intervals between beats), and generally causes the most dramatically high heart rates of any tachycardia (often ~280–300 bpm in dogs). The abnormal P′ morphology will be consistent throughout every beat of the tachycardia. Unlike sinus tachycardia, the onset and termination of SVT from normal sinus rhythm are typically abrupt.

Treatment of SVT is directed at prolonging AV nodal conduction time such that the supraventricular circuit is extinguished, allowing normal SA depolarization to resume control of heart rate and rhythm. Vagal maneuvers (such as manual pressure on the globes, nasal philtrum, or carotid sinus) can be attempted to slow AV nodal conduction. Vagal maneuvers may cause transient conversion to normal sinus rhythm, confirming the diagnosis of SVT. Diltiazem is the first-line medical treatment for SVT; it is generally given as small IV boluses until conversion to sinus rhythm occurs, and continued as a continuous rate infuser (CRI) if needed (see Table 3.6). Long-term management typically involves oral diltiazem. Other drugs that may be considered in some cases include sotalol or atenolol (see Table 3.6). Radiofrequency ablation is also available in select veterinary centers for dogs with SVT secondary

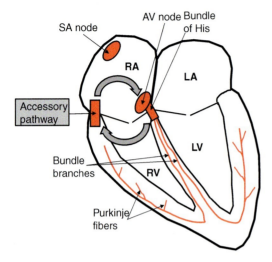

Fig. 3.11. Schematic representation of cardiac conduction system with a bypass tract between the right ventricular free wall and the right atrium. An impulse conducted antegrade through the AV node may return to re-activate the atria via the retrograde accessory pathway; that impulse can then be conducted again through the AV node in a re-entrant loop of SVT. LA, left atrium; LV, left ventricle; RA, right atrium; RV, right ventricle.

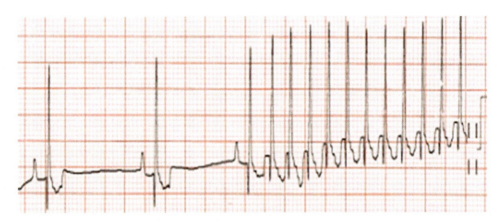

Fig. 3.12. Lead II ECG (25 mm/s, 10 mm/mV) showing normal sinus rhythm with onset of supraventricular tachycardia. The heart rate in SVT is approximately 300 bpm. The onset of the SVT from normal sinus rhythm is abrupt. The SVT is regular (R–R intervals are identical). The QRS complexes in SVT are identical to this patient's normal sinus complexes (narrow and positively deflected in lead II). During the tachycardia, no obvious P waves are noted. However, there is an irregularity in the S–T segment of every beat during SVT that likely represents a P′ wave.

to accessory pathways. Isolated SVPCs may not require treatment, particularly if overall average heart rate remains relatively normal.

Atrial fibrillation

Atrial fibrillation (AF), as distinguished from other supraventricular tachyarrhythmias, is caused by *multiple* disorganized wavefronts of electrical activation within the atria. This chaotic electrical activity prevents organized atrial depolarization and contraction and bombards the AV node with rapid stimulation, leading to an irregular tachycardia. As a rule, AF occurs in patients with large atria. Dogs and cats with AF typically have significant structural heart disease causing severe left atrial enlargement. Large animals and some giant breed dogs can develop AF in the absence of structural heart disease.

AF is readily recognized on ECG as an irregular tachycardia (see Fig. 3.13). Since the irregularity in rhythm can be more difficult to discern at higher heart rates, use of calipers or a ruler can facilitate comparison of R–R intervals. Normal P waves are not present. Variable baseline undulations can be seen, which depending on their level of organization may appear as irregular fibrillation waves ('f-waves'). In atrial flutter, which can be conceptualized as a variant of AF, the baseline appears as rapidly oscillating positive and negative deflections ('sawtooth' waves). The QRS complexes in AF are the same as sinus complexes for that patient, since the abnormal impulses in AF originate in the atria.

Once the wave of depolarization reaches the AV node, conduction to the ventricles occurs normally through the specialized conduction system (as outlined in Fig. 3.1), unless concurrent conduction block is present. In dogs and cats, AF is typically a permanent (rather than intermittent) rhythm, meaning that patients do not alternate between AF and normal sinus rhythm.

Since dogs and cats with AF usually have significant cardiac disease, diagnosis and treatment of the underlying structural heart disease (including congestive heart failure, if present) is a priority. For directed treatment of AF, rate control (decreasing ventricular response rate) is accomplished using drugs that slow AV nodal conduction. Options include calcium channel blockers (diltiazem), β-blockers (atenolol), or digoxin (a positive inotrope with parasympathomimetic properties; see Table 3.6). For patients with severe structural heart disease or CHF, β-blockers are generally avoided due to their negative inotropic effects. Diltiazem and digoxin are often used in combination, and the combination of both drugs been shown to offer superior long-term rate control in AF compared to either drug alone. In patients with AF and CHF, the initial goal is to reduce heart rate to approximately 160 bpm in the hospital (a rate that maximizes cardiac output). For chronic management, the goal is to reduce heart rate to more physiologic rates (~100–110 bpm at home). Rhythm control (electrical cardioversion to normal sinus rhythm) can be considered for patients with 'lone' AF (no evidence of structural heart disease).

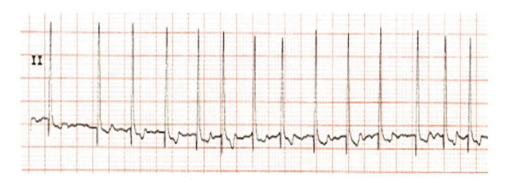

Fig. 3.13. Lead II ECG (25 mm/s, 10 mm/mV) showing atrial fibrillation. The heart rate is approximately 160 bpm. The rhythm is irregularly irregular (beat-to-beat variation in R–R interval that does not follow a clear pattern). QRS complexes are normal (narrow and upright in lead II). There is baseline undulation with no clear P waves visible. T waves are visible as positive deflections at a consistent interval after each QRS complex, and should not be confused with P waves.

Basic algorithm for differentiating tachyarrhythmias

In an emergency setting, tachyarrhythmias are the most common rhythms to cause hemodynamic compromise and require urgent treatment. The following algorithm can help to differentiate the four common tachycardic rhythms (sinus tachycardia, AF, VT, and SVT) using ECG findings (see Fig. 3.14).

1. *Is the tachycardia regular (all R–R intervals the same) or irregular (variation in R–R interval)?* As a rule, tachycardias are perfectly regular EXCEPT for AF. Exceptions include polymorphic ventricular tachycardia or paroxysmal SVT or VT alternating with sinus rhythm.
2. *Is QRS complex morphology 'normal'?* QRS complexes in VT are wide and bizarre. In all other tachycardias, the impulse originates above the ventricles, so QRS complexes should be identical to normal sinus complexes (narrow and upright in lead II, unless there is a concurrent bundle branch block or other intraventricular conduction abnormality).
3. *What is the morphology and timing of the P waves?* In ST, P waves of normal morphology occur consistently before every QRS complex at a normal P–R interval. In AF, P waves are absent, and instead baseline undulation or f waves may occur. In VT, normal P waves may be variably seen, but have no consistent relationship to QRS complexes. In SVT, atypical P′ waves can occur before, during, or after the QRS; however, P′ morphology will be consistent throughout the tachycardia.

Common bradyarrhythmias in small animals

Atrioventricular block

AV block is not truly a distinct cardiac 'rhythm,' but instead describes ECG manifestations of delayed or interrupted AV nodal conduction that usually occur within the context of an underlying sinus rhythm. That is, the SA node depolarizes and the impulse is conducted through the atria to cause a P wave as usual, but the impulse is either delayed or completely blocked at the level of the AV node. AV block is classically categorized by 'degrees' (1st-, 2nd-, and 3rd-degree AV block). *First-degree AV block* is essentially a sinus rhythm characterized by a prolonged P–R interval; each P wave is still eventually conducted through the AV node and results in a QRS complex. *Second-degree AV block* refers to a situation where the AV node is able to conduct some impulses but blocks others; this results in a situation where some P waves are conducted normally (resulting in P–QRS–T complexes), but other P waves are not conducted (see Fig. 3.15). *Third-degree AV block* occurs when the AV node is incapable of conducting any electrical impulses; all P waves are blocked at the level of the AV node, and the patient is sustained by a junctional or *ventricular escape rhythm* (see Fig. 3.16). Third-degree AV block necessarily involves AV dissociation because there is no relationship between P waves and QRS complexes.

There are two potential causes of AV block: (i) fibrosis or other structural disease of the AV node itself; or (ii) increased vagal tone causing physiologic delay AV nodal conduction. In general, *low-grade AV block* (1st degree and low-grade 2nd degree, where over half of P waves are conducted) is caused by high vagal tone. In contrast, *high-grade AV block* (3rd degree and high-grade 2nd degree, where less than half of P waves are conducted) is caused by structural disease of the AV node. An *atropine response test* (administration of atropine subcutaneously, with repeat ECG performed 20–30 minutes later; see Table 3.6) can differentiate whether a bradyarrhythmia such as AV block is caused by high vagal tone versus structural disease of the conduction system. A vagally mediated bradyarrhythmia will be *atropine-responsive*, meaning that the resulting rhythm will be normal sinus rhythm or sinus tachycardia at a rate of 140–160 bpm with normal P–R intervals and no nonconducted P waves. In contrast, AV block caused by structural AV nodal disease will be *non-atropine-responsive*, meaning that administration of atropine will not change the rate, rhythm, or degree of AV block.

Low-grade or atropine-responsive AV block typically does not require any directed treatment; similar to sinus bradycardia, this rhythm is either a manifestation of either increased vagal tone (see Table 3.2) or drug administration (especially sedatives such as opioids or α2-agonists). In contrast, high-grade AV block (which is generally non-atropine-responsive) is a medical emergency in dogs. Dogs with high-grade AV block are at high risk for their ventricular escape rhythm degenerating into ventricular fibrillation, causing sudden cardiac death; permanent pacemaker implantation (transvenous or epicardial) is indicated as soon as feasible.

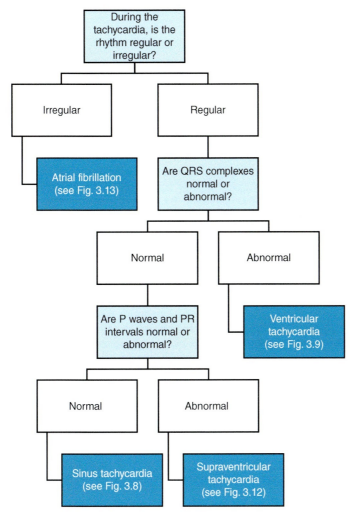

Fig. 3.14. Algorithm for ECG diagnosis of tachyarrhythmias.

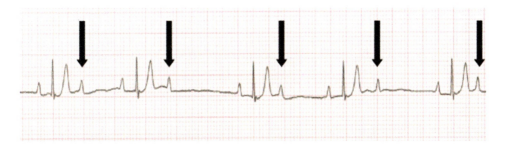

Fig. 3.15. Lead II ECG (25 mm/s, 10 mm/mV) showing sinus rhythm with 2nd-degree AV block. The sinus rate (P wave rate) is 100 bpm, while the ventricular rate (actual heart rate) is approximately 50 bpm. Every other P wave is conducted normally through the AV node to result in a normal P–QRS–T complex, while alternate P waves are not conducted (blocked; see arrows).

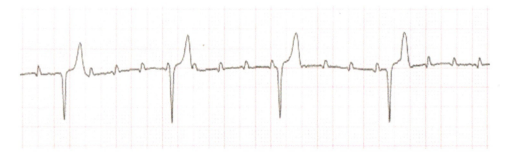

Fig. 3.16. Lead II ECG (25 mm/s, 10 mm/mV) showing 3rd-degree AV block. The sinus rate (P wave rate) is approximately 180 bpm, while the ventricular rate (actual heart rate) is 40 bpm. No P waves are conducted through the AV node. The QRS complexes are ventricular escape complexes. There is no relationship between P waves and QRS complexes.

Sinus node dysfunction / sick sinus syndrome

Sinus node dysfunction (SND) and sick sinus syndrome (SSS) refer to a spectrum of abnormalities of SA node function leading to intermittent failure of the SA node to depolarize. These rhythms are characterized on ECG by an underlying sinus rhythm (usually sinus bradycardia or sinus arrhythmia) with periods of *sinus arrest*, meaning rhythm pauses (with no SA node activity) lasting longer than two of the patient's 'normal' R–R intervals (see Fig. 3.17). These periods of sinus arrest may be terminated by another sinus-origin complex, or by an escape complex originating from the AV node (*junctional escape complex*) or ventricles (*ventricular escape complex*). Sometimes, this arrhythmia involves alternation between bradyarrhythmia/sinus arrest and paroxysms of SVT (termed *bradycardia–tachycardia syndrome*). This suite of ECG findings is referred to as SND in asymptomatic patients, whereas patients displaying symptoms of this bradyarrhythmia (typically syncope) are diagnosed with SSS.

Similar to AV block, there are two potential causes of SND/SSS: fibrosis or other structural disease of the SA node itself, or increased vagal tone causing physiologic decrease in rate of SA node depolarization. As with AV block, an *atropine response test* can differentiate structural SA node disease versus high vagal tone (see above and Table 3.6). ECG characteristics, including frequency or duration of sinus arrest, do not predict atropine response. Miniature Schnauzers, West Highland White Terriers, Dachshunds, and Cocker Spaniels are overrepresented in this condition, particularly older female dogs within these breeds.

Unlike high-grade AV block, SND/SSS is *not* an emergency; sudden cardiac death has not been reported with this condition. SND (asymptomatic) does not require any directed treatment, regardless of atropine response. Symptomatic SSS generally warrants treatment to decrease frequency of syncope. Most patients with SSS will respond to oral positive chronotropes (such as theophylline, propantheline, or hyoscyamine; see Table 3.6), and atropine response does predict long-term response to medical management. Permanent pacemaker implantation is indicated for dogs with medically refractory SSS. Bradycardia–tachycardia syndrome, while uncommon, presents a particular treatment challenge. Medical management is problematic for such patients because positive chronotropes (to increase sinus rate and decrease periods of sinus arrest) may exacerbate SVT, while drugs such as diltiazem (to slow AV nodal conduction and resolve SVT) will also suppress SA node automaticity and may exacerbate periods of sinus arrest. Permanent pacemaker placement is the treatment of choice in symptomatic patients with bradycardia–tachycardia syndrome.

Atrial standstill

Atrial standstill is an important bradyarrhythmia to recognize in emergency practice because it can signal the presence of life-threatening electrolyte abnormalities. Atrial standstill is characterized electrocardiographically by the complete absence of P waves (see Fig. 3.18). In atrial standstill, the SA node is still firing and conducting the impulse to the AV node through specialized atrial tracts, leading to ventricular

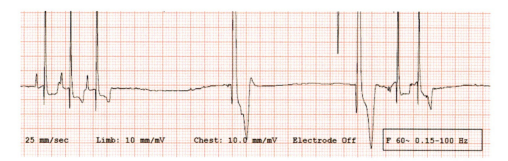

Fig. 3.17. Lead II ECG (25 mm/s, 10 mm/mV) showing sinus node dysfunction. The average heart rate is approximately 70 bpm. There is an underlying sinus arrhythmia with rhythm pauses exceeding two typical R–R intervals (periods of sinus arrest) terminated by ventricular escape complexes. The last two QRS complexes in this strip are not preceded by P waves and occur at an instantaneous heart rate of ~215 bpm, consistent with supraventricular premature complexes (SVPCs). This alternation of bradycardia/sinus arrest with SVPCs/supraventricular tachycardia is suggestive of bradycardia–tachycardia syndrome.

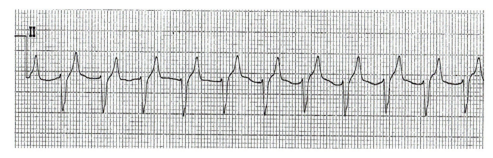

Fig. 3.18. Lead II ECG (25 mm/s, 10 mm/mV) showing atrial standstill in a cat with hyperkalemia. The heart rate is approximately 110 bpm. No P waves are visible. The QRS complexes are wide and bizarre, reflecting abnormal ventricular conduction. T waves are high amplitude. This rhythm can be distinguished from VT based on the heart rate (bradycardia) and complete absence of any atrial depolarization (no P waves).

depolarization; however, the atrial myocytes themselves do not depolarize. For this reason, atrial standstill is also sometimes called a 'sinoventricular rhythm.' Atrial standstill is sometimes confused for a ventricular rhythm because QRS complexes are wide and bizarre in both cases; however, recall that most ventricular rhythms are tachycardic, while heart rate in atrial standstill will be a relative bradycardia for that patient. Additionally, dissociated P waves are frequently visible in VT (see Fig. 3.9), while P waves are completely absent in atrial standstill.

There are two major causes of atrial standstill. The most common cause is severe hyperkalemia, for example, as seen in cats with urethral obstruction or dogs with hypoadrenocorticism. Hyperkalemia causes the resting membrane potential within cardiac myocytes to be less negative, which affects the ability of sodium channels to trigger an action potential. This leads to a suite of ECG findings including sinus bradycardia, diminished P wave amplitude, prolonged P–R interval, widened QRS complex, and increased T wave amplitude ('tall tented T waves'). Eventually, hyperkalemia 'paralyzes' sodium channels in atrial myocytes, leading to complete absence of P waves. The second and less common cause of atrial standstill is a primary atrial myopathy, believed to be an inherited cardiomyopathy in English Springer Spaniels and Labrador Retrievers.

Atrial standstill is a medical emergency. If caused by hyperkalemia, calcium gluconate is administered initially to re-establish the relationship between resting membrane potential and threshold potential in cardiomyocytes. This treatment is 'cardioprotective' and will improve the ECG abnormalities, but does not directly treat the electrolyte imbalance itself. Directed treatments to

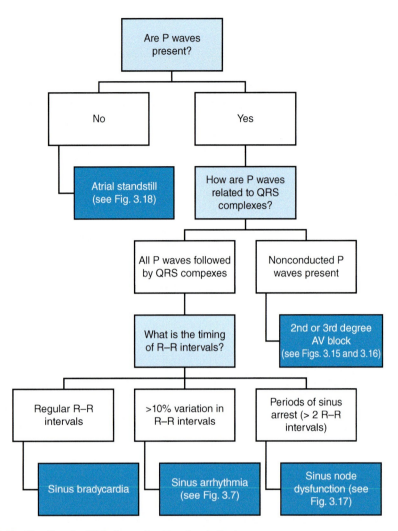

Fig. 3.19. Algorithm for ECG diagnosis of bradyarrhythmias.

drive excess potassium intracellularly include dextrose ± exogenous insulin, β2-agonists such as albuterol, and sodium bicarbonate; the underlying disease should then be addressed (see Chapter 8). For dogs with primary atrial myopathy, treatment of atrial standstill involves permanent pacemaker implantation.

Basic algorithm for differentiating bradyarrhythmias

The following algorithm can help to differentiate the five common bradyarrhythmias (sinus bradycardia, AV block, SND, atrial standstill arrhythmias, and sinus arrhythmia using ECG findings (see Fig. 3.19).

1. *Are P waves present?* The presence of P waves demonstrates that the atrial myocytes are capable of depolarization. Complete absence of P waves is suggestive of atrial standstill; all other bradyarrhythmias will have presence of at least some P waves.

2. *How are P waves related to QRS complexes?* If P waves are present, the next step is to determine their relationship to QRS complexes. If there are any P waves that are not followed by QRS complexes, this suggests that those P waves are not being conducted through the AV node to the ventricles. Presence of nonconducted P waves is characteristic

of AV block, either 2nd degree (some P waves conducted, some nonconducted) or 3rd degree (no P waves conducted).

3. *What is the degree of variation in R–R intervals?* If the bradyarrhythmia consists of normal P–QRS–T complexes of sinus origin, then the ECG diagnosis simply depends on the timing of R–R intervals. If R–R intervals are regular, the diagnosis is sinus bradycardia; if there is >10% variation in R–R intervals, the diagnosis is sinus arrhythmia. Rhythm pauses greater than two normal R–R intervals for that patient are termed 'sinus arrest' and are suggestive of sinus node dysfunction.

3.7 Case studies: Using an ECG monitor in Emergency Practice

Case study 1: Tachyarrhythmia in a Labrador Retriever

A 4-year-old male castrated Labrador Retriever presents for a 1-week history of abdominal distension and hyporexia and a single episode of syncope. Physical examination reveals a rapid, irregular heart rhythm; mucous membranes are pale and capillary refill time is prolonged; and femoral pulses are weak and variable. A grade III/VI right apical systolic heart murmur is auscultated. The patient is panting but eupneic, with normal lung sounds bilaterally. The abdomen is pendulous with a palpable fluid wave. The remainder of the physical examination is unremarkable. The ECG is shown in Fig. 3.20.

The first step in ECG interpretation is calculation of the heart rate (see Table 3.4). This patient has approximately 10 QRS complexes within the span of 15 large boxes (3 seconds) and 20 QRS complexes within the span of 30 large boxes (6 seconds), which corresponds to an average heart rate of 200 bpm. Instantaneous heart rates range from ~115 bpm (13 small boxes within the longest R–R interval) to ~300 bpm (5 small boxes within the shortest R–R interval). With this heart rate, the rhythm can be classified as a *tachyarrhythmia*.

The next step in ECG interpretation is asking a series of questions about the rhythm and P–QRS–T waveforms (see Table 3.5). Asking these questions sequentially yields the following information:

1. How many rhythms are present? *One rhythm*
2. Are the R–R intervals regular or irregular? *Irregular*
3. How are P waves and QRS complexes related? *No consistent P waves present*
4. Do P–QRS–T waveforms look normal or abnormal? *Normal (narrow and upright in lead II)*

Using these answers in conjunction with the algorithm shown in Fig. 3.14, this rhythm is identified as *atrial fibrillation*. Note that simply recognizing this rhythm as a tachycardia with irregular R–R intervals should already suggest atrial fibrillation as the most likely ECG diagnosis. The cardiovascular auscultation findings are consistent with this rhythm (irregular tachycardia, weak and variable femoral pulses).

Recall that in small animals, presence of atrial fibrillation generally suggests severe structural heart disease. This patient's clinical signs (syncope) and physical examination findings (heart murmur, suspicion of ascites) support this notion and suggest a diagnosis of right-sided congestive heart failure. Given this signalment (young Labrador Retriever), prioritized differential diagnoses would include congenital tricuspid valve dysplasia or dilated cardiomyopathy. Further diagnostic testing is indicated, including noninvasive blood pressure, thoracic radiographs, point-of-care thoracic and abdominal ultrasonography, point-of-care bloodwork (at minimum packed cell volume, total protein,

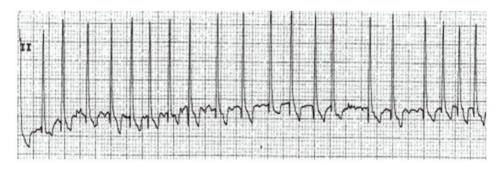

Fig. 3.20. Lead II ECG (25 mm/s, 10 mm/mV) from a Labrador Retriever with a history of abdominal distension and syncope.

BUN/creatinine, and electrolytes), and eventually a complete echocardiogram. In addition to management of the underlying structural heart disease and congestive heart failure (abdominocentesis, furosemide, pimobendan, and eventually an angiotensin-converting-enzyme inhibitor ± spironolactone), this patient will require treatment for this tachyarrhythmia, as rapid atrial fibrillation compromises cardiac filling time and thus decreases cardiac output.

Treatment for atrial fibrillation is directed at *decreasing the ventricular response rate* by slowing AV node conduction. Drug options include calcium-channel blockers (diltiazem), β-blockers, or digoxin. This patient is suspected to be in congestive heart failure and presumably has severe underlying structural heart disease (likely involving decreased systolic function); therefore β-blockers should be avoided due to their significant *negative inotropic* properties. Diltiazem is very effective at slowing AV nodal conduction but is a weak negative inotrope; digoxin is less effective at slowing AV nodal conduction but is a weak *positive* inotrope. An initial goal in the emergency setting is a moderate decrease in heart rate to 150–160 bpm (the heart rate that maximizes cardiac output in dogs). This can be accomplished either by diltiazem microboluses (0.05–0.2 mg/kg IV) or CRI (2–5 μg/kg/min), or digoxin loading (2.5 μg/kg slow bolus repeated hourly for 4 hours, for a total of 10 μg/kg; see Table 3.6). For long-term management, this patient will receive a combination of oral diltiazem (extended-release formulation, Diltiazem ER, 3–6 mg/kg PO q12h) and digoxin (3–5 μg/kg PO q12h; see Table 3.6), with the goal of decreasing heart rate to a more normal physiologic range (average daily heart rate < 125 bpm). The combination of digoxin and diltiazem has been shown more effective at heart rate reduction in atrial fibrillation compared to either medication alone.

Case 2: Bradyarrhythmia in a cat

An 8-year-old male castrated domestic shorthair cat presents laterally recumbent after having been lost outside for 2–3 days. Physical examination reveals dull mentation, pale mucous membranes with prolonged capillary refill time, and weak but synchronous femoral pulses. Rectal temperature is 97.0°F (36.1°C). Auscultation reveals a regular rhythm with no heart murmur and normal breath sounds. The patient is painful on abdominal palpation (growls and tries to bite). The remainder of the triage physical examination is unremarkable. The ECG is shown in Fig. 3.21.

The first step in ECG interpretation is calculation of the heart rate (see Table 3.4). This patient has approximately 6 QRS complexes within the span of 15 large boxes (3 seconds) and 12 QRS complexes within the span of 30 large boxes (6 seconds), which corresponds to an average heart rate of 120 bpm. This heart rate in a sick cat can be classified as a *bradyarrhythmia*.

The next step in ECG interpretation is asking a series of questions about the rhythm and P-QRS-T waveforms (see Table 3.5). Asking these questions sequentially yields the following information:

1. How many rhythms are present? *One rhythm*
2. Are the R–R intervals regular or irregular? *Regular*
3. How are P waves and QRS complexes related? *No P waves are present*
4. Do P–QRS–T waveforms look normal or abnormal? *All QRS complexes are abnormal (wide and bizarre, negatively deflected in lead II, with large T waves of opposite polarity to QRS complexes)*

Using these answers in conjunction with the algorithm shown in Figure 3.19, this rhythm is identified as *atrial standstill*. This ECG diagnosis is critically important in the triage assessment of this

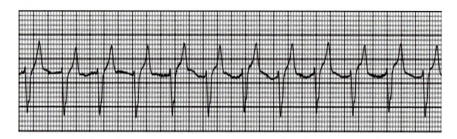

Fig. 3.21. Lead II ECG (25 mm/s, 10 mm/mV) from a domestic shorthair cat presenting with evidence of circulatory shock and abdominal pain.

patient. Recall that the most common cause of atrial standstill is hyperkalemia; in cats, the most common cause of clinically significant hyperkalemia is urethral obstruction. Taken together with physical examination findings of pain on abdominal palpation and evidence of circulatory shock, this patient likely has a life-threatening urethral obstruction requiring emergent medical management and de-obstruction. Additional diagnostic testing that should be performed urgently include point-of-care bloodwork to confirm presence and severity of hyperkalemia (as well as measurement of other electrolytes, packed cell volume/total protein, and BUN/creatinine), point-of-care abdominal ultrasound to confirm presence of enlarged turgid bladder, and abdominal radiographs to screen for presence of urolithiasis.

The most urgent immediate treatment for this patient is calcium gluconate; emergency dose is 100 mg/kg (or 1 mL/kg of a 10% solution), given slowly over 5–10 minutes. Calcium gluconate re-establishes the relationship between resting membrane potential and threshold potential in cardiomyocytes, and will improve ECG appearance (QRS complexes will become narrower, heart rate will increase, and P waves will begin to reappear). While calcium gluconate treats the life-threatening cardiac conduction disturbances associated with this electrolyte abnormality, further treatment is needed to treat the hyperkalemia itself (dextrose ± exogenous insulin, β2-agonists such as albuterol, etc.; see Chapter 8). Additional diagnostic testing therapy for urethral obstruction (intravenous crystalloid fluid therapy, urethral catheterization and de-obstruction) should be pursued.

Note that recognition of this ECG appearance as atrial standstill (rather than ventricular tachycardia) is vital to appropriate diagnosis and treatment of this patient. A misdiagnosis of ventricular tachycardia might have prompted lidocaine therapy, which (in addition to the risk of severe side effects in cats) would likely have slowed or extinguished this patient's ventricular depolarization completely, leading to cardiac arrest. The key to recognition of atrial standstill is the heart rate of 120 bpm in a cat, allowing the operator to focus on differentiating among bradyarrhythmias, rather than tachyarrhythmias.

Bibliography

Buczkowski, T., Janusek, D., Zavala-Fernandez, H., et al. (2013. Influence of mobile phones on the quality of ECG signal acquired by medical devices. *Measurement Science Review* 13, 231–236.

Cote, E., Ettinger, S.J. (2017) Cardiac arrhythmias. In: Ettinger, S.J., Feldman, E.C., Cote, E. (eds) *Textbook of Veterinary Internal Medicine*, 8th ed. Elsevier, St. Louis, Missouri, USA, pp. 1176–1200.

Cote, E., Harpster, N., Laste, N.J., et al. (2004) Atrial fibrillation in cats: 50 cases (1979-2002). *Journal of the American Veterinary Medical Association* 225, 256–260.

Finster, S.T., DeFrancesco, T.C., Atkins, C.E., et al. (2008) Supraventricular tachycardia in dogs: 65 cases (1990–2007). *Journal of Veterinary Emergency and Critical Care* 18, 503–510.

Gelzer, A.R.M., Kraus, M.S., Rishniw, M., et al. (2009) Combination therapy with digoxin and diltiazem controls ventricular rate in chronic atrial fibrillation in dogs better than digoxin or diltiazem monotherapy: a randomized crossover study in 18 dogs. *Journal of Veterinary Internal Medicine* 23, 499–508.

Gelzer, A.R.M., Kraus, M.S., Rishniw, M., et al. (2010) Combination therapy with mexiletine and sotolol suppresses inherited ventricular arrhythmias in German Shepherd dogs better than mexiletine or sotolol monotherapy: a randomized cross-over study. *Journal of Veterinary Cardiology* 12, 93–106.

Kraus, M., Gelzer, A., Rishniw, M. (2016) Detection of heart rate and rhythm with a smartphone-based electrocardiograph versus a reference standard electrocardiograph in dogs and cats. *Journal of the American Veterinary Medical Association* 249, 189–194.

Marriot, H.J.L., Conover, M.B. (1998) *Advanced Concepts in Arrhythmias*, 3rd ed. Mosby, St. Louis, Missouri, USA.

Menaut, P., Belanger, M.C., Beauchamp, G., et al. (2005). Atrial fibrillation in dogs with and without structural or functional cardiac disease: a retrospective study of 109 cases. *Journal of Veterinary Cardiology* 7, 75–83.

Meurs, K.M., Spier, A.W., Wright, N.A., et al. (2002) Comparison of the effects of four antiarrhythmic treatments for familial ventricular arrhythmias in Boxers. *Journal of the American Veterinary Medical Association* 221, 522–527.

Miller, M.W. (1999) Electrocardiography. In: Fox, P.R., Sisson, D., Moise, N.S. (eds) *Textbook of Canine and Feline Cardiology*, 2nd edn. Saunders, Philadelphia, Pennsylvania, USA, pp. 67–106.

Moise, N.S. (1999) Diagnosis and management of canine arrhythmias. In: Fox, P.R., Sisson, D., Moise, N.S. (eds) *Textbook of Canine and Feline Cardiology*, 2nd ed. Saunders, Philadelphia, Pennsylvania, USA, pp. 331–385.

Rishniw, M., Porciello, F., ERb, H.N., Fruganti, G. (2002) Effect of body position on the 6-lead ECG of dogs. *Journal of Veterinary Internal Medicine* 16, 69–73.

Santilli, R.A., Perego, M., Crosara, S., et al. (2008) Utility of 12-lead electrocardiogram for differentiating paroxysmal supraventricular tachycardias in dogs. *Journal of Veterinary Internal Medicine* 22, 915–923.

Schrope, D., Kelch, W. (2006) Signalment, clinical signs, and prognostic indicators associated with high-grade second- or third-degree atrioventricular block in dogs: 124 cases (January 1, 1997–December 31, 1997). *Journal of the American Veterinary Medical Association* 228, 1710–1717.

Smith, D.N., Schober, K.E. (2013) Effects of vagal maneuvers on heart rate and Doppler variables of left ventricular filling in healthy cats. *Journal of Veterinary Cardiology* 15, 33–40.

Stern, J.A., Hinchcliff, K.W., Constable, P.D. (2013) Effect of body position on electrocardiographic recordings in dogs. *Australian Veterinary Journal* 91, 281–286.

Tilley, L.P. (1992) *Essentials of Canine and Feline Electrocardiography*, 3rd edn. Lippincott Williams & Wilkins, Philadelphia, Pennsylvania, USA.

Ware, W.A. (2011) Overview of electrocardiography. In: Ware, W.A. (ed.) *Cardiovascular Disease in Small Animal Medicine*. Manson Publishing, London, UK, pp. 47–67.

Ward, J.W., DeFrancesco, T.C., Tou, S.P., *et al.* (2016) Outcome and survival in canine sick sinus syndrome and sinus node dysfunction: 93 cases (2002-2014). *Journal of Veterinary Cardiology* 18, 199–212.

Wess, G., Schulze, A., Geraghty, N., Hartmann, K. (2010) Ability of a 5-minute electrocardiography (ECG) for predicting arrhythmias in Doberman Pinschers with cardiomyopathy in comparison with a 24-hour ambulatory ECG. *Journal of Veterinary Internal Medicine* 24, 367–371.

Wright, K.N., Knilans, T.K., Irvin, H.M. (2006) When, why, and how to perform cardiac radiofrequency catheter ablation. *Journal of Veterinary Cardiology* 8, 95–107.

4 Pulse Oximetry

KRISTEN A. MARSHALL[1]* AND AIMEE C. BROOKS[2]

[1]*University of Tennessee, Knoxville, Tennessee, USA;* [2]*Purdue University College of Veterinary Medicine, West Lafayette, Indiana, USA*

4.1 Physiology

Oxygen (O_2) is carried in the blood in two forms: free gas dissolved in the plasma measured as a partial pressure (PO_2) and molecules reversibly bound to hemoglobin (Hb). Greater than 98% of the total oxygen in the blood is bound to Hb within red blood cells. The percentage of all available Hb-binding sites that are saturated with oxygen in arterial blood is called the SaO_2. When a pulse oximeter is used to estimate this saturation it is called the SpO_2. In this chapter, we will be focusing on the portion of oxygen that is bound to Hb. For more information about measurement and interpretation of PO_2, please see Chapter 5.

Each hemoglobin protein is composed of four protein subunits, with each subunit containing a heme and a globin portion (Fig. 4.1). The globin portion is made up of chains of amino acids that form spirals (helices), which give the protein its shape. Different types of globins will contain different amino acid sequences and lengths and are labeled by Greek letters. A complex of two α chains and two β chains is the most common globin configuration in adult mammals. Each globin chain is attached to a heme group that can interact with oxygen. Therefore, a fully saturated Hb protein is capable of carrying four oxygen molecules.

Hb exists in several different forms – which variety is determined by the amino acid composition of the α and β subunits. For example, adult human Hb contains two α and two β subunits, while fetal human Hb contains an α subunit and a γ-type β subunit. Abnormalities in the protein structure of Hb subunits as a result of genetic abnormalities can cause disease states in humans. The most commonly understood example of this is sickle cell anemia. Alpha- and β-subunit mutations likely exist in veterinary patients, but are poorly described.

The 'heme' portion of Hb is a porphyrin ring bound centrally to ferrous iron (Fe^{2+}; Fig. 4.2). The chemical structure of porphyrins contain many conjugated double bonds, which allow these compounds to absorb light within the visible spectrum, giving them color. This is why many similar porphyrins such as myoglobin (red) and chlorophyll (green) are varyingly colored, as are the breakdown products of heme (bilirubin; yellow, biliverdin; green, stercobilin; brown). Variation in the conformation of the porphyrin affects the wavelength of visible light that it absorbs. For Hb, this creates the visible difference between red arterial blood (containing oxygen, porphyrin, and Fe^{2+}) and purple venous blood (containing Fe^{2+} and porphyrin only). This variability in light absorption between oxygenated Hb (OxyHb) and deoxygenated Hb (DeOxyHb) is the basis for pulse oximetry and is how the eye can distinguish the presence of DeOxyHb as cyanosis.

Cyanosis is defined as a bluish discoloration of mucous membranes from the presence of an abnormal amount of DeOxyHb. Detection of cyanosis is subjective and dependent on variables such as ambient lighting (harder to detect with fluorescent lighting) and the visual acuity of the observer. In general, it is necessary to have a DeOxyHb concentration of ≥5 g/dL, consistent with a SpO_2 of <85%, to be able to visually detect cyanosis. Therefore, cyanosis may not be detected in severely anemic animals, especially if they do not have more than 5 g/dL of total Hb present in their body. These patients would likely die from hypoxemia before enough DeOxyHb is present for cyanosis to be observed. A general rule of thumb is that

---

* Corresponding author: kmarsh23@utk.edu

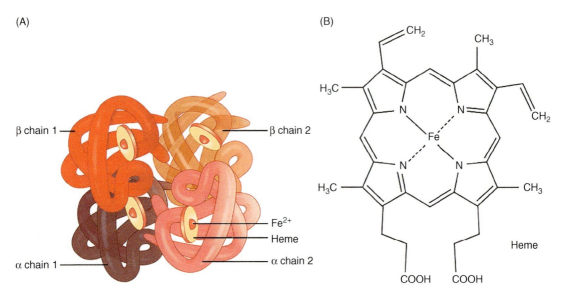

Fig. 4.1. A diagram of the structure of (A) hemoglobin and (B) heme. Note the two alpha and two beta globin chains, each with their associated heme subunits for oxygen binding. Open source Illustration from Anatomy & Physiology, Connexions https://commons.wikimedia.org/wiki/File:1904_Hemoglobin.jpg. (accessed 3 August 2019).

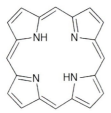

Fig. 4.2. The chemical structure of a porphyrin ring. Several varieties of porphyrin rings exist and are capable of binding with different metal ions. Porphyrins containing iron molecules are called heme. Open source illustration from https://commons.wikimedia.org/wiki/File:Porphyrin.svg (accessed 3 August 2019).

cyanotic animals can be presumed severely hypoxemic without further testing necessary (e.g. 'blue is bad'), but the lack of cyanosis does not necessarily indicate normal oxygen saturation ('pink is not necessarily OK').

Normally in nature, when Fe^{2+} reacts with O_2 it produces ferric iron (Fe^{3+}) as an *irreversible* oxidation reaction. A simple example of this reaction is rust on a cast iron skillet. However, the interaction between the iron molecule in heme and oxygen must be fully reversible under normal physiologic conditions to allow for easy uploading of oxygen in the lungs and offloading at the tissues. Oxygen can only bind to Hb in the ferrous (Fe^{2+}) state; an irreversible change to Fe^{3+} would render the molecule useless for carrying oxygen and the Hb would become non-functional as an O_2-transport protein. Therefore, to allow the Fe^{2+}–O_2 binding to be *reversible* in vivo, the globin portion of Hb contains approximately 20 amino acid residues that help to stabilize this interaction.

The most important of these amino acids is histidine which donates a negative charge to stabilize the Fe^{2+}–O_2 complex, changing the conformation of the surrounding globin proteins beyond just that single binding site and also affecting the other three binding sites within the same Hb complex. This protein conformation with one O_2 molecule binding to Fe^{2+} is termed a 'relaxed state' (RHb). In this relaxed state, Hb's affinity for oxygen increases by 150%, which facilitates rapid binding of the other three heme sites to O_2 molecules. In contrast, when no oxygen is bound to any Fe^{2+}, Hb undergoes a conformational change which disrupts the porphyrin ring structure. This results in Hb entering a 'tensed' state (THb). The structure of THb inhibits oxygen binding at any site; therefore, DeOxyHb has a low affinity for oxygen. This means that any given Hb protein in the blood prefers to be either fully saturated as OxyHb (four O_2 molecules) or fully desaturated (DeOxyHb, no O_2).

The term 'SaO_2' refers to the percentage of total Hb-binding sites bound to oxygen. Due to the conformational changes described above, Hb tends to either be fully bound (oxygen on all four sites – OxyHb – or deoxygenated). In other words, if 100 Hb proteins had a SaO_2 of 75%, it would typically indicate 25 were fully desaturated as DeOxyHb and 75 were fully saturated as OxyHb, as opposed to all 100 proteins each having three out of four binding sites filled with oxygen.

Oxyhemoglobin dissociation curve

How many Hb are fully saturated as OxyHb is determined by the partial pressure of oxygen in the plasma (PaO_2). Oxygen diffuses from the alveolus into the plasma first and then loads onto Hb. Conversely, when oxygen diffuses from the plasma into the tissues, oxygen is released from the Hb to replenish the plasma and allow for continued oxygen diffusion into tissues. The oxygen–hemoglobin dissociation curve (Fig. 4.3) describes the relationship between the SaO_2 and the PaO_2.

The dissolved oxygen (PaO_2) is the independent variable and is determined by lung function (see Chapter 5). The sigmoid shape of the OxyHb dissociation curve is due to the cooperation of the four oxygen binding sites on the Hb molecule. As the PaO_2 increases, SaO_2 rises rapidly as depicted by the steep slope of the curve. On the upper 'flatter' part of the curve, what seem to be small changes in SaO_2 (e.g. 95% to 90%) actually represents larger significant changes in oxygen concentration in the blood. As the curve becomes steeper, relatively small losses of lung function affecting PaO_2 can result in relatively large changes in SaO_2. The top of the curve is flattened because once all Hb molecules are fully saturated (SaO_2 = 100%), no matter how much the PaO_2 is increased, no further gain in SaO_2 is possible.

For patients who are breathing room air and therefore are still within the sigmoidal portion of the curve, the relationship between SpO_2 and PaO_2 allows SpO_2 to be used as a surrogate marker of PaO_2. For example, in a patient breathing room air with a pulse oximetry reading of 95%, it can be assumed that the PaO_2 is approximately 70 mmHg. The relationship between the dissolved oxygen and Hb-bound oxygen has significant clinical implications for the total oxygen content able to be carried in the blood as depicted in Box 4.1.

The oxygen–hemoglobin dissociation curve is a way to use the SpO_2 to approximate the PaO_2

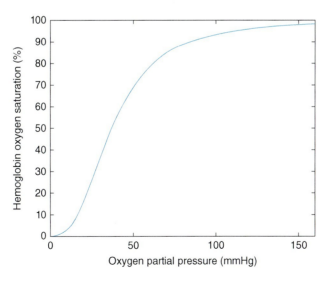

Fig. 4.3. The oxygen–hemoglobin dissociation curve describes the relationship between the percentage of Hb binding sites that are saturated with oxygen (SaO_2) and the partial pressure of oxygen in arterial blood (PaO_2) measured in millimeters of mercury (mmHg). Open source illustration from https://www.researchgate.net/figure/Hemoglobin-Binding-Curve-Hemoglobin-oxygen-saturation-as-a-function-of-partial-pressure_fig10_309876232 (accessed 3 August 2019).

Box 4.1. The impact of various scenarios on the total oxygen content of arterial blood (CaO_2).

The total oxygen content of the blood is calculated by the following equation:

$$CaO_2 = (Hb \times 1.34 \times SaO_2) + (PaO_2 \times 0.003)$$

Hb, hemoglobin in g/dL; SaO_2, the % saturation of arterial Hb as a decimal; and PaO_2, partial pressure of oxygen in arterial blood in mmHg.

1. For a normal canine patient with a normal hemoglobin of 15 mg/dL (equivalent to a PCV of ~45%) breathing room air (SpO_2 97%, PaO_2 100mmHg), we can solve this equation:

    $$CaO_2 = (15 \times 1.34 \times 0.97) + (100 \times 0.003) = \mathbf{19.8\,mL/dL}$$

    A normal CaO_2 is generally around 20 mL/dL

2. This normal patient is given 100% O_2, raising the PaO_2 to 500 mmHg. At this point according to the oxyhemoglobin dissociation curve, SaO_2 will be fully saturated at 100%:

    $$CaO_2 = (15 \times 1.34 \times 1) + (500 \times 0.003) = \mathbf{21.6\,mL/dL}$$

    While this is certainly a higher number than in point 1, raising the PaO_2 by five times (from 21% room air to 100% oxygen) only raised the CaO_2 by 1.2 mL/dL, or about 6%. This is because the Hb was already fully saturated at room air. Hemoglobin-bound oxygen contributes the largest volume to the total oxygen content. Therefore, when the hemoglobin is already saturated, raising the FiO_2 will only increase the dissolved oxygen content of the blood (the PaO_2), which has a much smaller impact on the total blood oxygen content than the amount of O_2 bound to Hb.

3. For a severely anemic patient with a hemoglobin of 3.3 mg/dL (PCV 10%) breathing room air (SpO_2 98%, PaO_2 100 mmHg):

    $$CaO_2 = (3.3 \times 1.34 \times 0.98) + (100 \times 0.003) = \mathbf{4.6\,mL/dL}; \text{ severely low}$$

4. If we provide the patient in point 3 with 40% oxygen supplementation and raise his PaO_2 to 200 mmHg with a SaO_2 of 100%:

    $$CaO_2 = (3.3 \times 1.34 \times 1) + (200 \times 0.003) = \mathbf{5.02\,mL/dL}; \text{ still severely low}$$

    Despite doubling the PaO_2, the CaO_2 only increased minimally. This is because the minimal amount of hemoglobin in this anemic dog is already fully saturated. The oxygen supplementation is only bolstering the dissolved plasma oxygen content (PaO_2) and not greatly improving the total oxygen content. This is why supplementing oxygen in a severely anemic animal cannot overcome the need for red blood cell transfusion.

5. In a patient with a normal Hb (15 mg/dL) who is hypoxemic (SpO_2 90% and PaO_2 60 mmHg):

    $$CaO_2 = (15 \times 1.34 \times 0.9) + (60 \times 0.003) = \mathbf{18\,mL/dL}; \text{ below normal}$$

6. Supplementation of the patient in point 5 with oxygen raises the PaO_2 to 80 mmHg, causing a concurrent rise in the SaO_2 to 95%

    $$CaO_2 = (15 \times 1.34 \times 0.95) + (80 \times 0.003) = \mathbf{19.3\,mL/dL}; \text{ closer to normal}$$

    Note that it is not the rise in PaO_2 that caused the majority of this change; the elevation from 60 to 80 mmHg added only 0.06 mg/dL to the total. However, because increasing the PaO_2 also increases the SaO_2 (Fig. 4.3), the total oxygen content carried by hemoglobin also increased, contributing the most to the increase in the total oxygen content.

when breathing room air. However, as shown in the curve, above a PaO_2 of about 100 mmHg, SaO_2 is no longer a good surrogate for PaO_2 (and by extension lung function). Once the patient's lungs hit the plateau depicted in Fig. 4.3, all the Hb-binding sites are saturated with oxygen and any additional oxygen diffusing from the lungs must remain in the dissolved pool. For example, in a patient with normal lungs and breathing 100% O_2 as when under general anesthesia, the expected PaO_2 should be approximately 400–500 mmHg but the SaO_2 will be 100%. If that same patient loses 50% lung function and the PaO_2 drops to 250 mmHg, the SaO_2 will still be 100%. In fact, for patients breathing higher concentrations of O_2, a decreasing SaO_2 is a *late* indicator of a significant loss of lung function, and is insensitive for detection of earlier, milder losses of lung function.

The oxygen–hemoglobin dissociation curve can also be shifted either left (increased Hb affinity for O_2) or right (decreased Hb affinity for O_2; see Fig. 4.4). As seen by the dashed lines in Fig. 4.4, when the curve is shifted to the right, the same PaO_2 correlates with a decreased SaO_2 versus the normal curve. For a left shift, it is the opposite; the same PaO_2 correlates with an increased SaO_2 versus normal. Factors that will right shift the curve include increased concentration of hydrogen ions (H^+; i.e. decreased pH), CO_2, and temperature. A practical example of this occurs in skeletal muscles during exercise. Exercise increases the amount of CO_2, H^+, and temperature, right shifting the curve and reducing the affinity of Hb for oxygen. The goal is to improve offloading of oxygen in the metabolically active tissues. Conversely, decreases in H^+ ions, increased pH, decreased CO_2, and decreased temperature cause the curve to be shifted to the left. These circumstances improve uptake of oxygen onto Hb and are similar to what occurs in the pulmonary capillaries where oxygen diffuses first into the plasma and is then loaded onto the Hb.

While very small shifts in the curve may happen even within different tissue beds, larger systemic abnormalities in pH or temperature can cause more global effects on oxygen delivery in the body. The reason that this is important is that shifting of the curve makes the 'normal' expected relationship between PaO_2 and SaO_2 invalid. For example, practitioners should be aware that in a patient who has an extreme fever, the curve will be shifted to the right and the SaO_2 will be lower than expected given the measured PaO_2 (Fig. 4.4). In this sort of setting, the best option for a clinician is to measure the PaO_2 directly rather than trying to predict it from the SaO_2 reading.

Abnormal hemoglobin forms

Methemoglobin

Oxidative damage to red blood cells can cause the formation of methemoglobin (MetHb). The damage results in the iron molecule at the core of the heme being converted from the ferrous (Fe^{2+}) to the ferric state (Fe^{3+}). In this state, MetHb is unable to bind to oxygen. Because some oxidative damage is always occurring in nature, red blood cells contain

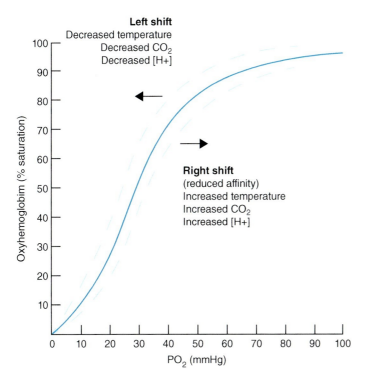

Fig. 4.4. Shifts in the oxyhemoglobin dissociation curve. The normal curve is depicted in the solid line, with the dotted lines indicating either right or left shifting caused by the listed factors. PO_2, partial pressure of oxygen; [H^+], hydrogen ion concentration; CO_2, carbon dioxide. Open source illustration from https://litfl.com/oxygen-haemoglobin-dissociation-curve/. (accessed 3 August 2019).

an enzyme called methemoglobin reductase, which reduces the iron back to the ferrous state. Normally, this mechanism maintains very low levels of MetHb in the blood. However, if this system is overwhelmed, as seen with various conditions including toxicities (see Table 4.1), high levels of MetHb can impair oxygen delivery by essentially creating a functional anemia. Because the change from Fe^{2+} to Fe^{3+} impacts the electrochemical structure of the porphyrin ring, it changes the wavelengths of light absorbed by the molecule, giving blood with a high content of MetHb a brown appearance.

Carboxyhemoglobin

The most common abnormal form of Hb encountered in veterinary medicine is carboxyhemoglobin (COHb). This results from inhalation of carbon monoxide (CO), a compound that binds to Hb with an affinity approximately 200–250 times greater than oxygen. This high-affinity binding means the Hb molecules that have CO bound at one site will remain in the relaxed state, increasing the affinity for binding O_2 at the other open sites. This also causes the OxyHb dissociation curve to shift to the left (Hb binding oxygen more readily).

OHb is detrimental in two ways. First, CO binds to a place that should be occupied by O_2, resulting in less O_2 overall in the blood. Secondly, by shifting the oxygen–hemoglobin dissociation curve to the left, COHb reduces offloading of any O_2 present on the Hb to the tissues. Since the iron-binding site on Hb is occupied by CO and the porphyrin ring is not changed versus normal, COHb absorbs very similar wavelengths of light as OxyHb. Therefore, the blood color with COHb is red, despite the fact that patients may have only a small amount of actual O_2 bound to Hb and decreased delivery of O_2 to tissues.

Table 4.1. Common causes of methemoglobinemia in veterinary medicine.

Medications	Toxins
Acetaminophen	Skunk musk
Benzocaine	Onions
Prilocaine	Garlic
Lidocaine	Naphthalene (mothballs)
Metoclopramide	
Sodium nitroprusside/nitroglycerin	
Hydroxyurea	

4.2 How Does Pulse Oximetry Work?

Pulse oximetry (aka 'pulse-ox') is a noninvasive, continuous monitoring modality that uses two wavelengths of light to estimate the SaO_2 in pulsatile arterial blood. Red light (wavelength 660 nm) and near infrared light (940 nm) are projected into tissues via a light-emitting diode (LED) on the pulse-ox probe. This light penetrates into tissues easily. Oxygenated Hb absorbs greater amounts of infrared light and less red light compared with deoxygenated Hb. How much light of each wavelength is absorbed vs how much was transmitted is detected by the photodiode sensor on the probe. The Lambert–Beer law states that the concentration of a substance is proportional to the absorption of light of a specific wavelength by the substance and the distance through which the light travels. Therefore, the differential light absorption between OxyHB and DeOxyHb can be used to calculate the amount of OxyHb versus DeOxyHb that is present.

As the light travels through the tissue bed, it will be absorbed by Hb in the arterial, capillary, and venous blood. To differentiate the Hb in arterial blood from these other areas, the pulse-ox probe must be placed in an area where arterial pulsation can be detected by the sensor. The sensor detects the absorption of light in these non-pulsatile areas as a 'static' signal, and the absorption of light in the arterial blood as an alternating signal (Fig. 4.5). It then uses a ratio of these signals and compares this ratio to proprietary formulas stored within the machine to calculate the SpO_2. It is crucial that the pulse-ox be able to detect an accurate pulsatile flow to be able to distinguish arterial Hb saturation from the Hb within other tissues.

Probe types

Two types of pulse oximetry probes are commonly used in veterinary medicine. Transmission probes (Fig. 4.6) are the type of probe commonly placed on a human finger or earlobe. The tissue is sandwiched between the LED and sensor portions of the probe. This type of probe is commonly placed on the tongue, lip, vulva, prepuce, toe webbing, flank, or ear of small animal patients. The tissue must be thin enough to allow light transmission (i.e. no thicker than can comfortably fit within the 'clip' of the transmission probe), but well-perfused enough to give a good pulsatile signal. Therefore, mucous membranes (tongue, lip, prepuce, vulva) tend to work best.

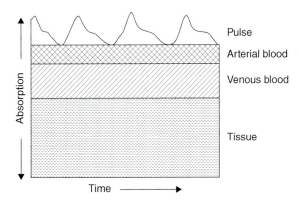

Fig. 4.5. Light passing through tissues will be absorbed by hemoglobin (Hb) in multiple compartments. By analyzing the ratio of absorption between the signal that varies with pulsatile flow versus the signal that is static, the pulse oximeter differentiates between the saturation of Hb in arterial blood and other tissues and reports only the saturation of the Hb in arterial blood. Therefore, detection of pulsatile flow is critical to the accuracy of the reading.

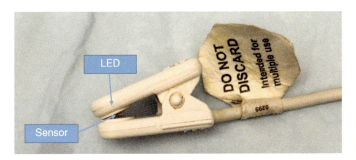

Fig. 4.6. Transmission pulse oximetry probe (Massimo, Irvine, California, USA). LED, light emitting diode.

Transmission probes are generally poorly tolerated for long-term use unless the patient is anesthetized or moribund since they fall off easily with movement. Also, transmission probes will gradually compress the tissue bed and can compress the vessels, reducing the all-important arterial blood flow and causing the probe to not give a reading. When using a transmission probe, the LED and sensor portions of the probe must be in correct alignment or the signal can be distorted, resulting in inaccurate measurements.

Reflectance probes (Fig. 4.7) have the LED and sensor on the same side of the probe. The emitted light is reflected off the bone and is then received by the sensor. To allow for proper reflection back to the sensor, the reflectance probe must either be placed over a flat bone (e.g. the forehead in humans or the ventral aspect of the first coccygeal bone in animals) or held at just the right angle to a more curved bone to allow proper reflection of the emitted light back to the sensor. The distance from the LED to the bone must not be any farther than the distance between the two sides of the transmission probe in order to allow the emitted light to reflect back to the sensor.

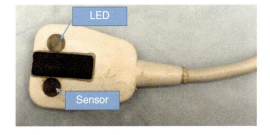

Fig. 4.7. Reflectance pulse oximetry probe (Massimo, Irvine, California, USA). LED, light emitting diode.

In anesthetized animals, reflectance probes can be used on the hard palate or within the esophagus. In awake animals, these probes can be used on the underside of the base of the tail, over the femoral artery/proximal femoral bone, on the dorsal surface of the metatarsus, or the plantar side of the carpus. Versions of reflectance probes made to be used intrarectally (pointed dorsally against the sacrum) can be used in asleep or awake patients depending on temperament. The advantage to reflectance probes is that they are sometimes better tolerated in awake animals for longer-term use (i.e. taped to the underside of a tail on a patient in the oxygen cage), and can be used on smaller patients where the larger transmission probe clips are too bulky for use. There is less pressure on the tissues than with the transmission probe clips as well, which may allow for longer use without occlusion of the arterial blood flow.

Gauging the accuracy of the pulse-ox readings

Accuracy of pulse oximetry results are generally gauged by observing the output on the pulse oximeter and correlating it to the patient. It is essential that probe is receiving a strong pulsatile blood flow signal. The signal quality can be reported on the pulse oximeter in a few different ways depending on the unit used. In some monitors the signal quality can be shown by bar indicators, where the greater number of bars, the better the signal quality (Figs 4.8 and 4.9). Other types of monitors display the actual plethysmographic tracing, similar to an arterial pressure waveform (Fig. 4.9). If the pulse oximeter displays a good-looking uniform waveform or high signal quality, it is more likely to be accurate (Figs 4.8 and 4.9).

To confirm the waveform is actually detecting the arterial pulse, the heart rate displayed on the pulse-ox should always be matched to the heart rate detected by an independent method (auscultation, pulse palpation, ECG, etc.) Any pulse oximetry reading in which the heart rate displayed on the machine does not match the patient's heart rate should be considered inaccurate (Figs 4.10 and 4.11). When initially attaching a pulse oximetry probe it is important to remember that it takes several heart beats for the sensor to assess the data from multiple waveform peaks, so the results are not instantaneous.

The results obtained from the pulse oximeter should always be correlated to the clinical status of the patient. For example, a patient who appears to be in significant respiratory distress with a pulse oximetry reading of 100% should ideally have their oxygenation status confirmed by an arterial blood gas before deciding that they do not need

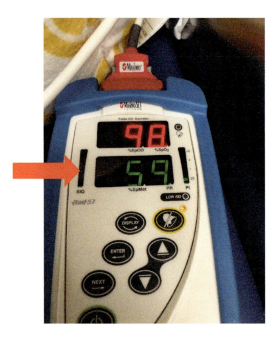

Fig. 4.8. A pulse oximetry unit (Massimo, Irvine, California, USA) demonstrating poor signal quality (SIQ) as shown by the red arrow.

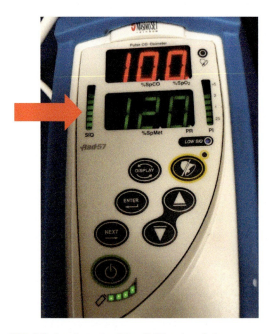

Fig. 4.9. A pulse oximetry unit (Massimo, Irvine, California, USA) receiving good signal quality (SIQ) as shown by the red arrow.

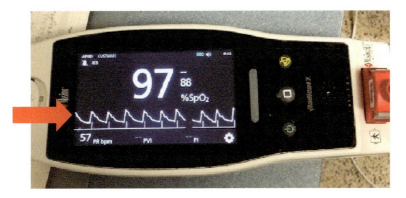

Fig. 4.10. A pulse oximetry unit (Massimo, Irvine, California, USA) displaying a plethysmographic tracing similar to an arterial waveform reading (red arrow). The waveform depicted in this image represents a good tracing and if the heart rate shown here matches the patient, the pulse oximetry reading is likely to be accurate barring other confounding variables (see Table 4.2).

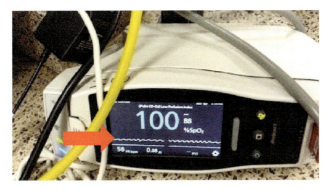

Fig. 4.11. A pulse oximeter displaying a weak waveform (red arrow). It is important to note in this photo that while the pulse oximetry value of 100% and a heart rate of 58 bpm are possibly within the normal reference range for a dog, the probe was not actually connected to a patient while it was displaying the readings shown in this photo, displaying a likely motion or time-delay artifact. This underlines the importance of ensuring a good waveform or signal quality along with heart rate on all patients prior to looking at the pulse oximetry reading.

oxygen supplementation. Similarly, anemic patients may have a normal pulse-ox reading but still be in need of oxygen to deliver to the tissues.

4.3 Indications for Pulse Oximetry

Patients frequently present to the emergency department for clinical signs consistent with respiratory distress. In that setting, it is important to differentiate between true hypoxemia and other conditions that can also cause a rapid respiratory rate such as pain, fear, stress, or acidosis. Pulse oximetry is a fast, minimally invasive way to screen for hypoxemia in these patients.

Patients with normal pulse-ox values (with strong signals that match their heart rates on the monitor, i.e. that are 'believe-able') should be suspected of having these 'look-alike' causes of tachypnea. Patients with 'believe-able' pulse-ox values <95%, with poor pulse-ox signals, or who have significant signs of respiratory abnormalities despite normal readings (e.g. significant work of breathing, abnormal upper airway noises, etc.) should be considered possibly hypoxemic until proven otherwise. Supply these patients with oxygen while additional diagnostics are performed to address the underlying cause.

If you are unsure if a patient is suffering from hypoxemia or are unable to believe the pulse-ox reading, perform an arterial blood gas (see Chapter 5). Patients who are cyanotic do not need to have pulse oximetry performed as the observer has already confirmed severe hypoxemia from visual examination. At that moment, these patients need emergent interventions, not exact measurements of the degree of hypoxemia.

Any patient undergoing heavy sedation or general anesthesia should have continuous monitoring with pulse oximetry. Patients who are heavily sedated to anesthetized are at high risk of hypoxemia, hypoventilation, or apnea for a variety of reasons. Continuous monitoring with pulse oximetry gives visual and auditory clues to the person monitoring anesthesia that desaturation is occurring and therefore can lead to life-saving interventions. It is important to remember that patients breathing high concentrations of oxygen are very far to the right on the flat portion of the OxyHb dissociation curve (see Fig. 4.3). As noted in Section 4.1, these patients can experience significant loss of lung function and reductions in PaO_2 long before they reach the sigmoidal portion of the curve and the pulse-ox will actually start to drop. Therefore, a reliably dropping pulse-ox in a patient breathing supplemental oxygen should be taken as a late indicator of a very serious oxygenation problem and immediately investigated.

4.4 Interpretation of Results

Pulse oximetry values are reported as a percentage. A normal SpO_2 in a patient breathing room air (FiO_2 = 21%) is generally between 96–98%, which corresponds to a PaO_2 on the OxyHb dissociation curve of 85–100 mmHg (see Fig. 4.2). Hypoxemia is defined as a PaO_2 less than 80 mmHg and severe hypoxemia as a PaO_2 of less than 60 mmHg. Therefore, patients with the correlating pulse-ox reading of <95% should be considered hypoxemic and <90% severely hypoxemic.

The pulse oximeter is generally accurate within ± 2–3% of the measured SaO_2 on an individual's arterial blood gas but becomes less accurate with worsening hypoxemia. In patients with a true SaO_2 <90%, the pulse oximeter may vary by as much as ± 5%. Therefore, readings should be interpreted more as trends within an individual patient and to classify general categories of hypoxemia rather than becoming fixated on a specific value. For example, a patient with a SpO_2 of 85% might actually be as low as 80% or as high as 90%; either way, this patient is severely hypoxemic and requires immediate intervention.

Patients breathing supplemental oxygen should have pulse-ox readings that are >98%. As mentioned in Section 4.1, pulse oximetry no longer correlates with PaO_2 once the PaO_2 is significantly greater than 100 mmHg and cannot be used as a surrogate for lung function outside of this range. Pulse oximetry values <95% indicate the need for oxygen supplementation as they correlate with PaO_2 values less than 80 mmHg (i.e. hypoxemia).

Pulse oximetry can be inaccurate for a variety of reasons as discussed in the next section. Any abnormal result that does not fit with the patient's presentation or physical exam should be confirmed with an arterial blood gas analysis, as this is the gold standard to diagnose hypoxemia. For more information about interpretation of arterial blood gas analysis, please see Chapter 5.

4.5 Pitfalls of Pulse Oximetry

Multiple factors can affect the accuracy of pulse oximetry in veterinary patients; these are outlined in Table 4.2. In general, anything that interferes with the pulse oximeter's ability to detect an accurate pulsatile light signal may cause interference. Additional patient factors that affect the accuracy of pulse oximetry are the presence of abnormal species of Hb; pulse oximetry cannot differentiate between MetHb, COHb, and OxyHb. Interestingly, the application of gauze sponges between the tongue and pulse-ox transmission probe has actually been shown to improve SpO_2 readings in both dogs and cats. It is hypothesized that the added thickness between the tongue and the LED and sensor on the probe improves contact pressure.

Hb alterations

It is important to remember that the pulse oximeter is an approximation of the percentage of Hb in arterial blood that is saturated with oxygen, NOT an approximation of the total arterial oxygen content. As outlined in Box 4.1, severely anemic patients can have significantly low arterial oxygen content despite fully saturated Hb.

Similarly, the presence of a normal amount of oxygen in the blood does not guarantee that tissues are adequately oxygenated. For example, cyanide toxicosis inhibits oxidative phosphorylation inside the cell, preventing extraction of oxygen from the blood into the cell. This will result in a high concentration of oxygen in both venous and arterial blood, as none leaves to enter the tissues yet the tissues are

Table 4.2. Possible causes of inaccurate pulse oximetry readings.

Abnormality	Example	Effect on SpO$_2$ reading
Carboxyhemoglobin	Patient in recent house fire	Spuriously high readings
Methemoglobin	Exposure to toxins or drugs (see Table 4.1)	Spurious readings in the 80s
Vasoconstriction	Hypothermia, shock, vasoconstrictive drugs	Reduced pulsatile signal, increased risk of motion artifacts, variable effects on readings
Vasodilation	Hyperthermia, SIRS/sepsis	Venous congestion may lead to venous pulsation and artifactually low readings as pulsing venous blood is misread as arterial
Excessive motion	Non-compliant patient	If interpreted as pulsation, may cause erroneous readings (both falsely high and low)
Pigmented tissues	Black pigment on gums/lips	Low signal quality as less light will reach the sensor (absorbed by pigment)
Other light sources/electrical energy detected by photodiode	Fluorescent lights, electrocautery	Variable effects if light is absorbed erroneously by sensor; better compensated for in newer units
Lack of pulsatile blood flow	Cardiac arrest, thrombosis of tissue bed	Other artifacts (e.g. motion) may be interpreted as pulsatile flow and give erroneous readings. Pulse oximetry should not be considered accurate in low flow/no flow states
Anemia	Blood loss, hemolysis	Generally accurate except at extremely low (<75%) saturation or anemic shock resulting in vasoconstriction
Intravenous dyes	Methylene blue	Spuriously low readings, pigment affects amount of light reaching the sensor
Hyperbilirubinemia/icterus	Hemolysis, liver disease	Generally accurate assuming minimal presence of other dyshemoglobinemias (e.g. COHb)
Shifted OxyHb dissociation curve	Changes in body temperature, acid–base status, hyper/hypoventilation	The correlation between SpO$_2$ and PaO$_2$ will be shifted (see Fig. 4.4); the practitioner must take this into account when interpreting SpO$_2$ values and using them to predict PaO$_2$
Arrhythmias	Atrial fibrillation, VPCs	Correlate with ECG, but if signal quality is good and SpO$_2$ reading is stable, generally do not affect accuracy of readings

COHb, carboxyhemoglobin; ECG, electrocardiogram; OxyHb, oxyhemoglobin; PaO$_2$, partial pressure of oxygen in plasma; SIRS, systemic inflammatory response syndrome; SpO$_2$, pulse oximetry; VPC, ventricular premature contraction.

hypoxemic. In this setting, despite all measured values being normal in the blood and mucous membranes appearing bright pink/red, the patient will still have a significant tissue oxygen derangement.

Dyshemoglobinemias, such as MetHb and COHb, are also particularly confounding to pulse oximetry. The two wavelengths of light emitted in traditional pulse oximetry cannot differentiate OxyHb from COHb. Pulse oximeters therefore measure COHb as OxyHb and will give spuriously high readings that do not reflect the true SaO$_2$. For example, if a patient has 80% OxyHb and 15% COHb, the pulse oximeter would read 95%, which is falsely inflated by 15%. In this setting, a PaO$_2$ MUST be measured to determine the amount of oxygen in the plasma available to tissues.

MeHb absorbs infrared and red light equally well, which is more infrared light than either OxyHb or DeOxyHb absorb. It also absorbs a similar amount of red light to DeOxyHb. Therefore, when there are significant MetHb levels in the blood (typically >30%), this can lead to a pulse oximetry machine reading in the 80–85% range, regardless of the actual amount of OxyHb. This might over or underestimate the true SaO_2 depending on the patient's clinical status. In this setting, a PaO_2 MUST be measured to determine the amount of oxygen in the plasma available to tissues. In order to definitively diagnose MetHb, co-oximetry (discussed below) or a MetHb assay should be performed.

Co-oximetry

Certain pulse oximetry units have the ability to measure abnormal Hb variants. The sensors on these units emit the standard wavelengths of light at 660 nm and 940 nm, but also emit two (or more) additional wavelengths at 500 nm and 1400 nm. These expanded wavelengths allow for the differentiation between MetHb, COHb, OxyHb, and DeOxyHb. These units are commercially available, although not widely used.

More commonly, co-oximetry is performed as part of arterial blood gas analysis, if the blood gas analyzer has spectrophotometric capabilities. To obtain the co-oximetry reading, the blood sample is hemolyzed and between four and eight different wavelengths of light are projected through the sample to measure OxyHb, DeOxyHb, COHb, and MetHb. The analyzer will typically display each as a % of the total Hb measured and calculate the percent oxygen saturation (SaO_2).

4.6 Case Studies

Case study 1: Do you trust this SpO_2 reading?

An 11-year-old female, spayed mixed breed dog presents for increased respiratory rate and effort. On physical examination she is quiet, alert and responsive, and is ambulatory with increased bronchovesicular sounds bilaterally. Her vitals include a temperature of 101.3°F (38.5°C), a heart rate of 190 beats/minute and a respiratory rate of 70 breaths/minute. Her mucous membranes are pink and moist. Your assistant reports that they performed a pulse oximetry measurement on your patient which revealed a SpO_2 of 45% and a heart rate of 180 beats/minute.

Do you believe this value? What would you do to troubleshoot to assess the accuracy of this value?

This is a significantly low SpO_2 reading, indicating very severe hypoxia barely compatible with life. This patient, while exhibiting signs consistent with respiratory distress (increased lung sounds and respiratory rate), is conscious and ambulatory which does not fit with the measured pulse oximetry reading. Assuming the patient is not also severely anemic, she would be expected to be cyanotic at a SpO_2 of 45% but her mucous membranes are pink.

Despite a heart rate that is 'close' to that of the patient, the poor correlation with clinical signs should make the practitioner consider this reading erroneous. This does not automatically mean we can assume the patient is oxygenating well, simply that we do not know her true level of oxygenation. Repeating the reading on a different tissue bed, making sure the probe is in place long enough to see good signal quality, troubleshooting for issues such as outlined in Table 4.2, or measurement of blood oxygenation (PaO_2) via arterial blood gas analysis could be considered in this patient to further assess whether or not hypoxemia is the cause of these clinical signs.

Case study 2: SpO_2 in a house fire patient

A 3-year-old female spayed domestic shorthaired cat presents after being rescued from a house fire. Her vital signs are as follows: temperature 101.0°F (38.3°C), pulse 220 beats/minute, respiratory rate 60 breaths/minute, mucous membranes pink, capillary refill time <2 seconds. She is obtunded and recumbent with increased respiratory effort. She has no obvious external burns but smells strongly of smoke. Her pulse-ox reads 98% with a strong signal matching her heart rate.

Does this patient require supplemental oxygen?

Given her history of recently being in a house fire, carbon monoxide, cyanide toxicity (commonly released from burning materials), and smoke inhalation are all possible concerns. While primary lung damage caused by smoke inhalation would normally lower the SpO_2, this may be masked by artificial elevation of the SpO_2 caused by COHb or cyanide toxicosis.

You perform a standard arterial blood gas and find a pH of 7.3, a PaO_2 of 90 mmHg, $PaCO_2$ of 32 mmHg, bicarbonate (HCO_3^-) of 15.2 mEq/L, base excess −9.9, and a SaO_2 of 96%. Lactate is moderately elevated at 4.0 mg/dL.

Does this patient require supplemental oxygen?

The normal PaO_2 tells you that the lungs are functioning well and severe compromise from smoke inhalation is unlikely at this point in time (but should be reassessed over time). However, if this analyzer is not performing co-oximetry, it cannot differentiate OxyHb from COHb, so the SaO_2 given by the analyzer may be confounded just like the pulse oximeter.

The elevated lactate (see Chapter 1) implies that the tissues are not receiving adequate oxygen/not able to utilize oxygen appropriately, consistent with decreased perfusion, COHb, or cyanide toxicosis.

At this point, you could perform co-oximetry (if available) to quantify the amount of COHb present, which would be useful in differentiating COHb from cyanide toxicosis. However, since short-term provision of oxygen is unlikely to harm this patient and is the mainstay of treatment for COHb toxicosis, high levels of O_2 should be provided to this patient to treat presumptive COHb toxicosis even if co-oximetry is not available. Oxygen therapy helps to out-compete the CO for the Hb binding sites and also helps to provide more oxygen to the plasma portion of the bloodstream.

Case study 3: Post-operative SpO_2 drop

A 6-month-old 3-kg miniature poodle undergoes a routine ovariohysterectomy at your clinic. During recovery/extubation, the patient appears to be in respiratory distress and diffuse crackles are ausculted in all lung lobes. The pulse oximeter throughout the procedure read 98%, but now reads 90% with a strong waveform that matches her heart rate.

What does the precipitous drop in the pulse-ox reading from anesthesia to recovery indicate?

While under general anesthesia this patient was breathing 100% oxygen, which should cause her PaO_2 to be between 400–500 mmHg. Her pulse-ox will read 98–100% as long as the PaO_2 is >100 mmHg (on the flat portion of the disassociation curve). Therefore, it is possible that her lung function was decreasing throughout the procedure, but this was not detected until she was removed from oxygen and placed back on room air since the pulse-ox reading would remain 100% even with significant alterations in lung function while she was receiving 100% oxygen. In fact, her pulse oximetry reading would not be expected to fall below normal while breathing 100% O_2 until her PaO_2 was <80 mmHg (i.e. >75% of lung function lost) All possible causes of iatrogenic respiratory compromise from intubation until present should be considered in this patient including but not limited to aspiration pneumonia, a pulmonary thromboembolism, pulmonary edema formation, severe atelectasis, and occult lung disease. In many cases, thoracic radiographs can lead to a diagnosis.

Further investigation revealed a math error resulting in the patient receiving 100 mL/kg/h of intravenous fluids during the procedure rather than 10 mL/kg/h. This led to fluid overload and pulmonary edema. The patient was treated with oxygen support and intravenous furosemide and made a complete recovery.

Bibliography

Auckburally, A. (2016) Pulse oximetry and oxygenation assessment in small animal practice. *In Practice* 38, 50–58.

Boron, W. (2012) Transport of oxygen and carbon dioxide in the blood. In: Boron, W., Boulpaep, E. (eds) *Medical Physiology*, 2nd edn. Elsevier, St Louis, Missouri, USA, pp. 672–684.

Brunelle, J., Degtiarov, A., Moran, R., et al. (1996) Simultaneous measurement of total hemoglobin and its derivatives in blood using co-oximeters: Analytical principles; their application in selecting analytical wavelengths and reference methods; a comparison of the results of the choices made. *Scandinavian Journal of Clinical and Laboratory Investigation* 56, 47-69.

Chan, E., Chan, M., Chan, M. (2017) Pulse oximetry: understanding its basic principles facilitates appreciation of its limitations. *Respiratory Medicine* 107, 789–799.

Duke-Novakovski, T. (2017) Basics of monitoring equipment. *Canadian Veterinary Journal* 58, 1200–1208.

Gewib, H., Timm, U., Kraitl, J., et al. (2017) Non-invasive multi wavelengths sensor system for measuring carboxy- and methemoglobin. *Current Directions in Biomedical Engineering* 3, 441–444.

Gracia, R., Shepherd, G. (2004) Cyanide poisoning and its treatment. *Pharmacotherapy* 24, 1358–1365.

Hackett, T. (2002) Pulse oximetry and end tidal carbon dioxide monitoring. *Veterinary Clinics of North America: Small Animal Practice* 32, 1021–1029.

Herrmann, K., Haskins, S. (2005) Determination of P_{50} for feline hemoglobin. *Journal of Veterinary Emergency and Critical Care* 15, 26–31.

Jubran, A. (2004) Pulse oximetry. *Intensive Care Medicine* 30, 2017–2020.

Mair, A., Taboada, F., Nitzan, M. (2017) Effect of lingual gauze swab placement on pulse oximeter readings in anesthetized dogs and cats. *Veterinary Record* 180, 49.

Marino, P.L. (2014) Systemic oxygenation. In: Marino, P.L. (ed.) *The ICU Book*, 4th edn. Wolters Kluwer, Philadelphia, Pennsylvania, USA, pp. 171–192.

Pachtinger, G. (2013) Monitoring of the emergent small animal patient. *Veterinary Clinics of North America: Small Animal Practice* 43, 705–720.

Proulx, J. (1999) Respiratory Monitoring: Arterial blood gas analysis, pulse oximetry, and end tidal carbon dioxide analysis. *Clinical Techniques in Small Animal Practice* 14, 227–230.

Rahily, L., Mandell, D. (2014) Methemoglobinemia. In: Silverstein, D., Hopper, K. (eds) *Small Animal Critical Care Medicine*, 2nd edn. Elsevier, St Louis, Missouri, USA, pp. 580–585.

Raschi-Sorrell, L. (2014) Blood gas and oximetry monitoring. In: Silverstein, D., Hopper, K. (eds.) *Small Animal Critical Care Medicine*, 2nd edn. Elsevier, St Louis, Missouri, USA, pp. 962–966.

Read, M., Rondeau, J., Kwong, G. (2016) Validation of noninvasive hemoglobin measurements using co-oximetry in anesthetized dogs. *Canadian Veterinary Journal* 57, 1161–1165.

Shamir, M., Avramovich, A., Smaka, T. (2012) The current status of continuous noninvasive measurement of total, carboxy and methemoglobin concentration. *Anesthesia and Analgesia* 114, 972–978.

Toffaletti, J., Rackley, C. (2016) Monitoring oxygen status. *Advances in Clinical Chemistry* 77, 103–123.

Thawley, V., Waddell, L. (2013) Pulse oximetry and capnography. *Topics in Companion Animal Medicine*, 28, 124-128.

Verhovsek, M., Henderson, M., Cox, G., *et al*. (2010) Unexpectedly low pulse oximetry measurements associated with variant hemoglobins: A systematic review. *American Journal of Hematology* 85, 882–885.

Vincent, J., Backer, D. (2004) Oxygen transport – the oxygen delivery controversy. *Intensive Care Medicine* 30, 1990–1996.

Yudin, J., Verhovsek, M. (2019) How we diagnose and manage altered oxygen affinity hemoglobin variants. *American Journal of Hematology* 94, 597–603.

5 Venous and Arterial Blood Gas Analysis

AIMEE C. BROOKS*

Purdue University College of Veterinary Medicine, West Lafayette, Indiana, USA

Venous blood gas analysis is often used as first-line 'stat' blood work to assess acid–base status, electrolytes, and (depending on the monitor) other parameters such as renal values and lactate. Arterial blood gas analysis is generally performed when assessment of the oxygenation/ventilation status of the patient is desired. As other chapters of this book (see Chapters 1 and 8) discuss point-of-care values such as lactate and electrolyte abnormalities, this chapter will focus on acid–base assessment and assessment of oxygenation/ventilation status. Indirect monitors of oxygenation and ventilation are discussed in Chapters 4 and 6, respectively.

5.1 Basic Physiology and Anatomy

Blood gas analysis: Acid–base

Acid–base: Traditional approach

The blood pH is inversely proportional to the concentration of hydrogen ions ([H+]) in the bloodstream; as [H+] goes up, pH goes down. Therefore, a decreasing pH is consistent with acid*emia* (more acidic blood) and an increasing pH with alkal*emia* (more basic or alkaline blood). The underlying process that causes the pH to go up or down is the –osis, e.g. an uncomplicated metabolic acid*osis* will result in acid*emia*.

The normal pH of most mammals is around 7.4. For dogs, the normal range of pH is 7.35–7.46, and for cats, 7.31–7.46, although these values will vary slightly by analyzer and readers should use the normal ranges provided for their machine. Values outside of these ranges should be considered abnormalities, with the more extreme deviations leading to more significant side effects. Severe acid–base abnormalities can cause significant dysfunction of the cardiovascular and neurological systems, and can result in organ failure and death.

When considering the pH, even small deviations from the normal range can be important. Since pH is a logarithmic scale, a change in pH from 7.4 to 7.1 indicates the amount of H+ in the system has doubled. Small changes can therefore have large effects; cellular enzymatic functions can be affected by pH deviations as small as 0.1 from the patient's normal baseline.

Because maintenance of normal pH within a tightly controlled range is so critical, the body has developed multiple buffering systems to help maintain pH within a normal range and mitigate the changes in pH that may occur with disease. The most important of these systems is the bicarbonate–carbonic acid system, commonly represented by the carbonic anhydrase equation (Box 5.1).

Box 5.1. Carbonic anhydrase equation.

$$CO_2 + H_2O \leftrightarrow H_2CO_3 \leftrightarrow H^+ + HCO_3^-$$

CO_2, carbon dioxide; H_2O, water; H_2CO_3, carbonic acid; H^+, hydrogen ion; HCO_3^-, bicarbonate.

The equation illustrates that carbon dioxide (CO_2), when combined with water, will form carbonic acid. This reaction is catalyzed by the enzyme carbonic anhydrase, allowing it to happen rapidly in the body. Carbonic acid quickly dissociates into hydrogen ion and bicarbonate. Because the body can

---

*Corresponding author: brook108@purdue.edu

rapidly change CO_2 levels by changes in breathing, this 'open' buffering system is extremely effective in keeping pH levels in the body near normal.

The classic Henderson–Hasselbalch equation (Box 5.2) describes how the relationship between the main components of this system (CO_2 and HCO_3^-) influence pH.

Box 5.2. Henderson–Hasselbalch equation.

$pH = 6.1 + \log[HCO_3^- / (0.03 \times PCO_2)]$ OR

$[H^+] = 24 \times PCO_2 / HCO_3^-$

HCO_3^-, bicarbonate; PCO_2, partial pressure of carbon dioxide dissolved in plasma.

The Henderson–Hasselbalch equation demonstrates that the pH of the body is determined by the *ratio* between HCO_3^- and PCO_2. That is, as the HCO_3^- content increases, pH will increase (alkalemia), and as the HCO_3^- content decreases, pH will also decrease (acidemia). Therefore, we think of HCO_3^- as acting as the main base in the body. Conversely, as PCO_2 content increases, pH will decrease (acidemia), and as PCO_2 content decreases, pH will increase (alkalemia). Hence, we think of PCO_2 as the main acid in the body.

The PCO_2 level is determined by alveolar ventilation (see below), and therefore it is representative of the *respiratory* side of acid–base assessment. Similarly, the HCO_3^- is regulated primarily by renal function, and therefore is representative of the *metabolic* side of acid–base assessment. Any process that changes the ratio between PCO_2 and HCO_3^- will alter the pH of the system (Box 5.2). For example, increasing PCO_2 *or* decreasing HCO_3^- will shift the blood towards acidemia, whereas decreasing PCO_2 *or* increasing HCO_3^- will shift the blood towards alkalemia. Common differentials for respiratory acidosis/alkalosis (aka hypoventilation and hyperventilation) are shown in Table 5.1. Common differentials for metabolic acidosis and alkalosis are shown in Tables 5.2 and 5.3, respectively.

When an acid–base abnormality occurs, the body attempts to compensate and bring the pH back toward normal by using the opposing system. For example, renal failure causes a primary *metabolic acidosis* because the body cannot excrete metabolic acids appropriately. This will cause a decrease in pH, which will trigger pH receptors in the carotid body and aortic arch that will stimulate ventilation. Increasing ventilation will drop the amount of PCO_2 (acid) in the blood (i.e. a *respiratory alkalosis*), bringing the pH closer to normal. Compensation can never bring the pH completely back to normal. Respiratory compensation for metabolic disorders happens quickly (within minutes) as changes in ventilation can occur rapidly. Metabolic compensation for primary respiratory disorders will take longer (2–5 days) as the kidneys must adjust the amount of acid retained or excreted in order to compensate.

Expected compensatory responses derived from healthy experimental dogs are shown in Table 5.4. To the author's knowledge, while these values are commonly extrapolated to cats, there are no published guidelines for expected compensatory responses in cats.

In traditional acid–base analysis as described above, both PCO_2 and HCO_3^- are viewed as independent variables and the ratio between the two determines the pH. On the respiratory side, this is fairly straightforward, as differentials for abnormalities in PCO_2 are synonymous with those for hypoventilation or hyperventilation (see Table 5.2). The weakness in simple traditional acid–base analysis comes with interpretation of the metabolic side of the equation. A strictly traditional approach does not allow differentiation between the many metabolic acids – both endogenous and exogenous – that HCO_3^- may be buffering. Therefore, additional analyses, including the non-traditional/semi-quantitative approach as described in the next section, have been developed in an attempt to better understand the underlying variables affecting the metabolic side of the equation.

Two modifications to traditional acid–base analysis involve using base excess (BE) and anion gap (AG) calculations to parse out the various causes of metabolic acidoses.

Acid–base: Modifications of traditional interpretation

BASE EXCESS One of the downsides of using HCO_3^- as the sole variable to assess the metabolic side of acid–base problems is that it can be influenced by PCO_2. As seen in Box 5.1, addition of PCO_2 to the system will shift the carbonic anhydrase equation

Table 5.1. Differentials for hyperventilation and hypoventilation.

Hypoventilation ($\uparrow PCO_2$)		Hyperventilation ($\downarrow PCO_2$)	
Anatomical location	Common causes	Physiological stimulation	Common causes
Central respiratory centers (brainstem)	Any significant CNS disease (trauma, inflammation/infection, neoplasia) Sedative or anesthetic drugs	Hypoxemia	(See Table 6)
Cervical spinal cord	Cervical IVDD, trauma	Stimulation of pulmonary receptors	Pneumonia, pulmonary edema, inhalation of irritants, pulmonary thromboembolism
Phrenic nerves/NMJ	NM diseases (myasthenia gravis) NM blocking drugs	Centrally detected stimuli: circulating drugs, metabolites, or cytokines	SIRS/sepsis, hyperadrenocorticism/steroids, liver disease, CNS diseases, exercise, heatstroke/hyperthermia
Diaphragm	Diaphragmatic hernia Respiratory muscle fatigue Excessive abdominal pressure (ascites, GDV, severe obesity)	Central: conscious perception of environment	Pain, stress, fear
Pleural space	Chest wall injury, severe accumulations of fluid or air	Iatrogenic	Excessive mechanical ventilation
Pulmonary compliance	Restrictive pleuritis, severe diffuse pulmonary disease		
Upper and lower airways	Airway obstruction, bronchoconstriction		

CNS, central nervous system; GDV, gastric dilatation volvulus; IVDD, intervertebral disc disease; NMJ, neuromuscular junction; NM, neuromuscular; SIRS, systemic inflammatory response syndrome.
Adapted from Dibartola, S.P. (ed.), *Fluid, Electrolyte and Acid–Base Disorders in Small Animal Practice*, 4th edn. Elsevier, St. Louis, Missouri, USA.

Table 5.2. Common differentials for metabolic acidosis.

High anion gap[a]	Normal gap (hyperchloremic)
Lactate (including D-lactate)	GI loss of bicarb (vomiting, diarrhea)
Uremia (retention of phosphates and sulfates)	Renal loss of bicarb/acid retention (renal tubular acidosis, carbonic anhydrase inhibitors)
Ketones	
Ethylene glycol/ethanol/methanol	Iatrogenic administration of chloride (NaCl, KCl, etc.)
Salicylate intoxication	Excess free water
(Other less common toxins such as paraldehyde, iron, cyanide, etc.)	Rebound post chronic respiratory alkalosis
	IV nutrition
Inborn errors of metabolism	Hypoadrenocorticism

[a]Using the traditional approach to define metabolic acidosis as a low pH caused by a low bicarbonate, causes of metabolic acidosis can be further subdivided into 'high-gap' versus 'normal gap' (hyperchloremic) metabolic acidosis by calculation of the anion gap (see the text). This helps the clinician sort which differentials are more likely the underlying cause of the metabolic acidosis. While there are many mnemonic aids used to recall causes for metabolic acidosis, the author prefers the mnemonic 'LUKES' as shown in bold for the commonly encountered clinical abnormalities causing an elevated anion gap.
Cl, chloride; GI, gastrointestinal; K, potassium; Na, sodium; IV, intravenous.
Adapted from Dibartola, S.P. (ed.), *Fluid, Electrolyte and Acid–Base Disorders in Small Animal Practice*, 4th edn. Elsevier, St. Louis, Missouri, USA.

to the right, producing both HCO_3^- and H^+. To overcome this influence, the mathematical concept of BE was developed. Base excess is a value calculated by the analyzer to represent the amount of base that must be theoretically added or removed from 1 L of oxygenated whole blood that has been normalized to 37°C and a PCO_2 of 40 mmHg in order to restore the pH of the sample to 7.4.

Table 5.3. Common differentials for metabolic alkalosis.

Gastric losses of chloride
Furosemide/diuretic therapy
Rebound post hypercapnia
Primary hyperaldosteronism
Hyperadrenocorticism
Administration of exogenous bicarbonate or products broken down into bicarbonate (lactate, acetate, gluconate, citrate, ketones)
Phosphorus binders
Severe hypokalemia or hypomagnesemia causing persistent hypochloremia
Free water deficit (aka "contraction alkalosis")
High dose penicillin administration

Adapted from Dibartola, S.P. (ed.), *Fluid, Electrolyte and Acid–Base Disorders in Small Animal Practice*, 4th edn. Elsevier, St. Louis, Missouri, USA.

Table 5.4. Expected compensation for primary acid–base abnormalities.

Primary acid–base disorder	Expected compensation[a]
Metabolic acidosis	↓ PCO_2 of 0.7 mmHg per each 1 mEq/L ↓ in HCO_3^- (±3)
Metabolic alkalosis	↑ PCO_2 of 0.7 mmHg per each 1 mEq/L ↑ in HCO_3^- (±3)
Respiratory acidosis (acute, <24 hours)	↑ HCO_3^- of 0.15 mEq/L per each 1 mmHg ↑ in PCO_2 (±2)
Respiratory acidosis (chronic, >2–5 days)	↑ HCO_3^- of 0.35 mEq/L per each 1 mmHg ↑ in PCO_2 (±2)
Respiratory alkalosis (acute, <24 hours)	↓ HCO_3^- of 0.25 mEq/L per each 1 mmHg ↓ in PCO_2 (±2)
Respiratory alkalosis (chronic, >2–5 days)	↓ HCO_3^- of 0.55 mEq/L per each 1 mmHg ↓ in PCO_2 (±2)

[a]These values are derived in healthy laboratory dogs and have not been validated in cats or ill dogs.
Adapted from In: Silverstein, D.C., Hopper, K. (eds), *Small Animal Critical Care Medicine*, 2nd edn. Elsevier, St. Louis, Missouri, USA.

Therefore, a patient with no acid–base abnormalities should have a BE of zero. While the reader should always use the normal values provided by their analyzer, a BE of 0 ± 3 would generally be considered normal. Since BE corrects for abnormal PCO_2 levels, it is considered to be a more 'pure' representation of the metabolic side of acid–base assessment in the presence of concurrent respiratory abnormalities.

ANION GAP Another modification to traditional analysis is the AG. The equation shown in Box 5.3 the difference between the major cations (positively charged molecules) and anions (negatively charged molecules) in the blood.

> **Box 5.3. Anion gap calculation.**
>
> AG = (Na^+ + K^+) − (HCO_3^- + Cl^-)
>
> Cl, chloride; HCO_3^-, bicarbonate; K, potassium; Na, sodium.

Due to the laws of electroneutrality, there must always be an equilibrium between cations and anions. This can be shown visually in a representation called a Gamblegram (Fig. 5.1). The anions and cations not included in the AG equation are often called 'unmeasured' despite the fact that many can be measured with modern analyzers. The unmeasured anions (UA) include molecules such as albumin and phosphate, whereas the unmeasured cations (UC) include molecules such as calcium and magnesium. Because the UA slightly exceed the UC in health, there is a normal AG range of 12–24 in the dog and 13–27 in the cat. An increasing AG almost always results from an increase in UA. This is often due to the presence of a 'new' anion such as lactate or ketones. Various toxins (ethylene glycol) and drugs (aspirin) will also act as anions and create an increased AG. Common differentials for high AG metabolic acidosis are shown in Table 5.2.

NON–TRADITIONAL ACID–BASE INTERPRETATION A common complaint of traditional acid–base analysis is that, while it helps define the acid–base abnormality, it does not necessarily help the clinician determine the underlying cause. This limitation led

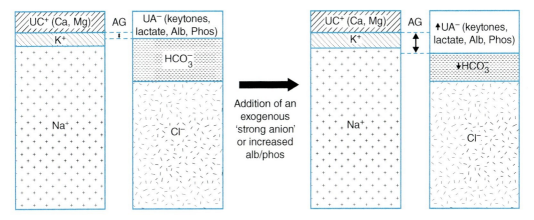

Fig. 5.1. *Gamblegram of a high-gap metabolic acidosis.* The left-hand paired boxes represent the normal Gamblegram in health with the positive cations on the left and negative anions on the right. Due to electroneutrality, the columns must always be the same height. Therefore, any change in the size of one box must be adjusted for by an equal change in the buffer (bicarbonate; HCO_3^-) box to compensate. Changes that result in an increase in size of the HCO_3^- represent metabolic alkalosis, and decreases in the HCO_3^- box size represent metabolic acidosis. This figure shows how an increase of an 'unmeasured' anion such as lactate will force a decrease the HCO_3^- box, representing an acidosis. The anion gap is visually represented as an increased difference in height between the UC and UA boxes. The right side of this figure displays a high-gap metabolic acidosis; common differentials can be found in Table 5.2. Alb, albumin; Cl, chloride; Ca, calcium; K, potassium; Mg, magnesium; Na, sodium; Phos, phosphorus; UA, unmeasured anions; UC, unmeasured cations.

to the development of alternative methods of acid–base assessment. While there are many versions of these methods, for simplicity this chapter will group discussion of them all (e.g. Stewart-Fencl-Figge, semi-quantitative) under the heading of the 'nontraditional' approach.

In the nontraditional approach, bicarbonate is considered a *dependent* variable whose level is influenced by buffering other acids or bases. This is different than the traditional approach, which considers the absolute amount of bicarbonate relative to CO_2 as a primary independent variable. For example, in the traditional approach, a normal-gap (hyperchloremic) metabolic acidosis is defined by a low HCO_3^- level. In the nontraditional approach, the primary cause of the acidosis would be attributed to an excess of chloride (the independent variable), and the drop in HCO_3^- as a secondary effect as HCO_3^- is being 'used up' as a dependent buffer. Taking it one step further, the non-traditional approach can independently calculate the impacts of multiple analytes such as electrolytes on the overall pH. This is advantageous because it allows the clinician to see when competing metabolic processes are masking each other.

Another advantage of the non-traditional approach is that it allows the clinician to assess the effect of total body water on acid–base status. Intuitively, it makes sense that changes in body water would affect pH. The pH of the body is 7.4, while the pH of water is 'neutral' on the pH scale at 7.0. Therefore, the body is slightly alkaline as compared to water. The addition of more water to the system is acidifying, and removal of more water is alkalinizing. Using sodium levels as a surrogate for total body water (see Chapter 8), the non-traditional approach allows the clinician to parse out the metabolic side of the analysis, including the impact of water, in much more detail.

Therefore, to perform non-traditional acid–base analysis, one must measure additional analytes above and beyond the PCO_2 and HCO_3^-. These include sodium, chloride, albumin, phosphorus, and lactate. Mathematical equations (Table 5.5) are then used to calculate the impact of each variable on acid–base status, with negative values indicating an acidifying effect, and positive values an alkalinizing effect. The sum of these values can then be subtracted from the BE. Any 'left over' BE unexplained by these five analytes implies an 'unmeasured' acid or base in the system (e.g. ketones). Case studies 1 and 2 contrast the use of the traditional approach to the non-traditional approach of acid–base analysis, and Fig. 5.2 shows an example of how counterbalancing abnormalities not seen with traditional analysis would be seen with non-traditional analysis.

Table 5.5. Calculations for non-traditional (semi-quantitative) acid–base analysis.

Effect	Formula[a]
Free water effect	Dogs: $0.25[(Na_p) - (Na_r)]$ Cats: $0.22[(Na_p) - (Na_r)]$
Corrected chloride	$Cl_p \times (Na_r/Na_p)$
Chloride effect	$Cl_r - Cl_{corrected}$
Phosphate effect	$0.58 (Phos_r - Phos_p)$
Albumin effect	$3.7 (Alb_r - Alb_p)$
Lactate effect	$-1 \times lactate_p$
Sum of effects	Free water effect + Cl effect + Phos effect + Alb effect + lactate effect
Unmeasured anion effect	Base excess − sum of effects

[a]Subscript p = patient value; subscript r = median value of analyzer reference range for that analyte. Calculated values that result in positive numbers will have alkalinizing effects, while those resulting in negative numbers will have acidifying effects.
Alb, albumin; Cl, chloride; Na, sodium; Phos, phosphorus.
Adapted from In: Silverstein, D.C., Hopper, K. (eds), *Small Animal Critical Care Medicine*, 2nd edn. Elsevier, St. Louis, Missouri, USA.

Blood gas analysis

Ventilation

The amount of air cycled through the lungs per minute is called the minute ventilation, and is the product of respiratory rate and tidal volume of each breath. Ventilation refreshes the gas in the alveolus, replenishing oxygen for diffusion into the blood and removing accumulated CO_2.

CO_2 is produced during aerobic metabolism in cells and is carried via the venous circulation back to the lungs for excretion. It is a very soluble gas that equilibrates rapidly between body compartments, blood, and the alveolar space. Because it equilibrates so rapidly, as long as circulatory flow is adequate, the level of CO_2 in the blood and the level in the alveolus can be assumed to be equal. Therefore, the level of CO_2 in the bloodstream is directly proportional to alveolar ventilation. This is why we use partial pressure of carbon dioxide (PCO_2) levels in the blood as the gold standard measurement of effective alveolar ventilation. A normal arterial PCO_2 ($PaCO_2$) level is approximately 40 mm Hg, with venous PCO_2 ($PvCO_2$) usually only slightly higher at ~45 mmHg. Significant differences between arterial and venous CO_2 imply issues with circulation in the tissue bed sampled, issues with generalized circulation (e.g. recent cardiopulmonary arrest), or sampling error.

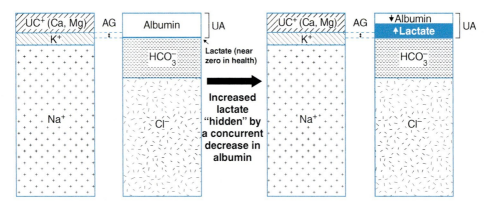

Fig. 5.2. *Gamblegram of elevated lactate/high anion gap masked by concurrent hypoalbuminemia.* As shown in Fig. 5.1, increasing lactate should normally increase the anion gap. However, as shown in the boxes to the right, a concurrent decrease in albumin will mask the expected increase in AG by maintaining the original 'size' of the UA box. In traditional acid–base analysis, no abnormalities would be noted even with calculation of the anion gap because these counterbalancing effects resulted in an unchanged bicarbonate level. The non-traditional approach measures the impact of albumin and lactate independently, revealing even the 'hidden' effects of counterbalancing abnormalities to the clinician. Cl, chloride; Ca, calcium; K, potassium; Mg, magnesium; Na, sodium; UA, unmeasured anions; UC, unmeasured cations.

The ventilatory rate is driven primarily by $PaCO_2$ levels sensed by receptors in the brain. Peripherally, PaO_2 and pH levels sensed within the carotid bodies and aortic arch also influence the ventilatory drive. Other factors such as mental/emotional status, temperature (primarily in dogs), lung irritant receptors, etc. can also influence breathing (see Table 5.1, hyperventilation). These signals will be summated within the respiratory centers in the brainstem, which will send signals down the cervical spinal cord to the paired phrenic nerves, which exit the spinal cord around segments C5–C7 (up to C4 in cats). The paired phrenic nerves innervate each crus of the diaphragm, the main muscle of breathing. Contraction of the diaphragm results in expansion of the thoracic cavity and a drop in intrathoracic pressure (it becomes more negative relative to atmosphere). This results in a concurrent drop in alveolar pressure as the lungs expand, drawing air down the airways and into the alveolus. In health, expiration happens as a result of relaxation of the diaphragm and elastic recoil of the lungs passively expelling air. With increased respiratory drive, accessory muscles of respiration (e.g. intercostals, abdominal musculature) will also be activated, increased the work of breathing.

Any pathology affecting these normal pathways needed for ventilation can result in hypoventilation and elevated $PaCO_2$ (see Table 5.1). In contrast, hyperventilation means $PaCO_2$ levels will be low, and therefore CO_2 is not stimulating the increase in breathing. Instead, other stimuli such as those outlined in Table 5.1 must be driving the hyperventilation in the face of an already low $PaCO_2$.

Oxygenation

With each breath, the alveolus is refreshed with gas. In a patient breathing room air, this gas is composed of 21% oxygen, 78% nitrogen, and 1% other miscellaneous gases. Dalton's law of partial pressures states that the total pressure (barometric pressure (Pb) = 760 mmHg at sea level) must equal the sum of the partial pressure of each gas making up the mixture. Therefore, room air is approximately 160 mmHg O_2, 593 mmHg N_2, and 7 mmHg other

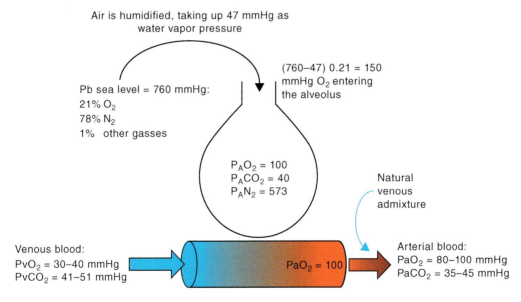

Fig. 5.3. Alveolar gas exchange breathing room air (21%) at sea level (barometric pressure (Pb) = 760 mmHg). As gas enters the airways, it is humidified, adding 47 mmHg of water vapor pressure to the total gas mixture. Once gas enters the alveolus, CO_2 diffuses into the alveolus from the bloodstream, further 'diluting' the alveolar oxygen content (P_AO_2). Oxygen diffuses from the alveolus into the bloodstream; increasing oxygen content of the capillary blood (PaO_2) is denoted as a blue to red gradient. Oxygen is taken up by hemoglobin (Hb), saturating the Hb in red blood cells. Even in health, a small amount of natural venous admixture occurs, mixing deoxygenated venous blood with the maximally oxygenated blood leaving the lungs (see text). This causes a slight drop in the oxygen level between the Alveolus and arterial blood (the A–a gradient).

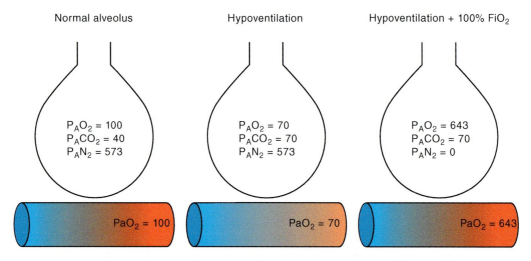

Fig. 5.4. Hypoventilation as a cause of hypoxemia. In the center alveolus, the gas is not being refreshed often enough with a new breath, resulting in a dropping P_AO_2 and rising P_ACO_2 as compared to the normally ventilated alveolus on the left. As seen on the right, administration of oxygen will displace the inert nitrogen in the alveolus, which greatly increases the diffusion gradient for oxygen and improves movement of oxygen into the blood. However, note that P_ACO_2 is still elevated and this patient still needs ventilation support to correct this. Hypoventilation as a cause of hypoxemia should be oxygen responsive as long as the patient is not completely apneic.

gasses. As air is warmed and humidified by passing through the airways, some partial pressure 'space' is taken up by water vapor, decreasing the partial pressure of oxygen entering the alveolus to approximately 150 mmHg. Once within the alveolus, the presence of a new gas (CO_2) means that the partial pressure of *alveolar* oxygen (P_AO_2) drops further to around 100–110 mmHg. (Fig. 5.4). This oxygen will then dissolve down its concentration gradient into the plasma of the pulmonary capillaries. This is now the partial pressure of oxygen in arterial blood (PaO_2). A common real-world analogy is to think of PaO_2 in plasma as similar to the CO_2 'fizz' in soda pop. The total amount of gas in the liquid is the main determinant of the pressure, but other factors such as temperature (see Section 5.4) can affect solubility and hence the partial pressure of the gas. This is important to remember as it is the pressure, not the total amount, of the gas that is reported by the analyzer.

A normal PaO_2 in a healthy patient breathing room air is generally between 80–100 mmHg. This is slightly lower than the 100–110 mmHg present in the pulmonary capillary blood. This is because as fully oxygenated pulmonary capillary blood makes its way through the left side of the heart into systemic circulation, a small amount of normal venous admixture occurs. The term 'venous admixture' refers to the idea that venous (desaturated) blood is mixing with the arterial (saturated) circulation without passing an alveolus to become oxygenated. This venous blood drops the overall oxygen content on the arterial side. In health, this venous admixture comes from the bronchial circulation and some of the cardiac venous return. This difference between the pulmonary arterial blood and pulmonary capillaries is the normal A–a gradient which should be < 20 mmHg (see Box 5.6 and Fig. 5.4). In diseased lungs or pathological shunts, an increased pathological amount of venous admixture (see Figs 5.6 to 5.9) dilutes the arterial oxygen content, resulting in hypoxemia.

Since oxygen is not a very soluble gas, not enough O_2 can be carried as PaO_2 alone to supply the tissues' oxygen needs. Therefore, the body has evolved hemoglobin (Hb) as a transport vehicle to carry more oxygen in the bloodstream; in fact, the majority (>98%) of the oxygen in blood is carried bound to Hb. Each Hb molecule can carry up to four oxygen molecules and each red blood cell contains approximately 270×10^6 molecules of Hb. The collective saturation of all the Hb in the bloodstream is referred to as the SaO_2 and is reported as a percent. The relationship between PaO_2 and SaO_2 is depicted graphically as the oxyhemoglobin disassociation curve; more information about this curve/relationship can be found in Chapter 4.

Oxygen levels in arterial blood can never exceed levels in the atmosphere unless the patient is breathing supplemental oxygen. Hypox*emia* (low level of oxygen in arterial blood, i.e. low PaO_2) is the common clinical oxygen abnormality, but should be distinguished from *tissue* hyp*oxia* (oxygen debt at the level of the tissues). For example, severe anemia (low Hb) will not affect the PaO_2 that dissolves into the blood from the lungs, and therefore the patient will not be hypox*emic* as measured on an arterial blood gas. However, without enough Hb to hold and carry O_2 in the blood to tissues, there will still be significant tissue hyp*oxia*.

Increasing the amount of oxygen in the alveolus will improve diffusion into the blood, as will increasing the surface area available for diffusion. Conversely, increasing the thickness of the tissue (e.g. fibrosis) through which the oxygen must pass will worsen diffusion. For example, providing supplemental oxygen means the 'space' in the alveolus that was previously composed of mostly nitrogen and a little bit of oxygen will now be replaced with all oxygen. This will greatly increase the partial pressure difference between the alveolus and bloodstream, and drive more oxygen into the blood (Fig. 5.5). Conversely, a disease such as pulmonary fibrosis that thickens the membrane and increases the distance across which oxygen must diffuse (i.e. a *diffusion impairment*) will cause less oxygen to pass from the alveolus into the blood, resulting in hypoxemia (Fig. 5.6). Because increasing the oxygen gradient between the alveolus and blood will improve diffusion, hypoxemia from a diffusion impairment is still very oxygen responsive.

Causes of hypoxemia are commonly divided into five physiological categories. These categories, disease examples of each, and supplemental oxygen responsiveness of each category, are outlined in Table 5.6 and Figs 5.4 to 5.9. For more detail, please see recommended supplemental texts.

5.2 How the Monitor Works

Sample collection and handling

Whole blood anticoagulated with lithium heparin is used for blood gas analysis. An appropriate blood to heparin ratio is important as overheparinization can lead to inaccurate results (see Table 5.7). Therefore, it is strongly recommended to use blood gas syringes that contain lyophilized heparin and to fill syringes to manufacturer's recommended volumes. The dried 'balanced' heparin that comes in designated blood gas syringes contains physiologic amounts of electrolytes to compensate for heparin's known ability to bind cations, especially calcium, so that the heparin itself does not distort the patient's measured electrolyte values. If the dilution of the sample with heparin exceeds 19%, then significant changes in PaO_2, $PaCO_2$, and pH as well as dilution of electrolyte values may be seen (see Table 5.7). For accurate measurement of ionized calcium (the variable most affected by heparin dilution), the final concentration should be <15 U heparin per mL of blood.

If dedicated blood gas syringes are not available, an evacuated syringe technique using liquid heparin (1,000 U/mL), and 22 g needle on a 3 mL syringe has been described by Hopper *et al.* (2005). After drawing 0.5 mL heparin into the syringe, it is evacuated completely, then 3 mL of air drawn in and forcibly expelled three times. This technique resulted in 0.04 mL of heparin remaining, which, when 1 mL of blood was added to this syringe, created a 4% dilution of the blood sample with heparin. This technique produced acceptable clinical readings for all variables, with the exception of low readings for ionized calcium and minor decreases in chloride.

Venous samples can be obtained from any vessel, but will reflect the status of the tissue bed they are draining. As such, samples obtained from a central

Table 5.6. Physiological differentials for hypoxemia (low PaO_2) and their expected degree of oxygen responsiveness.

Cause of hypoxemia	Disease example	Oxygen responsive?
Low inspired FiO_2/ low barometric pressure	Altitude Empty oxygen cylinder	Yes
Hypoventilation	See Table 5.1	Yes (still need to fix primary ventilation disorder)
Diffusion impairment	Pulmonary fibrosis	Yes
V/Q mismatch	Pneumonia, pulmonary edema	Variable
Right to left shunt	Reverse PDA	No

Further information can also be found in Figs 5.4 to 5.9.
PDA, patent ductus arteriosus in the heart.
Adapted from *West's Respiratory Physiology: The essentials*, 10th edn.

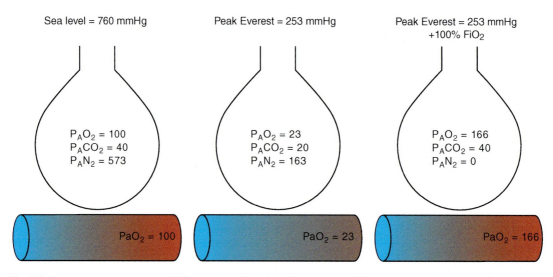

Fig. 5.5. Low barometric pressure (PB) or low fraction of inspired oxygen (FiO_2) as a cause for hypoxemia. A normal alveolus is shown at the left with values in the alveolus representing humidified air after 47 mmHg water vapor pressure has been added (see Fig. 5.3). When either the PB or FiO_2 decreases (center), the driving force (diffusion gradient) moving the oxygen across from the alveolus into the blood will decrease, resulting in less O_2 moving into the capillary blood and a low PaO_2. Despite compensatory hyperventilation to drop the P_ACO_2, the small oxygen gradient across the alveolus to the blood will result in hypoxemia. Addition of oxygen displaces nitrogen in the alveolus, which greatly increases the diffusion gradient for oxygen. Therefore, low PB/FiO_2 as a cause of hypoxemia is expected to be very oxygen responsive.

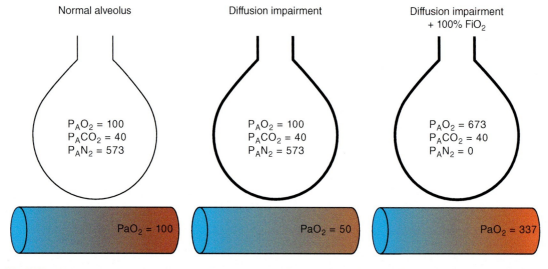

Fig. 5.6. Diffusion impairment as a cause of hypoxemia. While the amount of oxygen that enters the center alveolus is normal, there are barriers (increased tissue thickness/distance, decreased surface area) that result in decreased oxygen diffusion into the capillary blood. However, when the patient is given additional oxygen to breathe, the nitrogen in the alveolus is replaced by O_2 and the pressure differential between the alveolus and capillary blood will greatly increase. This increased gradient will drive more O_2 across into the blood despite the impaired diffusion barrier. Diffusion impairment as a cause of hypoxemia should therefore be oxygen responsive.

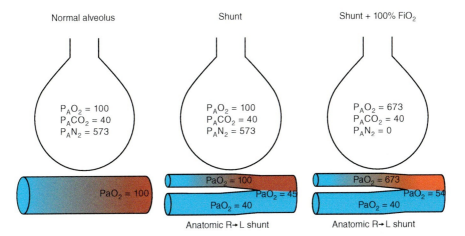

Fig. 5.7. Anatomic shunt as a cause of hypoxemia. Venous blood traveling through an aberrant vessel or opening between the right and left sides of the circulation will allow large amounts of venous blood to bypass oxygenation by the lungs. The degree of hypoxemia created will depend on how much venous admixture the shunt contributes to the total amount blood flow out of the left side of the heart. While the addition of oxygen can increase the oxygen content of the blood that does pass an alveolus (shown as increased 'redness' below the right alveolus), this is not enough to overcome the effect of the shunt. This is because hemoglobin cannot be saturated >100% and the majority of oxygen in blood is carried bound to hemoglobin. The small amount of additional 'red' oxygenation achieved as increased PaO_2 cannot overcome the downward 'drag' or dilution that the blue desaturated venous blood has on total oxygen content. Therefore, shunt as a cause of hypoxemia should have minimal to no response to oxygen supplementation.

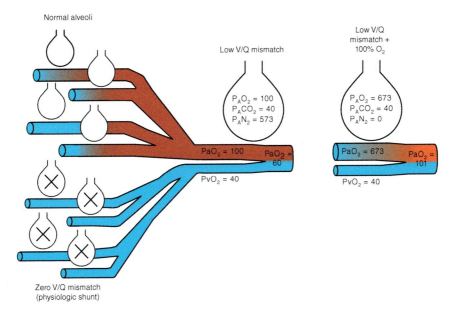

Fig. 5.8. Low ventilation/perfusion (V/Q) mismatch as a cause of hypoxemia. Alveoli that are not ventilated (V/Q = 0) as shown in the lower left essentially act as physiological shunts and can be considered similar to micro versions of the anatomical shunts discussed in Fig. 5.7. They will allow deoxygenated venous blood to bypass the lungs and mix with oxygenated blood on the left side of the heart, reducing overall oxygenation of the blood (e.g. increased venous admixture). Just as in Fig. 5.7 there is a limit to how much venous admixture can be overcome by addition of supplemental oxygen. Therefore, V/Q mismatch as a cause of hypoxemia is variably responsive to oxygen supplementation depending on the amount of venous admixture created, and becomes less response as V/Q mismatch worsens.

Venous and Arterial Blood Gas Analysis

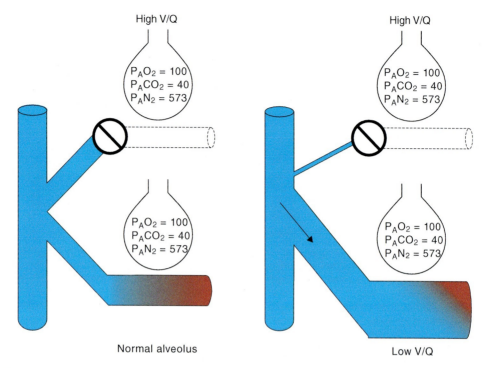

Fig. 5.9. High V/Q mismatch as a cause of hypoxemia. In high V/Q units, the alveolus is normally ventilated, but blood is blocked from flowing past that alveolus to perform gas exchange; a classic example is a pulmonary thromboembolism (PTE). However, this blood will find another route through the lungs and over-circulate adjacent alveoli as shown by diagram on the right. This alveolus can oxygenate some of this blood, but cannot keep up to oxygenate all of the 'diverted' blood. This essentially turns this previously normal unit into a low V/Q unit (ventilation is unchanged, but flow has increased). This results in hypoxemia as shown in Fig. 5.8. The response of these low V/Q units to oxygen will be similarly variable as in Fig. 5.8 depending on the degree of venous admixture created.

line are ideal as they reflect venous return from at least half of the body. Other venous sites can be used as long as there is not a specific disease (i.e. thromboembolism) affecting the tissue bed that would alter results compared to systemic blood. Venous samples can be used for acid–base analysis, but not for assessment of oxygenation status.

Arterial samples are more technically challenging to obtain, and are usually obtained from the dorsal pedal or femoral arteries, although coccygeal, auricular, and lingual arteries (in anesthetized patients) are also used. If repeated arterial sampling is needed, an arterial catheter should be placed. See Further reading section for techniques for arterial puncture and arterial catheter placement techniques. Arterial samples are needed for assessment of oxygenation.

For accurate pH, ventilation, and oxygen analysis, it is important that the sample not be allowed to equilibrate with air. Therefore, use of vented arterial blood gas syringes, careful avoidance of bubbles within the sample, and sealing the syringe prior to transport for analysis is important. Even in a sealed syringe containing no air bubbles, gas (carbon dioxide, oxygen) can still diffuse through plastic. Therefore, it is recommended to analyze samples within 15 minutes of collection.

Analyzer

Due to the need to analyze samples shortly after collection, blood gas analysis cannot be sent out and must be performed in-house. Various analyzers are available but generally fall into two categories: portable cartridge-based systems versus benchtop analyzers (see Chapter 1, Figs 1.5 and 1.6). Cartridge-based systems use single disposable cartridges to analyze each sample; the cartridge contains both the calibration solutions and the electrochemical sensors used for sample analysis. These analyzers

Table 5.7. Common pre-analytical factors that can affect blood gas analysis.

Confounder	Parameter affected, direction of change	Comment
Temperature	Temperature $\downarrow$ = $\downarrow$ PO_2 $\downarrow$ PCO_2 $\uparrow$ pH (Temperature $\uparrow$ will have the opposite effects)	Gas solubility increases at lower temperatures, allowing more gas to dissolve into liquid and decreasing the partial pressure. The subsequently decreased PCO_2 will inversely affect pH
Delay in analysis	For every hour delay at room temp: $\downarrow$ PO_2 by 2 mmHg/h $\uparrow$ PCO_2 by 1 mmHg/h $\downarrow$ pH 0.02–0.03/h All changes will be faster with increased WBC counts	Metabolism of O_2 and production of CO_2 by cells will continue within the blood, changing the levels in the sample (assuming an anaerobic environment)
$\uparrow$WBC	$\downarrow$ PO_2 over time	Increased cellular mass consumes oxygen more rapidly
Excessive heparin	$\downarrow$ pH $\downarrow$ HCO_3^- $\downarrow$ PCO_2 $\downarrow$ BE PO_2 – variable $\downarrow$ iCa	Dilution with excessive heparin will cause decreases in most variables; the PO_2 of liquid heparin itself is 150 mmHg (same as atmospheric PO_2) and so will raise or lower the patient value toward 150 mmHg depending on the patient's starting PaO_2 (e.g. whether patient receiving supplemental O_2 or not)
Pigmented/opaque substances in plasma	SaO_2 – variable effects	Methylene blue, cobalamin, very pronounced lipemia (e.g. TPN therapy), isosulfant blue, and fetal Hb can interfere with spectrophotometric measurements; endogenous pigments (bilirubin) should not
Anesthetic gas	$\uparrow$ PO_2	In older blood gas machines, anesthetic gas can be reduced by the Clarke electrode and spuriously detected as O_2
Air contamination (bubbles)	PaO_2 – variable $\downarrow$ PCO_2 $\uparrow$ pH	Values will equilibrate toward room air which should have PCO_2 of 0 and PO_2 of 150 mmHg at sea level. PaO_2 may be spuriously elevated or decreased depending on the FiO_2 breathed by the patient
Hemolysis	$\downarrow$ iCa $\downarrow$ PO_2 $\uparrow$ PCO_2	The exact reason hemolysis induces these changes in PO_2 and PCO_2 is unclear; there are suspected influences of cell-free hemoglobin and other intracellular molecules independent of influence of pH; this bias may be analyzer dependent

Cl, chloride; iCa, ionized calcium; K, potassium; TPN, total parenteral nutrition; WBC, white blood cells.

typically self-calibrate and bring the cartridge and sample up to temp (37°C) for analysis. They therefore need less maintenance and manual calibration of the machine. The cartridges contain set variables and are limited in what they will analyze. In addition, cartridge-based systems are generally less cost-effective if large volumes of samples are being run. However, they are generally small, portable, and battery-operated, making it easier to take them to the patient in the field.

In contrast, benchtop analyzers contain multi-use sensors and can measure a greater range of analytes than portable units. Some benchtop analyzers can measure bodily fluids in addition to blood and usually have panels that can be customized for each patient. These units are larger and are generally housed in a central area where samples are brought to them, such as a clinical pathology lab, or intensive care unit. While they are more cost-effective for high-throughput clinics, they generally require more manual calibration and maintenance.

Measurement of electrolytes is discussed in Chapter 8. For blood gas analysis, pH, PO_2, and PCO_2 are directly measured, and other variables

(SO_2, HCO_3^-, BE, etc.) are calculated. The pH is measured using a Sanz electrode, which consists of two electrodes; a silver–silver chloride 'measuring' electrode bathed in a solution of constant pH and surrounded by a H^+ sensitive glass membrane, and a silver–silver chloride or calomel (mercurous chloride) 'reference' electrode in a KCl solution that generates a steady voltage. When the sample passes by the membrane, it changes the H^+ concentration of the measuring electrode solution and the difference in voltage between the two electrodes is used to calculate the pH.

A Severinhaus electrode, used to measure PCO_2, works in a similar fashion. The reference electrode is identical to that in the Sanz electrode, but the measuring electrode is a platinum electrode within a pH sensitive glass membrane. The electrode is surrounded by a thin layer of bicarbonate solution contained within an outer membrane that permits CO_2, but not H^+, to diffuse in from the sample. When CO_2 diffuses into the bicarbonate solution, it creates carbonic acid which in turn disassociates to produce H^+ (see Box 5.1) which is detected by the measuring electrode. The voltage difference between the reference and Severinhaus electrodes is used to determine the change in pH, which is extrapolated to PCO_2 using the Henderson–Hasselbalch equation (see Box 5.2).

The PO_2 is measured using a Clarke electrode, which consists of a platinum cathode and a silver–silver chloride anode in an electrolyte solution, separated from the patient sample by an oxygen-permeable membrane. When oxygen contacts the cathode, it is reduced and draws electrons from the anode to the cathode to complete an electrical circuit. The current generated by this circuit is proportional to the amount of oxygen present.

Bicarbonate values are calculated using the Henderson–Hasselbalch equation (see Box 5.2) from the measured values of pH and PCO_2. Base excess is calculated from the PCO_2 and pH ± [Hb] using predetermined formulas. The SaO_2 is calculated on most analyzers from the pH, [Hb], and PaO_2. Analyzers with spectrophotometric capabilities (e.g. co-oximetry) can directly measure the SaO_2. See Chapter 4 for more information on co-oximetry.

Blood gas analyzers assess all samples at normal human body temperature (37°C). However, the partial pressure of gasses within the blood change with temperature. Think again of the analogy of a soda bottle: when the temperature rises, the gas becomes less soluble and the partial pressure of the gas inside the bottle will increase, leading to a large release of gas if the bottle is opened. The total *amount* of gas in the sealed container has not changed, but the proportion of gas in solution versus in the air will change. What is measured in blood gas analysis is the partial *pressure* (reported as $PaCO_2$ or PaO_2) of the gas in solution. The partial pressure will increase as temperature increases, and decrease as temperature decreases. Changes in temperature will also shift the oxyhemoglobin disassociation curve (see Chapter 4). Many blood gas analyzers will allow the user to input the patient's actual body temperature and will perform temperature corrections for PCO_2, PO_2, and SO_2. Although the formulas used to calculate these corrections are not linear, around normal body temperatures (37–38°C), PaO_2 will decrease by about 5 mmHg and $PaCO_2$ decrease by about 2 mmHg for every 1°C drop in body temperature. Therefore, unless body temperature changes are extreme, it is unlikely that temperature correction will change clinical decision making based on these small unit changes.

There is considerably controversy in the human literature as to whether using non-temperature-corrected values assuming a normal body temperature (e.g. 37°C, the 'alpha-stat' method) provides any different outcomes from using temperature-corrected values based on the patient's actual body temperature (the 'pH-stat' method). These controversies are more applicable to situations such as cardiac bypass or post-arrest–induced hypothermia, where temperatures are lowered to extreme levels. In addition, values considered 'normal,' whether temperature corrected or not, may be overshooting or undershooting the actual needs of the body at dysregulated temperatures. This is because when hypothermic the body utilizes less O_2 and produces less CO_2, and vice versa when hyperthermic. Currently, human medical literature seems to be leaning to the use of non-corrected (alpha-stat) values in adults, and corrected (pH-stat) values in pediatric patients, but this is still an area of much debate. There is no evidence in veterinary medicine as to the preferred method; each practice should decide whether to use temperature-corrected values or not to make medical decisions, and be consistent between clinicians.

5.3 Indications

Ideally, venous blood gas assessment to evaluate initial pH and electrolyte status should be performed in any truly emergent patient. As many blood gas panels also include renal values and hemoglobin levels, they can provide quick additional point-of-care information about the patient's disease processes.

Venous analysis can also be used as a reasonable surrogate for $PaCO_2$ in most patients. For example, if the $PvCO_2$ is 70 mmHg, one can reasonably infer that the $PaCO_2$ is likely to be around 65 mmHg and the patient is severely hypoventilating. Venous pH is generally 0.02–0.05 units lower than arterial because of the slightly higher PCO_2 content of venous blood. Assessment of $PvCO_2$ or $PaCO_2$ is important anytime a patient's ventilation status is in question. The ventilation status of a patient *cannot* be accurately determined by physical examination alone. For example, many clinicians will refer to animals with elevated respiratory rates (tachypnea) as 'hyperventilating.' However, it is important to remember that ventilation is a function of both respiratory rate and tidal volume. Therefore, patients with diseases that impair respiratory strength or drive (e.g. excessive sedation, see Table 5.1) can have inadequate ventilation (elevated PCO_2 values) even with a fast and shallow respiratory rate. Assessment of the $PaCO_2$ level is the gold standard method to quantify ventilation.

Arterial blood gas analysis is also commonly performed either to rule in/out hypoxemia as a true cause of a patient's underlying clinical signs or to assess severity and response to therapy in cases of respiratory disease. For example, if a patient presents on an emergency bases with an increased respiratory rate, this could be due to hypoxemia, or could be hyperventilation due to a 'lookalike' for respiratory distress, such as pain, compensation for a metabolic acidosis, hyperthermia, etc. (see Table 5.1). If initial screening tests and examination do not reveal an alternate explanation and/or pulse oximetry is not reliable in the patient, arterial blood gas analysis can be used to establish if hypoxemia is truly the cause of tachypnea.

In general, serial blood gas analysis (at least every 8–12 hours) should be considered in patients requiring oxygen and/or ventilator support. This data helps determine if oxygen supplementation levels are adequate, and assures adequate blood levels of PaO_2 and $PaCO_2$ as oxygen/ventilation support is weaned. However, due to increased cost and invasiveness as compared to SpO_2 and end tidal carbon dioxide ($ETCO_2$), arterial blood gas readings are typically performed intermittently and the results corroborated with those monitors (see Chapters 4 and 6) in each patient. In addition, methods such as the A–a gradient and P/F ratio (see Section 5.4) can be calculated from arterial blood gas data to help the clinician trend improvement or deterioration of lung function over time. Any major change in mechanical ventilator settings or patient stability should prompt reassessment of oxygenation and ventilation.

5.4 Interpretation of Findings

Blood gas analysis: Acid–base

Traditional acid–base analysis

1. Evaluate the pH. An elevated pH is an alkalemia, and a low pH an acidemia.
2. Determine what is causing the change in pH by looking at the PCO_2 and HCO_3^-. Remember that PCO_2 acts as an acid, so increased PCO_2 will cause a respiratory acidosis and decreased PCO_2 a respiratory alkalosis. The HCO_3^- acts as a base, so its influence will be opposite; increases in HCO_3^- will cause metabolic alkalosis, and decreases in HCO_3^- metabolic acidosis. The combination of these two forces will create the final '-emia' of the blood.
3. The third step is to determine if compensation is occurring. Compensation means the opposite process is trying to antagonize the pH change caused by the primary problem. For example, if the primary problem is a respiratory acidosis (increased PCO_2), the compensation will be a metabolic alkalosis (increased HCO_3^-). If the PCO_2 and HCO_3^- change in opposite directions, the disorder is considered a mixed disorder.
4. If it appears that compensation is occurring, the next step is to determine if compensation is appropriate or not. This is determined by the calculations in Table 5.4. If compensation is not adequate, the disorder is considered a mixed disorder (see Box 5.4).
5. If there is a metabolic acidosis, use the AG to further classify metabolic acidosis as 'high gap' or 'normal gap.' See Box 5.3, Case study 2, and Fig. 5.1 for further information about application of the anion gap.
   - An elevated gap implies the presence of additional anions not measured with the standard electrolytes. Common differentials for an elevated AG are shown in Table 5.2.
   - If the AG is normal, the chloride must be elevated to cause the metabolic acidosis. This is called either a 'normal gap' or 'hyperchloremic' metabolic acidosis. Common differentials for a hyperchloremic metabolic acidosis are shown in Table 5.2.

> **Box 5.4. Traditional acid–base analysis**
>
> Patient values:
>
> pH = 7.3 (normal = 7.4)
>
> PCO_2 = 25 mmHg (normal = 40 mmHg)
>
> HCO_3^- = 12 mmol/L (normal = 22 mmol/L)
>
> A pH of 7.3 is low = acidemia. The PCO_2 (acid) is *low* at 25 mmHg; the acidemia cannot be the 'fault' of the PCO_2. Therefore, a low HCO_3^- (base) of 12, indicating a metabolic acidosis, would be the culprit.
>
> Compensation: The body is breathing off PCO_2 (acid) to compensate for the metabolic acidosis created by the low HCO_3^-. The HCO_3^- is 10 points below normal. (22 − 12 = 10). To compensate, the PCO_2 should change 0.7 for every 1 point the HCO_3^- changes (see Table 5.1). 10 × 0.7 = 7. A normal PCO_2 of 40 − 7 = 33 ± 3 mmHg would be the expected compensation. This patient's PCO_2 of 25 is in excess of expected compensation, therefore it has a mixed disturbance of both metabolic acidosis and respiratory alkalosis.

Non-traditional (semi-quantitative) analysis

1. Evaluate the pH. An elevated pH is an alkalemia, and a low pH an acidemia.
2. Determine the respiratory aspect by evaluating the PCO_2. This is the same as in traditional analysis; elevations in PCO_2 will cause a respiratory acidosis and decreases in PCO_2 will cause a respiratory alkalosis.
3. Evaluate the metabolic aspect of the patient by mathematically calculating the contribution of electrolytes, protein, lactate, and water to the pH. Use the equations in Table 5.5, being sure to keep track of positive results (alkalinizing effect) or negative results (acidifying effect). Sum the output of each equation and subtract it from the BE calculated by the blood gas analyzer.
   - If the sum of the equations subtracted from the BE approaches zero, there are no 'unmeasured' acid–base influences. References for 'normal' unmeasured anions range up to ± 5.
   - If the difference between the equations and the BE is greater than 5, there are 'unmeasured influences' on the acid–base. These are generally toxins/drugs or errors of metabolism.
   - Case studies 1 and 2 in Section 5.4 illustrate the traditional and non-traditional approaches to acid–base analysis.

Blood gas analysis: Ventilation/oxygenation

Ventilation

1. Assess venous or arterial CO_2 levels. $PaCO_2$ values <35 mmHg are indicative of hyperventilation, 35-45 mmHg are considered normal, and values >45 mmHg are consistent with hypoventilation. Venous values will average about 5 mmHg higher than arterial values, assuming circulatory flow is adequate.
   - For example, if the $PvCO_2$ is 70 mmHg, one can reasonably infer that the $PaCO_2$ is likely to be around 65 mmHg and the patient is severely hypoventilating.
2. Patients who have a $PaCO_2$ >60 mmHg are severely hypoventilating and mechanical ventilation should be considered if the underlying cause of hypoventilation cannot be rapidly reversed (e.g. reversible sedatives).
   - Patients with excessive work of breathing (unable to rest) are in danger of exhaustion and respiratory arrest, and should also be considered candidates for ventilation. A PCO_2 level that is "normal" or rising in these patients is concerning for exhaustion and imminent respiratory arrest. See Case study 3.
3. Be aware that assessment of ventilation and assessment of the respiratory side of acid–base analysis are the same thing (assessment of PCO_2).

Oxygenation

1. Determine the fraction of inspired oxygen (FiO_2) and the barometric pressure (Pb). If the patient is breathing room air at sea level, FiO_2 = 21% and Pb = 760 mmHg.
2. Look at the PaO_2. The PaO_2 should be approximately four or five times the FiO_2. This relationship is the basis of the 'P/F ratio' (see Box 5.5).
   - Breathing room air at sea level, healthy lungs should create a PaO_2 of 80–100 mmHg in arterial blood. A PaO_2 of <80 mmHg is hypoxemia, with <60 mmHg considered severe hypoxemia.
   - A patient breathing 100% oxygen should have a PaO_2 of 400–500 mmHg.
   - At altitude, PaO_2 will drop proportionally as Pb decreases. The expected alveolar concentration of oxygen can be calculated

using the alveolar gas equation (Box 5.6). The measured arterial oxygen content (PaO$_2$) should not be less than 20 mmHg below the calculated alveolar content (P$_A$O$_2$). This is the 'A–a gradient' (Box 5.6).

3. If the patient is hypoxemic, consider which of the five physiological causes of hypoxemia is most likely (Table 5.6; see Figs 5.5 to 5.10).
   - As with most classification systems in medicine, there is often overlap with a single patient having hypoxemia due to multiple mechanisms simultaneously.
   - The most common cause of hypoxemia is V/Q mismatch.
   - Assess ventilation as previously discussed. Hypoventilation will cause hypoxemia as P$_A$CO$_2$ builds up and displaces P$_A$O$_2$ from the alveolus (see Fig. 5.5).
   - If the patient is hypoventilating, assessment of the A–a gradient (Box 5.6) can be helpful. A normal A–a gradient implies all hypoxemia can be attributed to the hypoventilation; fix the hypoventilation and the PaO$_2$ should normalize. An abnormal A–a gradient implies additional lung dysfunction on top of hypoventilatory hypoxemia. See Case study 2.
   - A 'quick and dirty' version of the A–a gradient is the 'rule of 120.' Breathing room air at sea level, the PaO$_2$ and PaCO$_2$ added together should be close to a sum of 120 or greater. If the sum is less than 120, there is lung dysfunction that cannot be explained by hypoventilation alone, and one of the other four causes of hypoxemia should also be considered.

4. Patients with a PaO$_2$ <60 mmHg despite normalized ventilation and traditional methods of maximal oxygen supplementation (FiO$_2$ 60%) are candidates for mechanical ventilation.

While these methods of oxygen assessment may provide useful clinical tools, studies in animals are lacking. In a study by Briganti *et al.* (2015), there

---

Box 5.5. Calculation of the P/F ratio.

PaO$_2$ / FiO$_2$ (as a decimal)

Normal lungs on room air: 100 mmHg / 0.21 = 476

Diseased lungs on 40% FiO: 100 mmHg / 0.40 = 250

The normal P/F ratio is 400–500.[a] The P/F ratio is used in humans to classify severity of acute respiratory distress syndrome (ARDS), with <300 consistent with mild ARDS, <200 moderate ARDS, and <100 severe ARDS.

[a]The P/F ratio does not take PCO$_2$ into account, so hypoventilation as a cause of hypoxemia will result in an abnormal P/F ratio even if there is no true lung pathology

---

Box 5.6. Calculation of the A–a gradient.

Alveolar gas equation → P$_A$O$_2$ = [FiO$_2$ (P$_B$ − P$_{H2O}$)] − (PaCO$_2$ / R)

Where FiO$_2$ is presented as a decimal (0.21 on room air), P$_B$ = barometric pressure in mmHg (760 at sea level), P$_{H2O}$ represents water vapor pressure in the airways, (generally assumed to be 47 mmHg), PaCO$_2$ is measured from the arterial blood gas, and R represents the respiratory quotient, a constant for which 0.8 is commonly used At sea level, breathing room air, the equation can be simplified to:

P$_A$O$_2$ = 150 − (PaCO$_2$ / R)

PaO$_2$ is measured from the arterial blood gas and subtracted from P$_A$O$_2$.

Normal P$_A$O$_2$ − PaO$_2$ (A–a gradient) should be <15–20 mmHg (FiO$_2$ 21%) or <50–110 mmHg (FiO$_2$ 100%)

What is a 'normal' A–a gradient becomes less clear as the FiO$_2$ increases. Some references state that for every 10% increase in FiO$_2$, the A–a gradient may increase by 5–7, while others list gradients up to 110 as normal at 100% FiO$_2$. Therefore, many clinicians will choose to use the A-a gradient only when the animal is breathing room air.

was poor correlation between the A–a gradient and P/F ratio with the actual degree of venous admixture measured in anesthetized horses. Therefore, in veterinary medicine, trends within an individual patient rather than exact values may be more reliable to assess progression of lung function.

5.5 Pitfalls of the Monitor

Sample handling/acquisition

The majority of errors in blood gas analysis are pre-analytical and result from improper sample handling or acquisition. If arterial samples are obtained by direct puncture rather than from a dedicated arterial line, they may contain venous or mixed venous–arterial blood and not accurately represent arterial values. In this case, comparison to values taken from a known venous sample and correlation with severity of clinical signs may help determine if the initial puncture was truly arterial. Venous values being used in lieu of arterial (e.g. $PvCO_2$, pH) may be inaccurate in low-flow hemodynamic states such as post-arrest, or if drawn from tissue beds that do not represent appropriate blood flow in the patient as a whole (e.g. from the hind limb of a feline thromboembolism patient). Similarly, if the sample introduced into the analyzer is not homogeneous, such as allowing sedimentation of red cells to occur without re-mixing immediately prior to analysis, values such as Hb and hematocrit (Hct) may be skewed.

Samples contaminated with fluids or medications (such as those collected inappropriately from central lines) can lead to false values. For example, samples contaminated with significant amounts of total parenteral nutrition or dextrose will have erroneously high blood glucose values. Other common pre-analytical errors and their expected effects are outlined in Table 5.7.

Monitor output

Appropriate quality control and maintenance is important for all instruments, but especially for noncartridge-based systems to ensure accuracy of results where multi-use electrodes must be appropriately maintained and replaced. Analyzers will give error readings rather than inappropriate results in most cases if samples are improperly loaded (not enough sample, air bubbles, fibrin clots, etc.). However, the presence of certain substances in the blood can be incorrectly perceived by the electrodes as normal analytes (see Chapter 8). For example, halogen ions such as bromide in patients receiving potassium bromide therapy will be detected as chloride by chloride-sensitive electrodes and give abnormally high chloride readings. Severely high salicylate levels (as in extreme toxicities) can do the same. If anion gap calculations or non-traditional acid–base analysis are being performed, incorrect electrolyte values will skew these calculations.

5.6 Case Studies

Case study 1: Traditional versus non-traditional acid–base analysis

A 10-year-old castrated male Labrador Retriever collapses during his first jog this spring. The owner initially took him home after the collapse, but the dog began to have bloody diarrhea and continued to have an increased respiratory rate and effort, so he is presented to the ER clinic 3 hours following the initial collapse event. On presentation, the dog is carried in by the owner, is mentally dull, has poor pulse quality, pale to cyanotic mucous membranes with a capillary refill time of 3–4 seconds, a heart rate of 180 bpm, temperature of 103.5°F (39.7°C), and stridorous upper airway noise. Petechiae are present on his ventral abdomen. A diagnosis of heat stroke and upper airway obstruction (presumed laryngeal paralysis) is made.

Oxygen is provided by mask, an intravenous (IV) catheter is placed, and the following venous blood gas and chemistry information is drawn from the IV catheter and analyzed on your stat bedside cartridge-based analyzer:

PCV/TP: 67%/9.2
Blood glucose: 29 mg/dL

Parameter (unit)	Patient value	Normal value[a]
pH	7.4	7.4
PvO_2 (mmHg)	30	35
$PvCO_2$ (mmHg)	55	45
HCO_3^- (mmol/L)	32.9	22
BE (mmol/L)	10	0
Na (mmol/L)	160	146
K (mmol/L)	5	4
Cl (mmol/L)	110	110

Continued

Parameter (unit)	Patient value	Normal value[a]
Albumin (g/dL)	2.1	3.1
Phosphorus (mg/dL)	7	3.9
Lactate (mmol/L)	7	<2

[a]Stated normal values used for calculations are the median of the analyzers' reference range. For example, if the range for sodium is 135–145, the median value used for normal is 140.

While a 0.5 mL/kg bolus of 50% dextrose diluted 1:1 with saline and an initial 30 mL/kg crystalloid bolus are started, the initial data is assessed:

Traditional approach

1. Evaluate the pH. Here, the pH is normal (7.4). This demonstrates one of the pitfalls of traditional acid–base analysis; by strictly following the 'rules' of acid–base analysis, a clinician might stop here and decide no acid–base abnormality is present. However, the savvy clinician chooses to assess each component that can contribute to acid–base abnormalities. Additional interpretation would be as follows:

2. Assessment of the respiratory side of the acid–base equation reveals an elevated $PvCO_2$ consistent with hypoventilation. This would be expected to cause an acidosis; the normal pH implies another alkalinizing process must also be happening. The hypoventilation should be addressed based on the likely differentials listed in Table 5.1. Given this patient's mentation and stridorous breathing, upper airway obstruction ± central respiratory depression and/or exhaustion of muscles of ventilation should all be considered possible causes of the hypoventilation.

3. Assessment of the metabolic side shows bicarbonate and base excess are also elevated which would be expected to cause a metabolic alkalosis. These processes are 'cancelling out' the respiratory acidosis, creating a normal pH. This would therefore be classified as a mixed disturbance. Further assessment of the list of differentials for metabolic alkalosis (see Table 5.3), indicates a free water deficit, as indicated by the elevated sodium level, is the most likely cause of the metabolic alkalosis.

Therapeutic interventions based on this analysis would include interventions to improve ventilation to resolve the respiratory acidosis (sedation and cooling, with possible intubation if necessary to improve upper airway obstruction), and treatment to improve perfusion (IV fluids). It is likely that the complexity of the metabolic aspect of acid–base would be missed on initial evaluation. Repeat blood gas analysis as each parameter was normalized would reveal the changing pH and might allow for further characterization of this dog's metabolic abnormalities.

Non-traditional approach

The assessment of the respiratory side of the acid–base equation is identical as above: an elevated $PvCO_2$ is consistent with hypoventilation and should be addressed based on the likely differentials listed in Table 5.1.

In order to assess the metabolic side of the acid–base equation, the given values are utilized in the equations listed in Table 5.5:

Effect	Formula	Patient value and median reference range value	Calculated effect
Free water effect	Dogs: $0.25[(Na_p) - (Na_r)]$ Cats: $0.22[(Na_p) - (Na_r)]$	$Na_p = 160$ $Na_r = 146$	3.5
Corrected chloride	$Cl_p \times (Na_r/Na_p)$	$Cl_p = 110$	$Cl_{corrected} = 100.4$ (see chloride effect in next row)
Chloride effect	$Cl_r - Cl_{corrected}$	$Cl_r = 110$ $Cl_{corrected} = 100.4$	9.6
Phosphate effect	$0.58 (Phos_r - Phos_p)$	$Phos_p = 7$ $Phos_r = 3.9$	−1.8
Albumin effect	$3.7 (Alb_r - Alb_p)$	$Alb_p = 2.1$ $Alb_r = 3.1$	3.7
Lactate effect	$-1 \times lactate_p$	$Lactate_p = 7$	−7
Sum of effects	Free water effect + Cl effect + Phos effect + alb effect + lactate effect		3.5 + 9.6 + (−1.8) + 3.7 + (−7) = 8
Unmeasured anion effect	Base excess − sum of effects	BE = 10	10 − 8 = 2

In this analysis, positive numbers indicate effects that will be alkalinizing (free water effect, chloride effect, albumin effect) and negative numbers indicate values that will be acidifying (phosphate, lactate). In contrast to traditional acid–base analysis, non-traditional (semi-quantitative) analysis demonstrates in this case that the metabolic side of the acid–base analysis is a mixed process (i.e. due to multiple underlying causes), and helps the clinician see what effect corrections of various values should have on acid–base status.

In this patient, a free water deficit (see Chapter 8) is causing a concentrating effect, which is 'correcting' the measured chloride to normal. This is hiding what is actually a significant hypochloremia that becomes apparent when the chloride is corrected. Combined with the hypoalbuminemia, these effects explain the alkalinizing forces of the metabolic assessment. Likely differentials in this patient include respiratory or renal losses of free water and hypoalbuminemia secondary to the systemic inflammatory response seen in heat stroke. These forces are masking the acidifying effects of a significant hyperlactatemia and moderate hyperphosphatemia, both presumably secondary to poor perfusion causing anaerobic metabolism and decreased glomerular filtration. When all effects (free water, chloride, phosphate, albumin, and lactate) are summed up and subtracted from the base excess, the unmeasured anion effect is <5, therefore there are unlikely to be any other significant unmeasured anions playing a role (such as toxins).

With both approaches, practitioners will recognize the respiratory abnormalities and be able to address the dog's hypoventilation. The non-traditional approach allows for a more nuanced breakdown of the contributions of each aspect of the metabolic disorders and might prompt more timely recognition of the free water deficit and chloride effects than with traditional analysis.

This patient was hospitalized in critical condition and required multiple interventions including plasma support for coagulopathy. He did make a full recovery and was discharged to his owners after 9 days of hospitalization.

Case study 2: Use of the anion gap in acid–base analysis

A 2.5-year-old spayed female domestic shorthair cat presents for lethargy and vomiting of one day's duration. On physical examination, the patient has no overt abnormalities. Abdominal imaging is within normal limits; a stat venous blood gas is run while full bloodwork is pending. The combined results of both are below:

Parameter (unit)	Patient value	Normal value[a]
pH	7.35	7.4
PvO_2 (mmHg)	35	35
$PvCO_2$ (mmHg)	21.2	45
HCO_3^- (mmol/L)	12	22
BE (mmol/L)	–13	0
Na (mmol/L)	153	153
K (mmol/L)	5.1	4.3
Cl (mmol/L)	120	122
Albumin (g/dL)	3.4	3.3
Phosphorus (mg/dL)	6.4	5.7
Lactate (mmol/L)	1.2	<2
Creatinine	3.5	
BUN	31	
Glucose	177	

[a]Stated normal values used for calculations are the median of the analyzers' reference range. For example, if the range for sodium is 148–157, the median value used for normal is 153.

Traditional analysis

1. Assess the pH. The pH is slightly acidemic.
2. Assess the PCO_2 and HCO_3^- to determine which is causing the acidosis.
   - $PvCO_2$ is low which would cause a respiratory alkalosis, so the pH is not the 'fault' of the respiratory side.
   - HCO_3^- is low which would cause a metabolic acidosis. This explains the pH. Therefore, this cat has a metabolic acidosis.
   - Is compensation adequate? For every 1-point change in HCO_3^-, pCO_2 should change by 0.7. 22 – 12 = 10 × 0.7 = 7. 45 – 7 = 38. The actual value of pCO_2 is much lower (21.2) than this expected value, so there is excessive hyperventilation beyond what is needed for compensation alone. This patient therefore has a mixed metabolic acidosis and respiratory alkalosis.
   - For a metabolic acidosis, assess the anion gap. AG = (153 + 5.1) – (120 + 12) = 26.1. This was considered elevated as compared to the reference range given for this chemistry analyzer (10–23), and approaches the upper end of general AG references for cats

(13–27). Of the LUKES differentials for high AG acidosis given in Table 5.2, uremia and toxins are most likely in this patient. While ketones have not been excluded, the normal glucose levels make this less likely. Further diagnostics would be needed to determine the underlying cause for uremia and screen for possible toxins.

Non-traditional approach

The assessment of the respiratory side of the acid–base equation is identical as above: a low $PvCO_2$ is consistent with hyperventilation and should be addressed based on the likely differentials listed in Table 5.1.

In order to assess the metabolic side of the acid–base equation, the given values are utilized in the equations listed in Table 5.5:

Effect	Formula	Patient value and median reference range value	Calculated effect
Free water effect	Dogs: $0.25[(Na_p) - (Na_r)]$ Cats: $0.22[(Na_p) - (Na_r)]$	$Na_p = 153$ $Na_r = 153$	0
Corrected chloride	$Cl_p \times (Na_r/Na_p)$	$Cl_p = 120$	$Cl_{corrected} = 120$, see next box
Chloride effect	$Cl_r - Cl_{corrected}$	$Cl_r = 122$ $Cl_{corrected} = 120$	2
Phosphate effect	$0.58 (Phos_r - Phos_p)$	$Phos_p = 6.4$ $Phos_r = 5.7$	–0.4
Albumin effect	$3.7 (Alb_r - Alb_p)$	$Alb_p = 3.4$ $Alb_r = 3.3$	–0.37
Lactate effect	$-1 \times lactate_p$	$Lactate_p = 1.2$	–1.2
Sum of effects	Free water effect + Cl effect + Phos effect + alb effect + lactate effect		$0 + 2 + (-0.4) + (-0.37) + (-1.2) = 0.03$
Unmeasured anion effect	Base excess – sum of effects	BE = –13	–13 – 0.03 = –13.03

The non-traditional assessment reveals a significant unmeasured anion effect (–13) as the main culprit of the acidosis. Given the concurrent azotemia, a renal toxin was highly suspected. On further questioning, the cat had access to a garage the prior day in which ethylene glycol was present. Despite supportive care with IV fluids and diuretics, the cat's urine output continued to decline and azotemia worsened (BUN 68, Creat 6.2) by the following day. Given the poor prognosis, at that point the owners elected humane euthanasia.

Using the AG to further assess the metabolic acidosis led to a possible diagnosis of a toxin such as ethylene glycol, but since uremia was also a differential for an elevated AG, the possibility of a toxin may still have been missed. Using non-traditional assessment, it becomes clear that the elevation in base excess is much greater than can be explained by the phosphate effect, which should be more elevated if uremia alone was causing the acidosis. A greatly elevated unmeasured anion effect leads the clinician more directly to a possible toxin present in the bloodstream as a likely cause of the acid–base abnormality.

Case study 3: Interpretation of oxygenation/ventilation status (use of the A–a gradient)

A 7-year-old castrated male Dachshund presents for progressive weakness and neck pain. Over the last 24 hours, despite appropriate pain management and strict cage rest, the dog has progressed to no longer being able to rise to walk. Because the dog cannot get up to eat or drink, the owner has been force-feeding food and water via syringe for the past 24 hours. The patient presents with the following initial exam parameters:

Temperature: 103°F (39.4°C); heart rate: 150 bpm; respiratory rate 70 breaths per minute, with a shallow rapid breathing pattern. Neurological exam reveals non-ambulatory tetraplegia with deep pain present in all four limbs and pain on palpation of the cervical spine. The remainder of the physical examination is within normal limits. The neurological localization is the cervical spinal cord segments C1–C5 and the patient is diagnosed with presumed intervertebral disk disease (IVDD) pending advanced imaging. A pulse oximeter placed on the patient while on room air reads 91%; with oxygen supplementation by mask, the reading improves to 97%.

Despite the elevated respiratory rate, it is important to remember that tachypnea ≠ hyperventilation. Ventilation is a product of BOTH rate and tidal volume, and this patient's cervical spinal cord disease is likely causing weakness of the diaphragm as well as generalized weakness of the limbs. Therefore, despite his tachypnea, this patient may be hypoventilating if he cannot generate an appropriate tidal volume with each breath. To assess the ventilation status, we must assess PCO_2 levels.

While $PvCO_2$ would likely be enough to help us assess ventilation alone, this patient was also hypoxemic on presentation, requiring oxygen supplementation. The next question is whether the hypoxemia is secondary to hypoventilation alone, or, is there another underlying lung issue (e.g. aspiration pneumonia secondary to syringe feeding or silent regurgitation) that is also contributing to hypoxemia? An arterial blood gas analysis would be preferred for assessing both questions in this dog.

The following arterial blood gas is obtained at sea level on room air:

Value (unit)	Patient value	Normal range
pH	7.25	7.35–7.45
PaO_2 (mmHg)	65	80–107 (FiO_2 21%)
$PaCO_2$ (mmHg)	56	34–40
HCO_3^- (mmol/L)	23.7	19–25
BE (mmol/L)	-2.7	0 ± 3

1. Assess the pH. The pH is acidemic.
2. Assess the $PaCO_2$ and HCO_3^- to determine which is causing the acidosis.
   - $PaCO_2$ is high which would cause a respiratory acidosis. This indicates hypoventilation. After assessing likely differentials for hypoventilation (Table 5.1), the most likely cause is a cervical spinal cord lesion.
   - HCO_3^- is normal; this should not cause an acidosis. Therefore, this is a primary respiratory acidosis.
   - Is compensation adequate? The history implies this is likely an acute (last 24 hours) change. Using the equations from Table 5.4, for every 1 mmHg that the $PaCO_2$ is elevated above normal, the HCO_3^- would be expected to rise by 0.15. Using 37 as a mid-range normal $PaCO_2$, 56 − 37 = 19 points above normal × 0.15 = 2.85. Therefore, if a mid-range normal HCO_3^- is 22, then 22 + 2.85 = 24.85 mmHg. The HCO_3^- of 23.7 mmHg is within 3 points of this expected value, therefore compensation is adequate. There is also no significant deflection of the BE to imply a concurrent metabolic component, therefore more advanced assessment of the metabolic side of this patient is not needed.
3. Assess the FiO_2. The blood gas was obtained on room air, so FiO_2 = 21%.
4. Assess the PaO_2. The PaO_2 is low at 65.
   - Of the five causes of hypoxemia, hypoventilation is already known to be present. Is there another cause of hypoxemia not explained by hypoventilation alone?
   - Perform the A–a gradient (see Box 5.5) for a patient breathing room air at sea level:
     A = 150 − ($PaCO_2$/R)
     A = 150 − (56/0.8) = 80.
     Therefore, the A–a gradient = P_AO_2 − PaO_2 = (80 − 65) = 15
     This is within acceptable limits and therefore all of this patient's current hypoxemia can be explained by hypoventilation.

Another approach using the 'rule of 120' shows that 65 + 56 = 121, therefore this patient was unlikely to have hypoxemia not explained by the hypoventilation.

Thoracic radiographs were normal and did not support any undiagnosed lung pathology. The patient was mechanically ventilated prior to and shortly after a ventral slot procedure for cervical IVDD. The dog was weaned from mechanical ventilation within 48 hours and was discharged home after an additional week of hospitalization. Following rehabilitation, the dog regained good ambulation with only minor residual conscious proprioception deficits.

Case study 4: Assessment of lung function in the hypoxemic patient

A 7-year-old castrated male mixed breed dog presents for a 1-week history of ocular discharge, skin lesions, and cough beginning in the last 48 hours. Temperature: 104.0°F (40°C); heart rate: 150 bpm; respiratory rate: 70 breathes per minute with harsh lung sounds diffusely.

Thoracic radiographs show a mixed nodular and diffuse interstitial pattern with enlarged tracheobronchial lymph nodes. A complete blood count showed a mild non-regenerative anemia, an inflammatory leukogram with a left shift, and mild thrombocytopenia. Cytology of one of the draining skin lesions showed pyogranulomatous inflammation and broad-based budding organisms consistent with *Blastomyces dermatitidis*. A diagnosis of disseminated blastomycosis was made. Treatment with itraconazole 5 mg/kg PO q12h and IV fluid support at 120 mL/kg/day to correct an estimated 5% fluid deficit in 24 hours were initiated. An arterial line was placed to allow for serial blood gas sampling. In the chart below, serial arterial blood gasses are shown along with degree of oxygen support. The bolded values are discussed further in the text below:

Value (unit) normal range]	Presentation	12 h	24 h	36 h	37 h
pH [7.35–7.45]	7.35	7.44	7.47	7.26	7.32
PaO_2 (mmHg) [4–5 × FiO_2]	**56**	**85**	72	**60**	192
$PaCO_2$ (mmHg) [34–40]	**22**	27	25	**40**	35
HCO_3^- (mmol/L) [19–25]	11.7	17.7	17.6	17.3	17.4
BE [0 ± 3]	−12.5	−5.7	−5.4	−8.5	−7.6
FiO_2 provided	21% (room air)	40% (bilateral nasal cannulas)	40% (bilateral nasal cannulas)	40% (bilateral nasal cannulas)	**100% (intubated and hand ventilated with anesthesia machine bag)**
P/F ratio [400–500]	267	**213**	**180**	**150**	192

1. Assess the pH. At presentation, the patient is acidemic. The $PaCO_2$ is low (hyperventilation) which should not cause an acidosis. The HCO_3^- and BE are also low, consistent with a metabolic acidosis. Using 22 as a normal HCO_3^- level, the HCO_3^- is 10.3 points below normal. Using the equations from Table 5.4, the PCO_2 should decrease by 0.7 for every 1 point the HCO_3^- is low if compensation is appropriate. 10.3 × 0.7 = 7.21. Therefore, the CO_2 should be approximately 33 mmHg (40−7.21). The measured CO_2 of 22 mmHg is lower than expected for compensation alone. Therefore, this patient has a *mixed metabolic acidosis and respiratory alkalosis*. Further information (electrolytes, lactate) would be needed for more in-depth assessment of the metabolic alkalosis using the non-traditional approach. For brevity, this remainder of this example focuses on the oxygenation/ventilation status of this patient rather than the acid–base component.

2. Assess $PaCO_2$. The $PaCO_2$ is low, consistent with hyperventilation. Causes of hyperventilation are likely multifactorial in this patient (Table 5.1), including hypoxemia, pulmonary receptor activation due to primary lung pathogen, and SIRS.

3. Assess PaO_2. The initial blood gas at presentation indicates severe hypoxemia (PaO_2 = 56 mmHg) on room air. The low $PaCO_2$ indicates that the patient is hyperventilating, therefore the low PaO_2 cannot be attributed to hypoventilation. As a confirmation of this information, you perform an A–a gradient (A–a = 66.5, significant lung pathology) or rule of 120 (56 + 28 = 78 which is <120) which again supports that the hypoxemia is separate from hypoventilation.

Bilateral nasal cannulas were placed in this dog at a setting of 100 mL/kg/min. Oxygen supplementation with bilateral nasal cannulas at 100 mL/kg/min of O_2 is presumed to generate a FiO_2 of approximately 40%. The PaO_2 in this dog improved to an acceptable level of 85 mmHg at the 12-hour mark on oxygen supplementation. All subsequent assessments of oxygenation must take this change in FiO_2 into account.

4. At 12 hours, lung function as represented by the P/F ratio declined slightly, but interpretation is complicated by the fact that the $PaCO_2$ also slightly increased. The patient's hyperventilation has been reduced because he is no longer hypoxemic. Because the P/F ratio does not take ventilation

into account, increases in $PaCO_2$ will decrease the ratio independently of actual diffusion functionality of the lung. This is because if you ventilate less (i.e. have a higher $PaCO_2$), you will move less air in and out of the alveoli and less oxygen diffuses into the blood, resulting in a lower PaO_2. This in turn lowers the P/F ratio. Therefore, it is difficult to say if there has been a true decline in lung function in the first 12 hours. An A–a gradient could be performed to more accurately assess this as compared to values at presentation, but would require taking the patient off oxygen supplementation to assess the blood gas at room air.

5. Moving from 12 to 24 hours, despite the $PaCO_2$ and FiO_2 remaining fairly static, the PaO_2 declines to 72 mmHg and therefore the P/F ratio also declines to 180, indicating a significant loss of pulmonary function.

6. At 36 hours, the $PaCO_2$ 'normalizes,' which is particularly concerning in an animal with prolonged increased respiratory effort as it most likely indicates the patient is fatiguing and is close to respiratory arrest. At this time point, this patient meets several criteria for requiring mechanical ventilation, including an inability to maintain a PaO_2 >60 despite maximal O_2 supplementation and excessive work of breathing leading to respiratory fatigue. Hence, the dog was intubated and hand ventilated via an anesthesia reservoir bag on 100% FiO_2. The P/F ratio improved to 192, similar to the previous 24-hour value (180), implying the decrease in P/F ratio at 36 hours was likely due to respiratory fatigue and relative hypoventilation rather than a true change in pulmonary function.

At this point, after discussing the necessity of initiating true mechanical ventilation with the owner, humane euthanasia was elected. Necropsy confirmed severe disseminated blastomycosis with lesions in all lung lobes, both eyes, multiple lymph nodes, skin, and bone.

Further Reading

Burkitt Creedon, J., Davis, H. (2012) *Advanced Monitoring and Procedures for Small Animal Emergency and Critical Care*. Wiley-Blackwell, Ames, Iowa, USA. A good resource with images on how to perform techniques including arterial blood sampling and arterial catheter placement.

Dibartola, S.P. (2012) *Fluid, electrolyte and acid–base disorders in small animal practice*, 4th edn. Elsevier, St. Louis, Missouri, USA. A comprehensive text reviewing acid–base physiology.

Silverstein, D.C., Hopper, K. (eds) (2012) *Small Animal Critical Care Medicine*, 2nd edn. Elsevier, St. Louis, Missouri, USA. Excellent concise reviews of acid–base analysis, ventilation, and oxygenation assessments.

West, J.B., Luks, A.M. (2016) *West's Respiratory Physiology: The Essentials*, 10th edn. Wolters Kluwer, Philadelphia, Pennsylvania, USA. An excellent review of the physiology behind ventilation and oxygenation disorders.

Bibliography

Baird, G. (2013) Preanalytical considerations in blood gas analysis. *Biochemia Medica* 23, 19–27.

Bateman, S. (2008) Making sense of blood gas results. *Veterinary Clinics of North America Small Animal* 38, 543–557.

Beaulieu, M., Lapointe, Y., Vinet, B. (1999) Stability of PO_2, PCO_2, and pH in fresh blood samples stored in a plastic syringe with low heparin in relation to various blood-gas and hematological parameters. *Clinical Biochemistry* 32, 101–107.

Bergman, L., Lundbye, J. (2015) Acid-base optimization during hypothermia. *Best Practice & Research Clinical Anaesthesiology* 29, 465–470.

Boron, W. (2009) Acid–base physiology. In: Boron, W.F., Boulpaep, E.L. (eds) *Medical Physiology*, 2nd edn. Saunders Elsevier, Philadelphia, Pennsylvania, USA, pp. 652–671.

Briganti, A., Portela, D.A., Grasso, S., et al. (2015) Accuracy of different oxygenation indices in estimating intrapulmonary shunting at increasing infusion rates of dobutamine in horses under general anaesthesia. *The Veterinary Journal* 204, 351–356.

Constable, P. (2014) Acid-base assessment: When and how to apply the Henderson-Hasselbalch equation and strong ion difference theory. *Veterinary Clinics of North America Food Animal* 30, 295–316.

DiBartola, S.P. (2012a) Introduction to acid-base disorders. In: Dibartola, S.P. (ed.) *Fluid, Electrolyte and Acid-Base Disorders in Small Animal Practice,* 4th edn. Elsevier, St. Louis, Missouri, USA, pp. 231–252.

DiBartola, S.P. (2012b) Metabolic acid-base disorders. In: Dibartola, S.P. (ed.), *Fluid, Electrolyte and Acid-Base Disorders in Small Animal Practice,* 4th edn. Elsevier, St. Louis, Missouri, USA, pp. 253–285.

Gonzalez, A., Waddell, L. (2016). Blood gas analyzers. *Topics in Companion Animal Medicine* 31, 27–34.

Haskins, S.C. (1977) Sampling and storage of blood for pH and blood gas analysis. *Journal of the American Veterinary Medical Association* 170, 429–433.

Hopper, K. (2015a) Traditional acid-base analysis. In: Silverstein, D.C., Hopper, K. (eds) *Small Animal Critical Care Medicine*, 2nd edn. Elsevier, St. Louis, Missouri, USA, pp. 289–295.

Hopper, K (2015b) Nontraditional acid-base analysis. In: Silverstein, D.C., Hopper, K. (eds), *Small Animal Critical Care Medicine*, 2nd edn. Elsevier, St. Louis, Missouri, USA, pp. 296–299.

Hopper, K., Rezende., M., Haskins, S. (2005) Assessment of the effect of dilution of blood samples with sodium heparin on blood gas, electrolyte, and lactate measurements in dogs. *American Journal of Veterinary Research* 66, 656–660.

Hopper, K., Epstein, S., Kass, P., *et al.* (2014) Evaluation of acid–base disorders in dogs and cats presenting to an emergency room. Part 1: Comparison of three methods of acid–base analysis. *Journal of Veterinary Emergency and Critical Care* 24, 493–501.

Jara-Aguirre, J., Meets, S.W., Wockenfus, A., *et al.* (2018) Blood gas sample spiking with total parenteral nutrition, lipid emulsion, and concentrated dextrose solutions as a model for predicting sample contamination based on glucose result. *Clinical Biochemistry* 55, 93–95.

Johnson, R.A., de Morais, H.A. (2012) Respiratory acid-base disorders. In: Dibartola, S.P. (ed.), *Fluid, Electrolyte and Acid-Base Disorders in Small Animal Practice*, 4th edn. Elsevier, St. Louis, Missouri, USA, pp. 287–301.

Knowles, T.P., Mullin, R.A., Hunter, J.A., *et al.* (2006) Effects of syringe material, sample storage time, and temperature on blood gases and oxygen saturation in arterialized human blood samples. *Respiratory Care* 51, 732–736.

Lippi, G., Fontana, R., Avanzini, P., *et al.* (2013) Influence of spurious hemolysis on blood gas analysis. *Clinical and Chemical Laboratory Medicine* 51, 1651–1654.

Toffaletti, J.G., Rackley, C.R. (2016) Monitoring oxygen status. *Advances in Clinical Chemistry* 77, 103–124.

6 Capnography

Laura A.M. Ilie*

Veterinary Specialty Center, Buffalo Grove, Illinois, USA

Capnography is the measurement of the partial pressure of carbon dioxide (CO_2) in exhaled respiratory gases at the end of expiration. The exhaled CO_2 in turn is an indirect assessment of the partial pressure of CO_2 in the arterial blood ($PaCO_2$) and as such provides insight into important life-sustaining systems including the respiratory, circulatory, and metabolic systems.

The measurement of the exhaled CO_2 has been used for many decades in human and veterinary medicine to assess the adequacy of ventilation under general anesthesia, appropriateness of intubation and, more recently, the efficacy of chest compressions during cardiopulmonary resuscitation (CPR).

6.1 Basic Physiology

Carbon dioxide is a metabolic byproduct produced when carbon is combined with oxygen as part of the body's energy-making processes. As it is formed, CO_2 diffuses from the tissues into the bloodstream and then is transported to the lungs where it diffuses into the alveoli. At the alveolar level, the red blood cells are 'unloading' CO_2. This carbon dioxide is then expelled through the breathing process (Fig. 6.1).

The $PaCO_2$ is carefully maintained by the body at an approximate constant pressure of 35–45 mmHg in non-sedated/anesthetized dogs and cats. This is because CO_2 plays an important role in homeostasis. Specifically, it acts as a buffer to maintain normal blood pH, plays an important role in the regulation of cerebral perfusion by regulating vascular tone, stimulates breathing in the brain's ventilator centers, and influences the affinity hemoglobin has for oxygen (O_2).

Measurement of the $PaCO_2$ concentration provides the clinician with useful information regarding the ventilation status of a patient. High $PaCO_2$ (hypercapnia) suggests hypoventilation while low $PaCO_2$ (hypocapnia) suggests hyperventilation.

The gold standard measurement of the $PaCO_2$ is performed by analyzing an arterial blood sample (see Chapter 5). Unfortunately, collection of arterial blood samples is not always easily achieved in small animals and can be associated with pain, thrombosis, and possible infection. Additionally, an arterial blood gas sample only provides a snapshot of the patient's CO_2 value at one point in time and requires repeat blood sampling to gage the animal's condition over time.

A noninvasive and indirect measurement of the $PaCO_2$ can be obtained by measuring the CO_2 level of the patient's expired breaths (i.e. end-tidal CO_2 ($ETCO_2$)) using a capnograph. In order to measure $ETCO_2$ the patient has to be intubated or to have a tight-fitting mask. If ventilation and perfusion are well matched, the $ETCO_2$ should be nearly equal to that of the $PaCO_2$ (i.e. 35–45 mmHg). Usually the $ETCO_2$ value is 2 to 5 mmHg less than that of arterial CO_2 because alveolar gases containing CO_2 will mix with dead-space gases containing no CO_2 in the anesthetic tubing, slightly reducing the $ETCO_2$ measurement versus the concentration of CO_2 in the alveolus. Conditions that may interrupt the transfer of CO_2 from the blood to the alveoli (i.e. pulmonary edema, hemorrhage, pneumonia, pulmonary embolism, emphysema) can lower the $ETCO_2$. In these situations, the difference between $PaCO_2$ and $ETCO_2$ levels can be increased.

In addition, $ETCO_2$ provides insight regarding the function of the circulatory system. For the CO_2 to travel from the cells to the alveolus, there must be appropriate cardiac output (CO) and at least relatively normal flow of blood through the heart and pulmonary system. If the CO is decreased in conditions like hypovolemia or poor cardiac output or the blood does not appropriately travel from the cells back to the alveolus (as occurs with vasodilatory shock or extreme vasoconstriction), the $ETCO_2$ will be low.

---

* Corresponding author: LIlie@vetspecialty.com

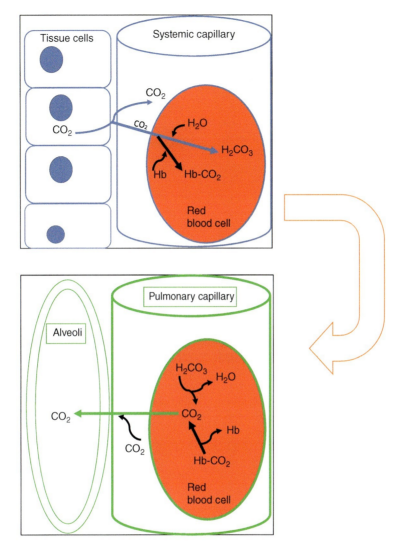

Fig. 6.1. Carbon dioxide metabolism. Carbon dioxide is a metabolic byproduct produced by the tissue cells. While some of the carbon dioxide remains dissolved in the plasma, most carbon dioxide diffuses into the red blood cells. In the red blood cell, it either binds to water molecules and forms carbonic acid or binds to hemoglobin to form carboxyhemoglobin. When the blood arrives in the lungs, the carbon dioxide diffuses into the alveoli. At the alveolar level, the red blood cells are 'unloading' CO_2 which is then expelled through the breathing process. CO_2, carbon dioxide; H_2CO_3, carbonic acid; H_2O, water; Hb, hemoglobin; Hb-CO_2, carboxyhemoglobin.

During CPR, measurement of $ETCO_2$ can reliably provide the clinician with information regarding the quality of chest compressions as well as an indirect assessment of the cardiac output and the blood flow through the heart and lungs.

In conclusion, measurement of the $ETCO_2$ provides the clinician with two important pieces of information: indirect evaluation of the patient's ventilatory status as well as information regarding the cardiac output and blood flow through the heart and pulmonary system.

6.2 How Capnography Works

There are two different ways to analyze the CO_2 concentration: plotted against time (time capnogram) or against expired lung volume during a respiratory cycle (volume capnogram).

The time capnogram gives an indication of the efficiency of ventilation. It is the most commonly used method because it is simple to use, evaluates both parts of the respiratory cycle (inspiration and expiration), and is an excellent tool for patient monitoring at bedside. The volume capnogram has its own benefits too: it allows a breath-by-breath quantification of the volume of lung ventilated, as well as the measurement of alveolar dead space, and physiological dead space. This means that the clinician can assess the degree of ventilation/perfusion (V/Q) mismatch. Different physiological concepts can be used (i.e. Bohr or Enghoff approach) to quantify the global V/Q mismatches. This method also allows separation of shunt fraction (blood passing by unventilated alveoli) and true dead space (air not available for gas exchange). The major limitations of volume capnograms include the requirement to use a mechanical ventilator and other elaborate equipment and it only provides information regarding the expiratory phase of the breathing cycle (as the expired CO_2 is plotted against expired lung volume).

This chapter will only focus on time capnograms.

A time capnograph provides a graphic representation (waveform) denoting the relationship of the $ETCO_2$ concentration to time. It also provides a measured value of the maximum level of $ETCO_2$ at the end of each breath. Changes in size, shape, and distribution of the waveforms are suggestive of underlying pathologic conditions while changes in the level of measured $ETCO_2$ reflect disease severity as well as response to treatment.

Capnometry is further classified based on the technique used to measure CO_2 concentration:

- *Qualitative capnometry*: provides a color-coded (colorimetric) capnogram representing the presence of CO_2 in the patient's breath.
- Quantitative capnometry: provides a numeric value for the measured CO_2 concentration. It can also provide a graphic form which is called 'quantitative capnography.'

Qualitative capnometry

Qualitative (colorimetric) capnographs are handheld devices which contain a pH-sensitive impregnated paper. If the exhaled gas contains CO_2, the color of the paper changes from purple to yellow. These devices are best utilized to confirm proper endotracheal intubation. The device is placed at the end of the endotracheal tube (ETT). If the color does not change, there is a high chance the ETT tube is in the esophagus and it needs to be repositioned. It is important to wait for six breaths before deciding if the ETT is properly placed.

Quantitative capnometry

There are multiple physical methods that can be used to *quantitatively measure* CO_2 : (i) infrared spectroscopy; (ii) molecular correlation spectroscopy; (iii) Raman spectrography; (iv) photo acoustic spectrography; (v) mass spectrography; and (vi) chemical colorimetric analysis spectrography.

The most commonly used principle is the measure of infrared light; therefore, this method will be described in more detail in this chapter. This principle uses the application of the Beer and Lambert Laws and infrared waves. This means that the quantity of infrared (IR) waveforms absorbed is proportional to the concentration of the infrared-absorbing substance. In other words, the quantity of infrared waveforms absorbed by CO_2 molecules is proportional to the concentration of CO_2 present in the expired gas. The higher the CO_2 concentration the higher the quantity of IR absorbed. This concept might seem difficult to follow, but it will be described in more detail below.

A capnograph using infrared spectroscopy contains three main components: (i) infrared source; (ii) sample chamber; and (iii) infrared detector.

The infrared source

As the name implies, the infrared source emits infrared waves. The infrared waves are absorbed by different gases present in the anesthesia circuit. Each gas absorbs infrared waves of different wavelengths. For example, CO_2 absorbs infrared wavelengths of 4.25 micrometers, nitrous oxide absorbs infrared wavelengths of 4.5 micrometers, while oxygen does not absorb infrared light.

Why is this important? Because knowing the wavelength absorption of a certain gas (in our case the CO_2), a device can be designed with an infrared source that will only emit that specific wavelength and only measure the concentration of that gas. If the source were to emit a wide spectrum of wavelengths, then it might measure the concentration of other gases that are not of importance and the final reading will not be accurate. Therefore, in most capnographs the infrared source is designed to emit wavelengths within very narrow limits. A graphic representation of the main components is found in Fig. 6.2.

Sample chamber

This chamber is made of sapphire, which allows the infrared waves to pass through. When the patient expires, the gas expired also passes through this chamber. The infrared waves will be absorbed by the expired CO_2 based on its concentration (i.e. the higher the expired CO_2 concentration, the higher the absorption of the infrared light). See Fig. 6.2.

Infrared detector

An infrared detector is located opposite to the infrared source (on the other side of the sample chamber). When infrared waves reach this detector, a signal will be transmitted to the monitor. The higher the number of infrared waveforms that reach the detector, the lower the CO_2 reading will be. This occurs because *many* infrared waveforms reaching the detector mean that *few* infrared waveforms have been absorbed by the passing CO_2 (therefore the concentration of CO_2 is low). For example, if the patient exhales a *high* concentration of CO_2, this will cause an *increase* in infrared absorption in the sampling chamber; therefore, a *low* number of infrared waves will reach the detector, indicating a *high* $ETCO_2$.

There is a proprietary algorithm that implements the information received by the detector to determine the exact $ETCO_2$ value displayed on the screen of the capnograph.

Quantitative capnographs are also classified based on the location of the infrared detector: (i) mainstream capnographs; or (ii) sidestream capnographs.

MAINSTREAM CAPNOGRAPHY In the mainstream capnograph, an airway adapter is inserted directly between the breathing circuit and the endotracheal tube. An infrared source and detector are attached to the airway adapter (sometimes it can be found as a single unit or as separate parts, see Figs 6.3 to 6.5).

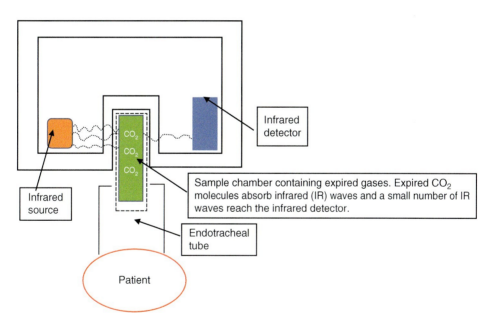

Fig. 6.2. Schematic representation of a capnograph using infrared spectrography with its three main components: infrared source, sample chamber and infrared detector. Note the infrared source is emitting infrared waves toward the sample chamber. The patient expires anesthesia gases, including CO_2. The infrared waves will be absorbed by the expired CO_2 molecules based on its concentration (i.e. the higher the expired CO_2 concentration, the higher the absorption of the infrared light). The infrared waves not absorbed by the CO_2 molecules will reach the detector and a signal will be transmitted to the monitor. The lower the number of infrared waveforms that reach the detector, the higher the CO_2 reading will be. CO_2, carbon dioxide.

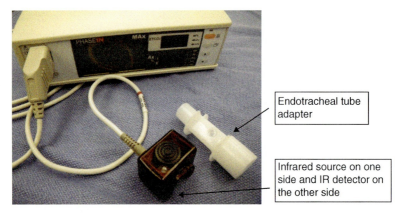

Fig. 6.3. Mainstream capnograph with separate infrared sensor (IR) as well as an endotracheal tube adapter. The endotracheal tube adapter fits inside the IR sensor. The smaller end of the endotracheal adapter attachs to the endotracheal tube of the patient, while the larger end connects to the anesthesia circuit.

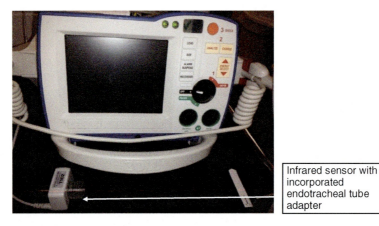

Fig. 6.4. Mainstream capnograph with endotracheal tube adapter incorporated within the infrared source/detector.

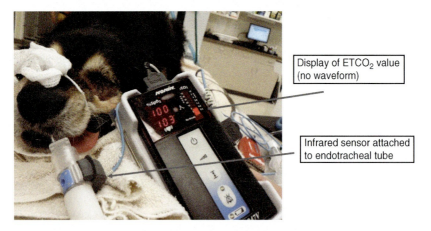

Fig. 6.5. Mainstream capnometer attached to a patient's endotracheal tube. Note that a waveform is not provided with this device.

The detector is attached to the monitor via an electrical wire.

SIDESTREAM CAPNOGRAPHY In sidestream capnography, the detector is in the main unit itself (away from the airway) and a very small pump aspirates gas samples (usually 50–150 mL/min, depending on whether the machine measures other gases) from the patient's airway through a small tube into the main unit. This sampling tube is connected to a T-piece inserted at the endotracheal tube or anesthesia mask connector (Fig. 6.6A). The gas that is withdrawn from the patient often contains anesthetic gases; the exhausted gas from the capnograph must be routed to a gas scavenger or returned to the patient's breathing system (Fig. 6.6B).

Each method of sampling comes with its own unique set of advantages and disadvantages. Mainstream technology generally produces more sharply delineated waveforms compared to a sidestream capnograph. In addition, since mainstream units do not remove gas from the anesthetic circuit, there is no need to separately scavenge anesthetic gases. Mainstream units are more durable than sidestream units, have fewer disposable components, do not require additional sample tubing, and tend to be reasonable in cost. Mainstream analyzers also provide instantaneous readings.

In contrast, sidestream capnographs have the unique advantage of allowing monitoring of non-intubated subjects by connecting the sidestream micro tube to a face mask or a nasal catheter line. When using nasal $ETCO_2$, it is unlikely that dilution of CO_2 will occur and it has been demonstrated that the general waveform is comparable to and representative of the $ETCO_2$ obtained from an endotracheal tube (as long as the patient breathes through its nose). When using a face mask, significant dilution of CO_2 is expected. This is because the samples of expired gas are mixed with the

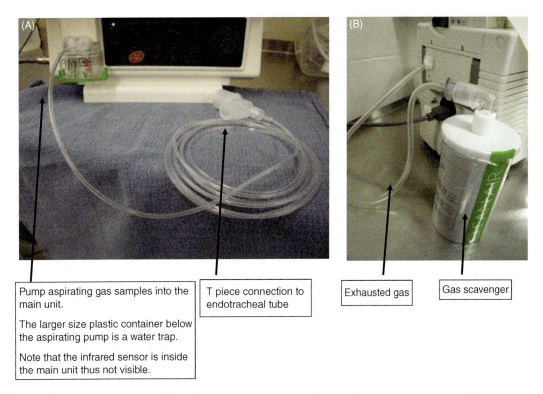

Fig. 6.6. Sidestream capnograph. (A) A sidestream capnographs with a small aspiration pump that takes a sample of expired gas directly from the patient's expired gas (which includes CO_2 and anesthetic gas) and brings it to the infrared sensor located inside the main unit. (B) After the gas sample is analyzed, the exhausted gas that has been sampled from the patient by the capnograph is routed to a gas scavenger to remove CO_2 and any waste anesthesia gases (such as isoflurane). CO_2, carbon dioxide.

atmospheric gases in the mask in addition to the fresh gas flow into the mask. This dilutes the concentration of CO_2 and leads to a falsely low $ETCO_2$ as compared to an intubated patient. However, knowing that there is CO_2 dilution, face mask–derived $ETCO_2$ readings can still be trended over time within a single patient and provide clinical information. It is noteworthy to mention that some capnography systems (like the Oridion systems) have a dual nasal and mouth sampling device that may give a better idea of real $ETCO_2$ in patients who are panting/breathing through their mouth.

Other advantages of sidestream capnographs include faster warm-up time than mainstream units, low dead space added to the circuit, and the capability to measure several respiratory gases at once including anesthetic gases. The line and adaptor that attach to the ETT are also lightweight which reduces the chance of kinking or disconnection of the system.

One other aspect of the sidestream capnograph that needs to be mentioned is that condensation from humidified gas and patient's secretions may develop and it can accumulate in the sampling line. This can lead to inaccurate $ETCO_2$ readings as it can affect the sampling cell function or sometimes cause occlusion of the sampling line. Frequent replacement of the sampling line may be required. To avoid this or to at least decrease the frequency of sampling line replacement, most units come with a water trap (see Fig. 6.7) located at the end of the sampling tube. Some units also have water permeable tubing such as Nafion® tubing. This tubing has a unique property to transfer moisture from one side of the membrane to the other. This is done chemically via differential vapor pressure (the water molecules move from a higher pressure to a lower pressure) and is therefore very selective for water molecules only. If there is high moisture pressure in the tubing, the water molecules will be transferred outside of the tubing and the gas that reaches the analysis chamber will be moisture-free and will not interfere with the CO_2 reading.

A microstream system has also been developed which is a variation of the traditional sidestream units. In the microstream technology there is no sensor at the airway. It uses laser-based molecular spectroscopy as the infrared emission source. The expired CO_2 travels along a thin tube before reaching the chamber where the detector is located. The microstream system allows for a smaller transition

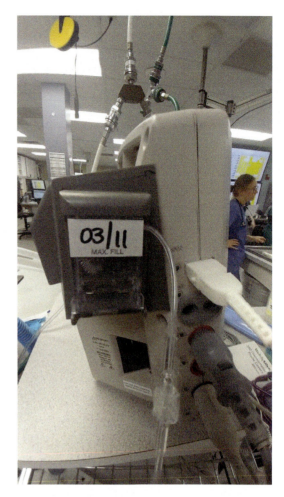

Fig. 6.7. Water trap sidestream capnograph. This is a sidestream capnograph and the water trap can be seen on the side of the machine.

period between the mouth and the detection chamber than traditional sidestream technology and thus a capnograph curve that is almost synchronized with the passage of air at the mouth. In addition, the microstream system has less dead space than traditional units (less than 0.5 mL of dead space), which makes this a useful $ETCO_2$ monitor for the small-sized patient. Other benefits of the microstream technology include a low-flow 50 mL/min sample rate, no dilution with supplementary oxygen, and no cross reaction with other gases. Using a low-flow sample rate is especially beneficial for our small-sized patients which tend to have a low tidal volume and a fast respiratory rate. Using a high-flow sampling rate (i.e. 150 mL/min used with classic capnographs) can result in erroneous $ETCO_2$ measurements and distorted waveforms. Also, low-flow sample rates minimize dispersion of gases in the sampling tubes and there is a less likely chance of aspirating condensed water and secretions minimizing the chances of occlusion.

6.3 Indications for Capnography in Small Animals

Anesthesia or heavy sedation

The use of a capnograph along with pulse oximetry, electrocardiogram, and blood pressure monitoring is recommended in every patient that undergoes general anesthesia or heavy sedation. Becoming familiar with the normal as well as abnormal waveforms provided by the capnograph, the clinician/technician can gain a rapid visual evaluation of ventilation in the anesthetized patient as well as detect problems encountered along the way. More detail regarding waveform interpretation is provided in Section 6.4.

Cardiopulmonary resuscitation

As mentioned at the beginning of this chapter, the measurement of $ETCO_2$ provides the clinician with two important pieces of information: an overview of the patient's ventilatory status as well as an idea of the cardiac output and the blood flow through the heart and pulmonary system.

Since $ETCO_2$ is proportional to pulmonary blood flow (the better the blood flow, the more CO_2 is delivered to the alveoli to breathe out), $ETCO_2$ can be used as a measure of chest compression efficacy during CPR assuming the ventilations administered are unchanging in rate and size of breath. During cardiopulmonary arrest there is no blood flow nor ventilation. When closed chest compressions are performed, very few alveoli are perfused because the blood flow to the lungs is low. By providing manual ventilation with an AMBU bag, many alveoli are ventilated but are not perfused. During this time the $ETCO_2$ will be low. If the blood flow to the lungs improves (CPR is successful and return of spontaneous circulation is achieved), more alveoli will be perfused and subsequently the $ETCO_2$ will increase.

During chest compressions in CPR, the goal value of $ETCO_2$ should be above 15–20 mmHg. Lower values have been associated with a significant decrease in the likelihood of the patient having return of spontaneous circulation. A declining or low $ETCO_2$ value during CPR may suggest rescuer fatigue or ineffective chest compressions by the rescuer. It should also alert the clinician to seek other factors contributing to declining cardiac output or which are rendering chest compressions less successful such as ongoing hemorrhage, cardiac tamponade, or pneumothorax.

Feeding tube placement

Although, radiography remains the 'gold standard' method to confirm proper placement of nasoesophageal/gastric feeding tubes, capnography can be used as an adjunct technique. The partial pressure of CO_2 in the stomach and esophagus is negligible. Therefore, the $ETCO_2$ value should be zero in correctly placed feeding tubes and higher if the tube is mis-placed in the airways.

Upper airway emergencies

Capnography may be beneficial in patients who require intubation to treat life-threatening upper airway obstruction or severe upper airway inflammation (i.e. brachycephalic syndrome, laryngeal paralysis, etc.). In most cases, these patients have received a large volume of sedation and/or anxiolytic drugs prior to and in order to facilitate intubation, including but not limited to propofol, opioids, benzodiazepines, alpha-2 agonists, and acepromazine. It is important to monitor the $ETCO_2$ in these patients to ensure that they are not hypercapnic as a result of respiratory depression from the sedation/anesthesia. If hypercapnia is noted, these patients may need manual or mechanical ventilation until the drugs wear off or can be reversed and their ventilatory drive returns.

Mechanical ventilation

In all patients being mechanically ventilated, it is useful to monitor paired $PaCO_2$ and $ETCO_2$ values. If the $ETCO_2$ is proved to be representative of the $PaCO_2$ by comparison to the arterial blood gas analysis in a particular patient, changes in $ETCO_2$ may be assumed to signify similar changes in $PaCO_2$. In that way the noninvasive $ETCO_2$ allows the patient to avoid numerous arterial punctures (if an arterial catheter is not in place already) and the expense of running multiple blood gas analyses. The capnograph also provides a continuous display of the $ETCO_2$ which allows for detection of sudden changes in the carbon dioxide values. It is important to remember that this relationship between $ETCO_2$ and $PaCO_2$ will only be valid if there are no major respiratory or hemodynamic changes in the patient. It is not recommended to use $ETCO_2$ solely to assess $PaCO_2$ without at least periodic comparisons to the arterial carbon dioxide value.

Measuring paired $PaCO_2$ and $ETCO_2$ values also allows the clinician to determine the difference between the arterial and end-tidal CO_2. This difference is referred to as the $P_{(a-ET)}CO_2$ gradient. The arterial to $ETCO_2$ gradient should be ≤ 5 mmHg in anesthetized normal dogs. The $P_{(a-ET)}CO_2$ gradient can provide the clinician with valuable information regarding the clinical progress of a critically ill patient; trends of this value may be used to assess improvement. Table 6.1 summarizes some of the causes of altered $PaCO_2$–$ETCO_2$ gradient.

Traumatic brain injury patients

Patients with traumatic brain injury require careful monitoring of their ventilatory status. Hyperventilation (low $PaCO_2$) leads to cerebral vasoconstriction which helps to preserve intracranial pressure while hypoventilation (high $PaCO_2$) can cause cerebral vasodilation which in turn can increase intracranial pressure.

Manual hyperventilation may be considered for intubated patients with severe neurologic decompensation or those at high risk of cerebral herniation. The recommended $ETCO_2$ target for this sub-category of patients is 30-35 mmHg. If manual hyperventilation is performed it should be limited to a duration of 4-6 hours (such as during advanced imaging like magnetic resonance imaging; MRI) to prevent excessive cerebral vasoconstriction and possible ischemic damage to the brain. It is not recommended to provide prophylactic hyperventilation during the initial resuscitation of patients with traumatic brain injury so as to avoid vasoconstriction that could impede oxygen delivery to damaged brain cells.

6.4 Interpretation of End-Tidal Carbon Dioxide

Clinical information can be obtained from three sources in CO_2 analysis: (i) numerical values of $ETCO_2$ (*capnometry*); (ii) shape of the waveform (*capnogram*); or (iii) the difference between $ETCO_2$ and $PaCO_2$ ($P_{(a-ET)}CO_2$ gradient).

Table 6.1. The most common causes of altered $P_{(a-ET)}CO_2$ gradient.

Increased $P_{(a-ET)}CO_2$ gradient	Examples
Ventilation perfusion mismatch	Acute respiratory distress syndrome Pulmonary infiltrates (edema, hemorrhage, pneumonia) Diffusion barrier preventing diffusion of carbon dioxide into the alveoli ($ETCO_2$ to be significantly lower than $PaCO_2$) Pulmonary thromboembolism Decreased lung perfusion and increased alveolar dead space causing $ETCO_2$ to be significantly lower than $PaCO_2$
Increased alveolar dead space	Chronic obstructive pulmonary-like disease Pulmonary thromboembolism These conditions tend to cause an incomplete alveolar emptying (i.e. chronic airway obstruction causes gas to be trapped in the alveoli not allowing complete gas exchange therefore the $ETCO_2$ reads low)
Decreased cardiac output	Heart disease Less delivery of carbon dioxide from the tissues to the alveoli for gas exchange resulting in low $ETCO_2$
Low patient tidal volume to equipment dead space	Increase in dead space ventilation Patient exhaling into dead space; CO_2 not measured by capnograph
Leak in the sampling system or around endotracheal tube	Exhaled gases lost from system False decrease in $ETCO_2$ value measured by capnograph

$PaCO_2$, arterial concentration of carbon dioxide (measured in mmHg); $ETCO_2$, end-tidal carbon dioxide concentration (measured in mmHg); $P_{(a-ET)}CO_2$, difference between arterial and end-tidal carbon dioxide concentrations.

In a clinical situation, it is important to interpret the information provided by capnometry (i.e. the numerical value of $ETCO_2$) along with capnography (the graphic representation of the waveform). Numerical values should be used as a tool in evaluation of *the overall ventilatory status* of the patient while the shapes of the waveforms *offer more specific diagnostic clues*.

Capnometry

There are four major causes for increases or decreases in the numerical values of the $ETCO_2$:

- cellular/metabolic reasons (changes in the rate of CO_2 production in the tissues) as seen with hypothermia, fever, seizures, etc.;
- variations in alveolar ventilation (secondary to pain, bronchospasm, drug therapy, etc.);
- alterations in pulmonary perfusion (changes in delivery of blood and CO_2 to the alveoli) as seen with cardiac failure, cardiac arrest, pulmonary thromboembolism, etc.; and
- technical malfunctions of the anesthesia machine.

Tables 6.2 and 6.3 summarize the most common causes of increased and decreased $ETCO_2$ values.

Capnogram

Understanding waveforms generated during ventilation and how to interpret them can provide a great deal of information, sometimes even making the difference between life and death for the patient. A normal capnogram shows a regular, nearly square waveform that represents the inhalation of CO_2-free gases during inspiration and the path of CO_2 from the alveoli to the mouth during expiration.

There is a very small volume of breath that does not participate in gas exchange (it is CO_2 free) called respiratory dead space. This anatomic dead space represents the total volume of the conducting airways from the nose or mouth down to the level of the terminal bronchioles. The dead space can be increased in intubated patients due to presence of endotracheal tubes that are too long or additional tubing added to the anesthesia circuit (i.e. choosing an anesthesia circuit that is too large for the size of the patient).

When the patient first starts to exhale, there will be no CO_2 detected by the capnograph because the gas from the dead space is exhaled first. As the exhalation continues, the concentration of CO_2 increases until it reaches a peak at the end of exhalation; then the CO_2 concentration drops to baseline as the patient starts to inhale CO_2-free gases. This can be seen best on a time capnogram (Fig. 6.8).

As seen in Fig. 6.8, a time capnogram has two important segments – inspiratory and expiratory – as well as two angles (alpha and beta). The expiratory segment of a time capnogram includes phase I, II and III, while the inspiratory phase includes phase 0 and the beginning of phase I.

Table 6.2. Most common causes of increased $ETCO_2$ values (greater than 50 mmHg).

Cause	Physiologic explanation
Cellular/metabolic	Increased muscle activity or metabolic rate caused by seizures, fever, or severe sepsis, leading to increased cellular CO_2 production
Variations in alveolar ventilation	Respiratory center suppression leading to decreased ventilation rate or depth: due to neurologic disease, head trauma, toxin/drug induced, pain Inability to perform full lung expansion: due to pleural effusion, pneumothorax Inappropriate intubation (i.e. bronchial intubation leading to ventilation of only one lung) Decreased manual ventilation rate or decreased respiratory rate during mechanical ventilation Partial airway obstruction (mass vs mucus plug vs ETT kinked vs other)
Alterations in pulmonary perfusion	Congestive heart failure – poor lung perfusion, thus poor gas exchange
Technical malfunction of the anesthesia machine	Expiratory valve malfunction (accumulation of expired gases including CO_2) Slow fresh gas flow (with non-rebreathing systems) leading to build-up of CO_2 in the system Exhausted CO_2 absorbent (rebreathing carbon dioxide)

$ETCO_2$, end-tidal carbon dioxide; ETT, endotracheal tube; CO_2, carbon dioxide.

Table 6.3. Most common causes of decreased $ETCO_2$ values (less than 30 mmHg).

Cause	Physiologic explanation
Cellular/metabolic	• Decreased metabolic and cellular function due to hypothermia, metabolic acidosis leading to decreased CO_2 formation
Variations in alveolar ventilation	• Pain or anxiety-induced tachypnea • Excessive manual ventilation or increased respiratory rate during mechanical ventilation • Bronchospasm, asthma, chronic bronchitis causing decreased gas exchange in the alveoli • Total airway obstruction blocking gas exchange in the alveoli • Apnea/respiratory arrest
Alterations in pulmonary perfusion	• Sampling line leak or obstruction in sidestream capnographs • Total airway obstruction or disconnected system • Malfunctioning ETT cuff (deflated or too small for patient's size) causing gas to be expired around the tube rather than going through the analyzer Inappropriate placement of the ETT (i.e. into the esophagus) • If a non-rebreathing system is used (patient smaller than 7 kg), the fresh gas flow may be too high, causing dilution of the expired gas and lowering the $ETCO_2$ • Increased dead space (especially in small-sized patients) causing carbon dioxide to stay in the system rather than pass through the capnograph • Accidental extubation
Technical malfunction of the anesthesia machine	• Expiratory valve malfunction (accumulation of expired gases including CO_2) Slow fresh gas flow (with non-rebreathing systems) leading to build-up of carbon dioxide in the system • Exhausted CO_2 absorbent (rebreathing carbon dioxide)

$ETCO_2$, end-tidal carbon dioxide; ETT, endotracheal tube; CO_2, carbon dioxide.

- *Phase I (respiratory baseline)*: this phase represents inspiration which means the CO_2 concentration should be zero. The expiration phase starts right before the end of this phase, but because it does not contain any expired CO_2 (due to the presence of dead space) it is displayed as a flat line.
- *Phase II (expiratory upstroke)*: as the name implies, in this phase the CO_2 concentration rises rapidly, and an upswing of the baseline will be seen. As the expiration progresses, the CO_2 from the alveoli will replace the 'CO_2 -free gas' previously present in the trachea and endotracheal tube and be sensed by the capnometer.
- *Phase III (alveolar plateau)*: as expiration continues, the alveoli become empty and the CO_2 level reaches a plateau level. Because not all the alveoli empty at the same exact time, the alveolar plateau phase is slightly sloped. This happens because the alveoli with a low ventilation:perfusion ratio (i.e. well perfused with blood but not ventilated as effectively) have a higher CO_2 concentration and usually empty late in the exhalation phase. The highest point of phase III corresponds to the actual $ETCO_2$.
- *Phase 0 (inspiratory downstroke)*: the CO_2 concentration rapidly declines to zero during inhalation as CO_2-free gas is drawn into the lungs, past the carbon dioxide sensor.
- *Alpha angle*: the angle between phase II and III is the α angle. This angle is typically considered to be an indirect representation of the ventilation: perfusion status of the lung. The slope and the height of phase III can be influenced by airway resistance, cardiac output, and CO_2 production, resulting in changes in the degree of the alpha angle. Normally this angle is between 100° and 110°. For example, an increase in alpha angle may suggest increased airway resistance (i.e. an obstruction from things such as asthma, bronchospasm, kinked endotracheal tube, etc.). The angle increases since it takes longer to expel the carbon dioxide-rich gas from the alveoli when there is airway spasm or other airway obstruction.
- *Beta angle*: the angle between phase III and the inspiratory downstroke is the β angle. This angle is usually about 90 degrees. This angle is used to assess the degree of rebreathing; it will increase as the rebreathing increases since it will take

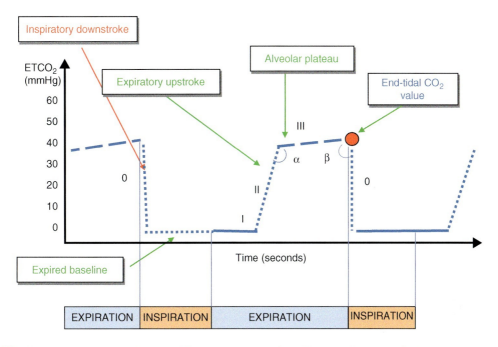

Fig. 6.8. Graphic representation of a normal time capnogram produced by mainstream or side stream capnography. Phase 0-Inspiration; Phase I- Anatomical dead space, expired baseline; Phase II- Expiratory upstroke (mix of dead space gas and alveolar gas); Phase III- Alveolar plateau; Alpha angle: Angle between phase II and phase III; Beta angle: Angle between phase III and descending limb of inspiratory segment.

longer to replace the CO_2 in the alveoli with fresh gas when there is rebreathing.

The shape of a capnogram from a healthy patient is very similar regardless of age, breed, or species. Lung pathologies or equipment malfunctions will change the appearance of the capnograph waveform. Any anesthetist (doctor or technician) needs to recognize normal from abnormal. Proper interpretation of capnographic waveforms during anesthesia will help the clinician identify life-threatening conditions and equipment malfunctions (i.e. leak, esophageal intubation, rebreathing of CO_2, loss of capnographic wave from disconnection of the anesthesia circuit, obstructed/kinked endotracheal tube or respiratory arrest hypercapnia/hypoventilation, and many more).

Commonly encountered abnormal capnographic waveforms

When interpreting a capnogram it is recommended to do so in a systematic way each time to make sure no important aspects are being overlooked. Evaluate the overall shape of the waveform, height, frequency, baseline as well as the rhythm of the waveform following the questions:

1. Is a waveform present?
2. What is the shape of the waveform? (steep, sloping, prolonged?)
3. What is the height of the waveform? (short, tall?)
4. How frequent are the breaths (too fast, too slow?)
5. What about the baseline? Where does it start? (is there rebreathing?)

Table 6.4 summarizes the most commonly encountered abnormalities in the capnographic waveform.

In patients undergoing endotracheal intubation, capnography can help to show that the trachea, and not the esophagus, has been successfully intubated. A series of successive, steady, normal capnographic waveforms must be seen to rule out esophageal intubation (Fig. 6.9). A similar graphic representation to Fig. 6.9 can be seen when there is disconnection of the anesthesia circuit or the endotracheal tube, occlusion, or disconnection of the sampling catheter (when a sidestream system is used) or if apnea is present.

Table. 6.4. Common abnormalities in the capnographic waveform.

Segment affected	Possible causes	Troubleshooting
Wave form	*Absent* – suggests disconnection of the breathing circuit; obstruction/kinking of the sampling line; cardiac arrest; esophageal intubation	Check patient's vital signs and start CPR if needed Check ETT connections Check sampling line Check proper placement of the ETT
Shape of the waveform	*Slant (prolonged) phase II or III* – suggests obstruction of the expiratory flow (i.e kinked ETT; bronchospasm; asthma) or leaks in the breathing system	Check ETT for obstruction/kinks Check breathing circuit and ETT cuff for leaks Consider a bronchodilator
	Slant (prolonged) phase 0 – suggests malfunction of the inspiratory valve when a closed-circuit system is used	Check inspiratory valve for malfunction
Frequency of the waveform	*Too fast* – suggests hyperventilation	Consider decreasing the respiratory rate if manually or mechanically ventilated or increase the depth of anesthesia if spontaneously breathing
	Too slow – suggests hypoventilation	Consider increasing the respiratory rate if manually or mechanically ventilated or reduce depth of anesthesia if spontaneously breathing
Inspiratory baseline	*Gradual elevation* – suggests rebreathing	Check sodalime as well as the inspiratory and expiratory valves Check the sidestream tubing and replace if needed
	Sudden elevation along with increased $ETCO_2$ – suggests contamination of the sampling cell with mucus or water	Disconnecting the sampling line and flushing it with air from a syringe can sometimes clear it, but it may be necessary to replace these components. Elevating the sidestream sampling line above the ventilator circuit helps to prevent the entry of condensed water. A humidity barrier such as Nafion® tubing is also useful
Height of the waveform	*Tall waveform* – suggests hypoventilation or increased metabolic rate	Consider increasing the respiratory rate
	Short waveform – suggests hyperventilation or a decrease in metabolic rate or cardiac output	Consider decreasing the respiratory rate

ETT, endotracheal tube; CPR, cardiopulmonary resuscitation; $ETCO_2$, end-tidal carbon dioxide.

Rebreathing of carbon dioxide is easily seen on the capnogram as an elevated baseline and increase in $ETCO_2$ value (Fig. 6.10). Causes for rebreathing include:

- expiratory valve malfunction;
- low fresh gas flow (in the non-rebreathing circuits);
- the carbon dioxide absorber (soda lime) is chemically exhausted (characterized by a change in color - usually becomes purple/blue when exhausted).

Capnograms can also help us identify if there is a total or partial obstruction of the ETT. If a partial obstruction is present, there will be a small or absent alveolar plateau noted as well as a prolonged inspiratory upstroke (Fig. 6.11). If a total obstruction is present, there will be no waveform as the gas sample cannot reach the sample chamber.

It is not unusual to have the ETT cuff inflated too much or too little. Ideally a Possey Cufflator™ should be used to properly measure the pressure in the cuff. The Possey Cufflator™ is an endotracheal tube inflator and manometer. It has an air vent button and inflator bulb to quickly adjust the ETT cuff pressure. The inflator's gauge on the manometer shows the recommended pressure range in centimeters of water (usually between 20–30 cm H_2O). Should there be a leak of air around the endotracheal

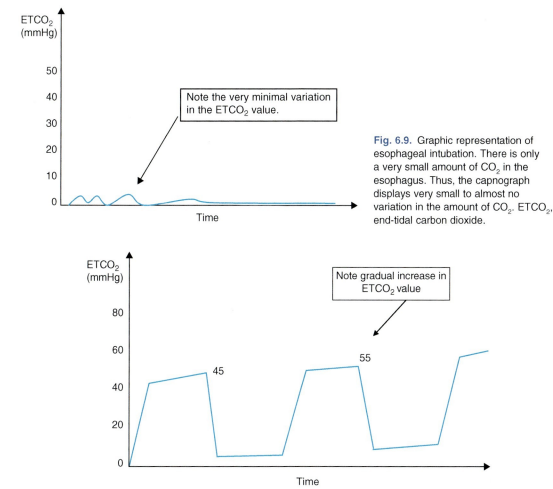

Fig. 6.9. Graphic representation of esophageal intubation. There is only a very small amount of CO_2 in the esophagus. Thus, the capnograph displays very small to almost no variation in the amount of CO_2. $ETCO_2$, end-tidal carbon dioxide.

Fig. 6.10. Graphic representation of hypercapnia and rebreathing. Note the $ETCO_2$ value increases with each breath and it is above 50 mmHg while rebreathing is noted as the presence of an elevated baseline. $ETCO_2$, end-tidal carbon dioxide; CO_2, carbon dioxide.

cuff, there will be a dilution of the $ETCO_2$ and the number will be artificially lowered. Graphically we will see a shorter alveolar plateau that blends in with the inspiratory downstroke (Fig. 6.12).

Common causes for hypoventilation leading to hypercapnia (increased $ETCO_2$ number) include sedation or an underlying condition affecting the respiratory center in the brain (neurologic disease, toxin, trauma, etc.). In those cases, the capnogram will display an increase in $ETCO_2$ (see Fig. 6.10).

A less commonly-seen change in the capnogram is cardiogenic oscillation. The end of phase III and phase 0 of the waveform undulates rather than going to a flat baseline as a result of the beating heart 'compressing' the lungs and altering the capnograph waveform. Cardiogenic oscillations are usually seen in mechanically ventilated patients and its presence suggests either superficial breaths (not deep enough) or not enough breaths per minute. If cardiogenic oscillations are seen in an anesthetized patient with spontaneous breathing, assisted or mechanical ventilation may be considered to improve the depth and quality of respirations (Fig. 6.13).

Shallow breathing or panting causes transient lowering of $ETCO_2$ because shallow breaths are

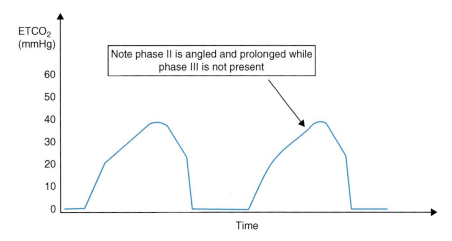

Fig. 6.11. Graphic representation of an obstructed endotracheal tube. In this case, the CO_2 cannot be easily expelled, thus the ascending slope (phase II) is prolonged and there is no alveolar plateau (phase III). There is no obvious alpha angle. This usually happens when the endotracheal tube obstruction is severe enough to prevent complete expiration of the gas during the expiratory phase by the time the next inspiratory phase occurs. Due to absence of phase III, the alpha angle is not obvious either. $ETCO_2$, end-tidal carbon dioxide.

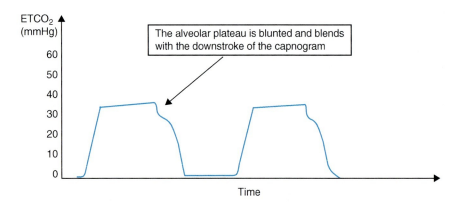

Fig. 6.12. Graphic representation of leak around the endotracheal tube cuff. If air leaks around the cuff, it will dilute the $ETCO_2$ making it a lower concentration. This will shorten the alveolar plateau as the CO_2 drops. Note a shorter alveolar plateau (phase III) and an undulating shape of phase 0. $ETCO_2$, end-tidal carbon dioxide.

largely dead-space ventilation. This can be distinguished from true decreases in $ETCO_2$ because the $ETCO_2$ will rise again after a deep inspiration when full gas exchange occurs.

A flat line may be seen when there is severe bronchospasm leading to complete obstruction, tracheal tube obstruction, obstruction of the sampling tubing, apnea, cardiac arrest, or a disconnected capnograph.

If an abnormal $ETCO_2$ value is obtained, evaluate the patient prior to attributing the abnormal value to equipment malfunction or a change in the patient's condition. If the patient is stable clinically, consider the possibility of malfunction of the anesthetic circuit or the capnograph or poor connection between capnograph and anesthesia circuit/patient.

6.5 Pitfalls of the Monitor

General comments

Capnography is valuable for monitoring a patient's respiratory status. However, capnograms must

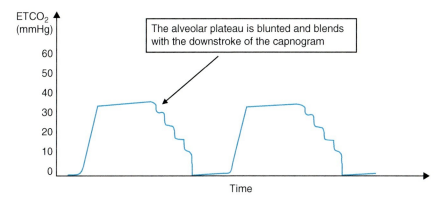

Fig. 6.13. Cardiogenic oscillations. Note the irregular shape of the phase III and phase 0. The wavy shape of phase 0 is due to the heart transmitting its vibrations to the lung and airway during inspiration. If cardiogenic oscillations are seen in an anesthetized patient with spontaneous breathing, assisted or mechanical ventilation may be considered to adjust the depth and rate of breathing. ETCO$_2$, end-tidal carbon dioxide.

always be interpreted in conjunction with other physiological variables and the clinical situation. The ETCO$_2$ does NOT replace arterial and venous blood gas analysis. As mentioned above, at constant ventilation the ETCO$_2$ will represent the ventilatory status of the patient as well as provide information about the cardiac output. If there is lung pathology present or the patient is very sick, the ETCO$_2$ will not accurately reflect the ventilatory status nor the cardiac output, necessitating measurement of the PaCO$_2$ as well as other parameters assessing cardiac output. The sicker the patient is, the more likely the perfusion to the lungs is negatively affected. Therefore, in critically ill intubated patients, the patient's PaCO$_2$ is *at least* as high if not higher than the displayed ETCO$_2$ measurement. It is therefore important to document the actual carbon dioxide concentration in the blood.

General equipment shortcomings

With all carbon dioxide analyzers, water can interfere with CO$_2$ analysis and lead to errors. Therefore, it is important to prevent condensation of moisture from the patient's expired breath on the analyzer (some units have a sensor within the airway adapter that contains a heater or other means to prevent condensation).

In addition, loose connections (especially important in the sidestream analyzer) can lead to falsely low ETCO$_2$ values. Always ensure that the sidestream sampling line is securely connected to the circuit and to the water trap on the capnograph and that the water trap is firmly attached to the machine.

Specific drawbacks

When using a *colorimetric capnogram*, there are some limitations. First, the pH-sensitive paper will respond to anything that changes its pH. Therefore, contamination with things such as vomitus will alter the color of the paper and not be appropriately representative of the ETCO$_2$. A colorimetric capnogram cannot be used during chest compressions in CPR as it will not provide a level of CO$_2$. The rescuer needs a numerical quantity of CO$_2$ exhaled with each breath in order to assess the quality of the chest compressions and to determine return of spontaneous circulation (ROSC).

When using a quantitative capnogram, each method of sampling (mainstream versus sidestream) comes with its own unique set of advantages and disadvantages. Disadvantages of the mainstream analyzers include increased dead space (the analyzer is part of the breathing circuit) and sometimes mild false elevation in CO$_2$ readings secondary to accumulation of condensation inside the unit. Also, the weight of the analyzer probe may cause accidental disconnection from the anesthesia circuit, especially with a small ETT.

Disadvantages of sidestream analyzers include a time delay in the waveform (allowing for the time to suction the gas sample from the anesthesia circuit and analyze it; this is done at a fixed rate per minute).

Also, as mentioned previously, sidestream units require connection to a scavenging system in order to remove inhaled anesthetic gases. As it removes inhaled anesthetic gas from the patient, there can uncommonly be inadvertent exposure of the environment and the staff to the gas. Finally, the small sampling tubing can become obstructed with water, blood or secretions and become non-functional.

In addition, small patients (less than 7 kg) are usually connected to a non-rebreathing anesthesia system which uses a high fresh gas flow. This can result in distortion of the sidestream capnograph waveform leading to an erroneously low $ETCO_2$ reading. Several options exist to overcome this limitation. One alternative is to use the lowest possible sampling rate on your monitor. A second option is to insert a catheter or needle into the ETT (Fig. 6.14). The catheter or needle technique may result in a more normal waveform as it is less distorted by the fresh gas flow. However, when using a catheter or needle, there can be disconnection at the site of insertion into the ETT or obstruction of the catheter or needle by secretions or bending. In rare cases, the ETT may have to be discarded after use if the catheter or needle has created a leak in the tube. A third alternative is to use an airway adapter that has an inner lumen with a small diameter (Fig. 6.15). The smaller diameter of the inner lumen reduces the dead space of the adapter as it fits perfectly to the ETT connector through which the patient's gas stream will pass. This adaptor is easier to use than an additional needle or catheter and carries a minimal risk of blockage or contamination by secretions. This type of airway adaptor is commonly used in exotics.

When using microstream technology, the biggest disadvantage is the need to replace the microstream tubing every 4–8 hours per the manufacturer's

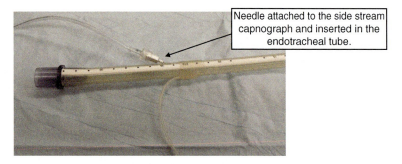

Fig. 6.14. Alternative to sampling between the endotracheal tube and the breathing system. The insertion of a needle into the endotracheal tube allows for a more accurate waveform and $ETCO_2$ value. By inserting the needle closer to the patient, it reduces dead space.

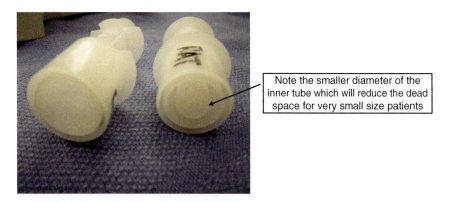

Fig. 6.15. Airway adapters for small size animals (exotics). The tube to the right has an inner lumen with a very small diameter, thus reducing the dead space significantly for small size patients. Compare to the adapter on the left side which does not have an inner tube and is commonly used for larger size dogs.

recommendations. In addition to the frequent changes, all attachments and tubing must be ordered directly from the manufacturer which can limit its availability.

6.6 Case Studies

Case study 1: The importance of close monitoring until patient is fully recovered

A 2-year-old male neutered healthy French Bulldog underwent soft palate resection, everted laryngeal sacculectomy and wedge resection of his nares. He was stable under anesthesia and was transferred to the recovery area. The nurse noticed it was taking him a very long time to wake up and she was unable to extubate him. His vital signs (heart rate, respiratory rate, systolic blood pressure, and oxygenation level via pulse oximetry (SpO_2)) were closely monitored and recorded to be within normal limits. He had received 0.1 mg/kg hydromorphone 1-hour prior.

When his $ETCO_2$ was checked it was found to be elevated (over 70 mmHg) (Fig. 6.16). The patient

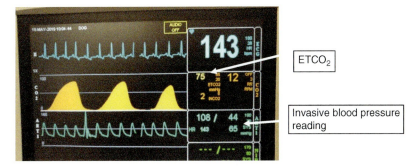

Fig. 6.16. Multiparameter monitor attached to an intubated patient recovering from anesthesia. Note the $ETCO_2$ is elevated (75 mmHg) while all other vital signs including invasive blood pressure and heart rate are within normal limits.

was manually ventilated and hydromorphone was reversed with naloxone. The patient's $ETCO_2$ improved and he was successfully extubated. Please note that elevated levels of carbon dioxide can act to make a patient continue to be anesthetized and in humans can cause drowsiness.

It is important to monitor every patient's vital signs (including $ETCO_2$, SpO_2, blood pressure, electrocardiogram, etc.) until the animal is fully recovered and able to swallow on its own.

Case study 2: The importance of serial $ETCO_2$ and $PaCO_2$ monitoring

A 13-year-old male neutered Brussels Griffon with a history of severe mitral and tricuspid valve regurgitation was recently diagnosed with a solitary lung mass in the right caudal lung lobe. A lateral right thoracotomy and a right caudal lung lobectomy were performed. The patient's PaO_2 2 hours after surgery on 4 L/min nasal oxygen was 50 mmHg. Mechanical ventilation was instituted due to severe hypoxemia. The patient's oxygenation level improved while receiving 100% oxygen supplementation and assist-controlled breathing with pressure support. The patient was closely monitored and serial readings of his $ETCO_2$, SPO_2, invasive blood pressure, and heart rate/rhythm were recorded. All his vital signs were within normal limits, including capnograph readings consistently between 45–50 mmHg. When an arterial blood gas was performed, the $PaCO_2$ was noted to be 82 mmHg. There were three possible reasons for the huge difference between the $ETCO_2$ reading and the actual $PaCO_2$ in this dog.

1. *Increased dead space*: it is possible that there were areas of the lung that were not perfused. Therefore, it is possible that the alveoli were not receiving carbon dioxide back from those areas. Alternatively, there could have been areas of the lung that were not well ventilated due to atelectasis and collapse of the airways leading to decreased gas exchange. Atelectasis is common in patients who have been in a particular position for a long period of time receiving surgery.

2. *Decreased cardiac output*: this patient has underlying heart disease and is recovering from anesthesia. Medications he received intraoperatively and postoperatively could have decreased his cardiac output and lung perfusion.

3. *Pulmonary thromboembolic event*: it is possible that this patient had a pulmonary thromboembolism postoperatively that decreased perfusion to the lungs and therefore impeded carbon dioxide delivery to the lungs. Postoperative patients, especially those with underlying diseases such as neoplasia or cardiac disease are hypercoagulable and more likely to produce blood clots.

In response to his condition, the dog's respiratory rate was increased from 20 to 28 and the $PaCO_2$ decreased to normal limits. This response to treatment made us believe the patient had poorly ventilated areas of his lungs such as occur with atelectasis, which improved with increased ventilation. An echocardiogram was also performed at this time and moderate pulmonary hypertension was present without further worsening of his cardiac function making decreased cardiac output less likely. A pulmonary thromboembolism could still not be ruled out.

This case demonstrates one of the limitations of $ETCO_2$ monitoring in anesthetized patients: the value of the displayed $ETCO_2$ informs the clinician that the $PaCO_2$ is *at least* the value of the recorded $ETCO_2$ but it is not uncommon for the blood $PaCO_2$ to be *higher* in critically ill patients. Therefore, it is very important to check the $PaCO_2$ not only when the patient's $ETCO_2$ reading is climbing but also periodically (at least every 8 to 12 hours) to ensure that the $ETCO_2$ is properly representative of the $PaCO_2$ reading even when the $ETCO_2$ remains constantly within normal limits.

7 Applications of Serial Focal Ultrasound Techniques in the Hospitalized Small Animal Patient

Danielle M. Hundley*

VCA Midwest Referral and Emergency Center, Omaha, Nebraska, USA

The use of abdominal focal assessment sonographically for trauma/triage/tracking (AFAST[3]) to document the incidence of traumatic canine hemoabdomen was first documented by Boysen *et al*. in 2004. Since this study, AFAST[3] has become a valuable resource in veterinary triage and serial monitoring in the critically ill patient. Ultrasound (US) in veterinary medicine is now used in numerous applications including but not limited to: AFAST[3], thoracic focal assessment sonographically for trauma /triage/tracking (TFAST[3]), veterinary beside lung ultrasound examination (VetBLUE), cage-side organ assessments for trauma triage and tracking (COAST[3]), US-guided vascular access, and US-based cardiac output monitoring. The purpose of this chapter is to give an overview of basic concepts and clinical applications of AFAST[3], TFAST[3], VetBLUE, and US-guided vascular access in the veterinary emergency and critical care patient for the non-radiologist veterinarian.

7.1 Ultrasound Fundamentals

Sound waves

Sound waves have variable wavelengths and amplitude with a frequency defined as the number of cycles repeated over a given time interval. The equation that describes the relationship between wavelengths and frequency is:

$$\text{wavelength (mm)} = \frac{\text{propagation speed}}{\text{frequency (MHz)}}$$

Therefore, a higher frequency results in a shorter wavelength than a lower frequency (assuming the static propagation speed [rate that sound travels through a medium in number of cycles per second (cycles/s or Hz)] remains the same). Frequencies commonly utilized in medical imaging vary between 3–12 MHz. In US imaging, the frequency of a probe determines the depth of penetration as well as the resolution/detail of the images acquired. An US probe with a higher frequency will have shorter wavelength and will thus have greater resolution/detail for tissues that are superficial and have less detail in deeper structures. An US probe with a lower frequency will have lower resolution/detail overall but will have deeper penetration because of the associated longer wavelength.

The amplitude and intensity of US waves decrease as they travel through tissue, a phenomenon known as *attenuation*. Given a fixed propagation distance, attenuation affects high-frequency US waves to a greater degree than lower frequency waves. This dictates the use of lower frequency transducers for deeper areas of interest, albeit at the expense of resolution.

Ultrasound probes are constructed of piezoelectric crystals. The exact alignment of these crystals varies based upon the function of the US probe. Commonly, during AFAST[3] assessments the US probe is a micro convex US probe, which is ideal for abdominal scanning due to its small footprint and wide scanning field.

Ultrasound images are constructed secondary to reflections of sound waves as they travel through tissues. Returning waves/echoes of the sound waves that return to the US probe cause vibration and create an electric current. The electric current, in

---

* Corresponding author: dhundley1@gmail.com

turn, generates the US images projected onto the monitor through the US machine's software.

Acoustic characteristics

A tissue's acoustic appearance is dependent upon several factors; the most important factor is the tissue's acoustic impedance. Acoustic impedance determines the level of sound wave reflection and thus the echogenicity of the tissues on the monitor. Ultrasound wave reflections are stronger at interfaces of tissues with variable acoustic impedances and weaker between tissues with similar acoustic impedances. As density of a tissue increases, the level of acoustic impedance increases. Imaging tissues with mild variation in acoustic impedance allows for examination of changes in echogenicity between tissues as well as intra-organ architecture comparison. If the difference between acoustic impedance is large (such as imaging from muscle to bone) then the US waves are reflected away and less detail is appreciated.

The ultrasound terms for describing white, gray, and black areas are hyperechoic, hypoechoic, anechoic, and isoechoic in comparison to their surrounding tissues. Hyperechoic imaging occurs when nearly all the US waves are returned to the US receiver, thus creating a bright white projection. This is often seen with bone, stone, and air. Hypoechoic imaging occurs when variable degrees of US waves are reflected to the receiver; this creates an image with varying shades of gray. Anechoic images occur when no US waves return to the receiver; this creates a pure lack of projection, shown as black. Examples of anechoic areas in the body include fluids such as urine, bile, and blood. Isoechoic images occur when tissues are the same shades of gray. Tissue echogenicity varies among organs and tissues.

Normal and abnormal tissues are described as hypoechoic and hyperechoic to their normal state or to other structures. Figure 7.1 shows the relative echogenicity of tissues and other materials. A mnemonic that the author uses to remember the order from hypoechoic to hyperechoic for core abdominal organs is 'My cat likes sunny places': My, renal medulla; cat, renal cortex; likes, liver; sunny, spleen; places, renal pelvis/prostate.

Setting the machine to obtain a diagnostic image

Control settings are utilized to regulate the intensity of echoes returning from varying depths. Echoes coming from tissue interfaces deep in the body are weakened and subsequently are darker/have less resolution due to attenuation. Echoes returning from superficial structures are higher in amplitude (better resolution) due to less attenuation than that of deeper structures. To try to maintain a uniform echogenicity of the entire organ, time-gain compensation, depth and frequency settings can be utilized to optimize an image.

The goal with US is to focus on one area of the abdomen or one organ at a time. Thus, it is important to adjust the *depth* of the image to focus on the organ of interest. Ideally the depth of the US beam should be adjusted so that the organ of interest is captured within the top three-quarters of the US viewing window.

The *frequency* should be at the highest frequency allowable to still see the deepest part of the organ of interest. Remember that the higher the frequency, the lower the penetration of the US waves. Thus, a higher frequency will have higher imaging quality for superficial structures.

The *gain* control electronically amplifies returning echoes (i.e. controls how bright the images are) and can be adjusted to create stronger echoes at all levels. Decreasing the gain results in an overall darker image. This control should be set carefully. If the gain is too high, the image is too bright and contrast resolution is decreased. If the gain is set too low, the image will be dark and information may be lost. It is tempting to set the gain too high if performing US examination in a room that is not dark enough, so always take ambient light and its effect on the screen into account when adjusting the gain.

Many newer machines (especially those utilized for bedside AFAST[3]/TFAST[3]/VetBLUE/COAST[3]) now have an image control function that will set correct gain and time-gain compensation control parameters automatically. Therefore, when using these machines for AFAST[3], TFAST[3], and VetBLUE, using standard abdominal settings and simply adjusting the depth of the image will be sufficient to obtain adequate images.

Artifacts

Ultrasound artifacts create echo signals that do not represent true tissue. Artifacts may be produced by improper equipment operation but are also inherent in ultrasound imaging techniques. Successful ultrasound interpretation depends on the ability to recognize the difference between real tissue signals and imaging artifact. Please see Table 7.1 for a description of different types of artifacts.

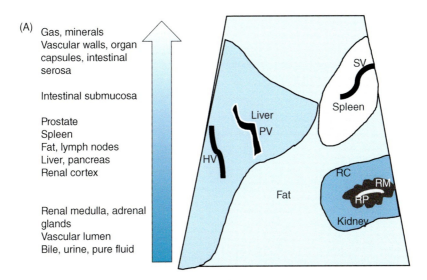

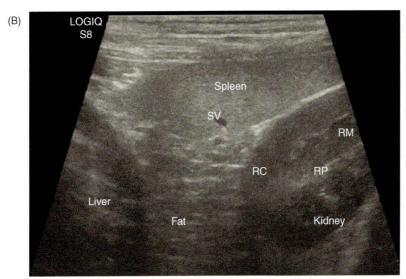

Fig. 7.1. (A) Graphic representation of variation of tissue echogenicity among organs and tissues. The appearance of structures on ultrasound varies based upon their echogenicity. This figure represents variations in echogenicity within the abdomen. The arrow shows variation in echogenicity from hypoechoic to hyperechoic (bottom to top of arrow). The structures listed to the left of the arrow are in order from hyperechoic to hypoechoic (top to bottom). The images to the right of the arrow directly compare the echogenicity differences between kidney, liver, spleen, and mesenteric fat. Within the structures labeled liver, the portal vein has thicker vascular walls than the hepatic vein, thus the portal vein walls appear more hyperechoic. (B) An US image of the spleen, kidney, liver, and mesenteric fat. HV, hepatic vein; PV, portal vein; RC, rental cortex; RM, renal medulla; RP, renal pelvis; SV, splenic vein.

7.2 How to Perform Bedside Ultrasound Examination

Ultrasound settings and patient positioning

When performing an AFAST[3], TFAST[3], and VetBLUE examination, standard abdominal settings with the ability to adjust depth is the best way to achieve adequate images. A curvilinear probe with a frequency range of 5–10 MHz is usually sufficient for most cats and dogs. When performing the AFAST[3], TFAST[3], and VetBLUE, the patient usually does not need to have any hair clipped. The transducer should achieve adequate skin contact by parting the fur and utilizing the combination of coupling gel ± alcohol. In patients that are hemodynamically unstable and could imminently arrest, the use of alcohol is discouraged as it is a fire hazard if a patient needs electrical defibrillation. Additionally, alcohol has the potential to damage some piezoelectric US transducers.

When performing bedside US-guided vascular access, the US setting should be changed to vascular imaging with the ability to adjust depth. Some machines may have a needle enhancement setting which may be helpful in seeing the needle during cannulation of vessels. Ideally a linear phase array

Table 7.1. Common ultrasound artifacts.

Artifact	Causes of artifact	How the artifact appears

Reverberation	Occurs when the ultrasound beam bounces back and forth between two highly reflective interfaces
	Occur within the tissue or between the tissue-transducer interface and another structure within the tissues
		Appear as regularly spaced echo signals NOT representative of anatomic structures:
		    Distance between each signal corresponds to distance between the two interfaces
		    Each reverberation signal weaker than the one preceding it
		Seen when imaging irregular lung surfaces, the gastrointestinal tract, and abscesses containing gas producing bacteria
		B-lines are an example in TFAST[3]
		Air artifacts during SR, HR, and CC views on AFAST[3]:
		    Air within the colon creates an air interface which US cannot pass through well
		    Results in dirty shadow within the far field

Acoustic shadowing	An absence or significant reduction of echo signal (reduced amplitude) occurring deep to a strongly reflective (i.e. gas), or absorptive (i.e. bone) interface
	Shadowing most pronounced when the structure is located within the focal zone of the transducer, high-frequency transducer is utilized
	Shadowing useful to diagnose renal and cystic calculi, other mineralized abdominal structures
		Mineralized structures present a black shadow seen distal to the structure:
		    Example: rib shadows during lung ultrasound
		Gas produces a 'dirty' or white shadow distally:
		    Example: gas within the colon during AFAST[3] (CC examination)
		    Bowel gas shadow may move with peristalsis

Refraction	Bending of the sound beam occurring on the margins of rounded organ structures. US beam strikes an object at angle other than 90° and the beam returns in a different position Sound wave deflected from its true path	Same effect as shadowing (seen as black areas distal to structure creating the artifact): Example: hypoechoic shadowing on cranial and caudal poles of a rounded mass or kidney mistaken as fluid Avoid artifact by moving US probe so beam is more perpendicular to the structure
Acoustic enhancement	Sound beam travels through tissue with no interfaces Attenuation occurs as beam passes through tissue → increases intensity of images distal to structure, creating falsely hyperechoic structure Example: fluid-filled structure (gall bladder, urinary bladder)	Beam attenuated to lesser extent as it passes through structure with no interfaces → louder/increased intensity echoes in tissue interfaces through which the beam passes Structures distal to things such as urinary bladder, gall bladder, cysts, and ascites are falsely hyperechoic; can be mistaken as hyperechoic lesion within surrounding tissues CC view during AFAST[3] predisposed to acoustic enhancement of the tissues deep to the urinary bladder

Continued

Table 7.1. Continued.

Artifact	Causes of artifact	How the artifact appears

Mirror image	Created by altered paths of reflected sound between interfaces
	Create the illusion of anatomic structures in areas where they are not actually located
	Example: highly reflective surface of the diaphragm → makes liver appear to be on both sides of the diaphragm (could be mistaken as a diaphragmatic hernia)
		DH view during AFAST[3], air-soft tissue interference between liver, diaphragm, and lungs creates mirror image
		SR view during AFAST[3] in very small dogs and cats:
		  Possible to image both kidneys in same US image
		  Can be misinterpreted as a false mirror image artifact

Slice thickness	US beam plane is near the edge of a cystic structure (e.g. gall bladder or urinary bladder), echoes are received from outside the structure due to beam's thickness. 'Filling-in' of the structure may occur → falsely simulates debris or causes a smaller cystic structure to appear solid	Simulates debris in normally anechoic structures Misrepresents a cystic structure as a solid structure Example: false mass or sludge effects within the urinary bladder Recognized by scanning in more than one plane, allowing resolution of the artifact

Side lobe	Stray echoes displaced laterally, outside the main beam, from US transducer
	Transducer is positioned over a fluid-filled structure and 'side beams' may encounter soft tissue structure outside the fluid structure:
	  US machine assumes side lobes originated from the main US beam within the fluid-filled structure
	  US machine places the echogenic signal within the fluid
		Side lobe artifact similar in appearance to slice thickness
		Creates the appearance of echogenic material within a fluid-filled structure:
		  Example: bowel gas near the gall bladder or urinary bladder creating a strong reflection confused with echogenic debris or calculi
		DH view during AFAST[3] predisposed to side lobe and edge shadowing artifacts:
		  Causes decreased clarity along luminal borders
		  Gives false appearance of sediment

AFAST[3], abdominal focal assessment sonographically for trauma/triage/tracking; CC, cystocolic; DH, diaphragmaticohepatic; HR, hepatorenal; SR, splenorenal; TFAST[3], thoracic focal assessment sonographically for trauma/triage/tracking; US, ultrasound.

probe with a minimum frequency of 7.5 MHz should be utilized as it has superior detail for superficial structures. However, a curvilinear probe with a frequency range of 5–8 MHz with an adjustable depth to less than 4 cm may also allow for sufficient imaging for vascular access. In contrast to other bedside imaging, when using an ultrasound-guided technique (UST) for vascular access, the patient needs to have fur clipped, the site should be aseptically prepared, and the US probe should be aseptically housed in a sterile cover such as a sterile glove filled with coupling gel. Alcohol can be applied to the skin to allow for contact between the skin and sterile US probe cover.

When completing the AFAST[3] and TFAST[3] examinations, a veterinary patient is typically placed in right lateral recumbency (Figs 7.2 and 7.3). This position is ideal because it allows for full assessment of the left kidney and gallbladder in nearly every examination. Right lateral is also a standard recumbency during triage for electrocardiogram assessment (see Chapter 3). Additionally, when performing abdominocentesis, right lateral recumbency minimizes the chance of mistakenly sampling the spleen by keeping it elevated and away from the more gravity-dependent free abdominal fluid.

In patients that are hemodynamically unstable or extremely stressed in lateral recumbency a modified sternal approach (Fig. 7.4) has been described for AFAST[3] and TFAST[3] (albeit not validated in veterinary medicine). In this approach, the cranial aspect of the patient is kept sternal while the caudal aspect of the patient is rotated to the desired right lateral recumbency. An AFAST[3] examination is not recommended to be performed in dorsal recumbency, primarily due to risks of exacerbating potential hemodynamic instability and respiratory compromise

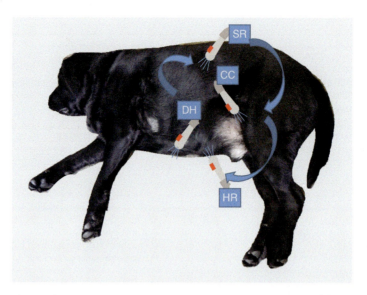

Fig. 7.2. Standard positioning for the abdominal focused assessment for trauma (AFAST[3]) examination. The AFAST[3] views are the following: diaphragmaticohepatic (DH), splenorenal (SR), cystocolic (CC), and hepatorenal (HR). The red marker on the US probe notes the direction the US transducer indicator should be placed during each examination point during the AFAST[3] examination. Often the US indicator is pointed cranially on the patient or to the operator's left as this correlates with the left-hand side of most US monitors..

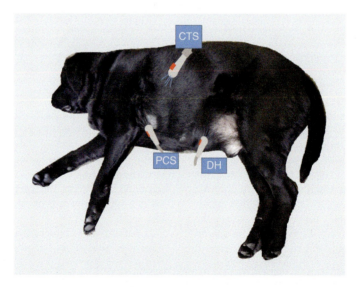

Fig. 7.3. TFAST[3] five-point protocol. The TFAST[3] is typically performed in right lateral recumbency in stable patients. In those that are dyspneic and intolerant of lateral recumbency, a modified sternal or standing approach has also been described. The TFAST[3] views consist of the left and right pericardial site (PCS) views, right and left chest tube site (CTS) and the diaphragmaticohepatic (DH) view. The red marker on the ultrasound (US) probe notes the direction the US transducer indicator should be placed during each examination point in the TFAST[3] examination

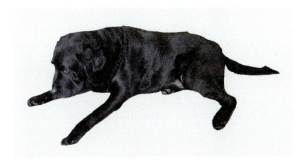

Fig. 7.4. Modified sternal recumbency for FAST scanning. In patients that are dyspneic or too stressed to be in right lateral recumbency, a modified sternal recumbency has been described to perform AFAST[3] and TFAST[3] procedures. In this recumbency, the thorax and forelimbs are in sternal recumbency while the hindlimbs are shifted into right lateral recumbency. This position hopefully allows the patient to be less stressed and allows for possible larger tidal volumes in respiratory compromised patients.

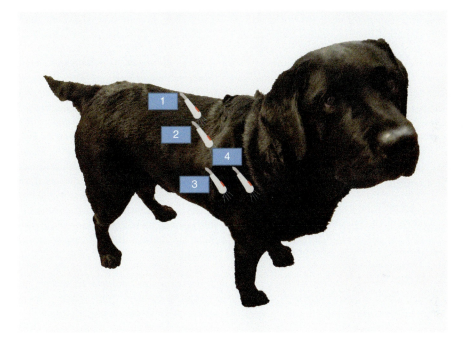

Fig. 7.5. VetBLUE protocol. The regions evaluated during the VetBLUE protocol are the following: (1) caudodorsal lung lobe region; (2) perihilar lung lobe region; (3) middle lung lobe region; and (4) cranial lung lobe region. All four regions are assessed on both the left and right hemithorax. The caudodorsal lung lobe is at the level of approximately the TFAST[3] CTS of the left hemithorax (directly dorsal to the xiphoid within the upper one third of the thorax at approximately the eighth to ninth intercostal space). The perihilar lung lobe region is a point within the central one third of the thorax between intercostal spaces six and seven. The middle lung lobe region is a point within the lower one-third of the thorax over the heart at the level of the fourth and fifth intercostal spaces. The cranial lung lobe region is a point within the ventral one third of the thorax cranial to the heart at approximately intercostal spaces two and three. Often the patient's thoracic limb needs to be extended cranially to achieve this view. The operator should repeat all four sites on the opposing thorax side to complete the VetBLUE protocol. For each site, the US operator can assess for the presence of A-lines with glide sign, B-lines, shred sign, tissue sign, nodule sign, and presence of pleural effusion. See text for more detail on these signs.

in trauma patients. Additionally, this position has not been validated for AFAST[3] examinations in the veterinary patient at this time.

When completing the VetBLUE protocol for lung ultrasound, the patient is typically placed in sternal recumbency or standing (Fig. 7.5). Dorsal recumbency is not recommended as many patients that are in respiratory distress are hemodynamically unstable and being placed into dorsal recumbency may be overly stressful and lead to possible decompensation of the patient.

If possible, fluid found on AFAST[3], TFAST[3], or VetBLUE should be sampled via US-guided centesis to further characterize the type of effusion. The fluid should be sampled because visualization of fluid alone cannot accurately characterize the type of fluid. If unable to safely sample scant amounts of effusion, a reassessment FAST[3] should be performed after fluid resuscitation. Any samples obtained should ideally be saved for culture, biochemical testing, and cytology. The details of abdominal and thoracic fluid analysis methods are beyond the scope of this chapter and the reader is referred to the Further Reading section for more information.

For ultrasound-guided jugular venous catheterization/blood sampling, the patient is typically placed in lateral recumbency but dorsal recumbency in stable animals has also been described. As mentioned above, dorsal recumbency is not recommended in hemodynamically compromised patients. If other vessels are being catheterized/sampled, whatever recumbency and style of restraint required for access to that vessel is acceptable.

The AFAST[3] examination

With the patient in right lateral recumbency, perform the examination in a clockwise order starting at the cranial aspect of the patient (Fig. 7.2). The AFAST[3] views are the following: diaphragmaticohepatic (DH), splenorenal (SR), cystocolic (CC), and hepatorenal (HR).

Diaphragmaticohepatic view

The DH view is used to survey for fluid around the liver and diaphragm as well as to evaluate the pleural and pericardial spaces. This is one of the places where fluid often accumulates first.

The DH view is obtained in the following way:

1. Utilizing the curvilinear probe, place the probe longitudinally (US indicator/notch pointed cranially) at the base of the patient's xiphoid process. The depth should be adjusted to visualize the liver, gall bladder, and diaphragm. The gall bladder can be assessed for contents and wall appearance, and the lobes of the liver and diaphragm can be evaluated for free fluid accumulation between them. Care should be made to not mistake the gall bladder for free fluid. The best way to do this is to move the US probe (i.e. 'fan' it) to see all sides of the gall bladder and look for the biliary tree extending out of the gall bladder.

A halo sign surrounding the gall bladder (gall bladder wall thickens and appears striated with alternating echogenicity – hypoechoic and then hyperechoic) is sometimes noted. This occurs with pericardial effusion, severe hypoalbuminemia, cholangiohepatitis, pancreatitis, right-sided heart failure, and canine anaphylaxis.

2. The US probe is then fanned to the left and right to evaluate other liver lobes. Always keep the diaphragm in view to look for effusion between the liver lobes and diaphragm. Make attempts to avoid the stomach during this component of the examination to help prevent edge shadowing artifact.

3. Move the US probe so the beam is directed cranially through the diaphragm into the thorax and increase the depth to extend the viewing window into the pericardial and pleural spaces to assess for fluid. This should be attempted in all patients but can prove challenging, especially in large breed patients, as the distance may exceed the maximum imaging window of the US. Viewing the pericardial and pleural spaces through this acoustic vantage point allows for less air artifact. In some veterinary patients, imaging of the heart through this view can be challenging because the heart may not lie on the diaphragm like it does in people. When this occurs, there can be an air interface between the diaphragm and the heart which can obscure imaging.

When suspicious of or differentiating between pericardial and pleural effusion, the operator should utilize at least one more additional TFAST[3] view, such as the pericardial sites (see TFAST[3] section below), to confirm the presence of pericardial or pleural effusion. If pericardial effusion is suspected, the operator should also use multiple TFAST[3] views to differentiate pericardial effusion from a dilated heart chamber to avoid a potentially life-threatening misinterpretation.

Lisciandro *et al.* in 2012 showed that nearly 88% of pericardial effusions were detected by the DH view and used the term 'race-track sign' to portray the presence of pericardial effusion. The race-track sign describes the smooth visible borders created by the pericardial sac and border of the myocardium that delineates the pericardial fluid within the pericardial sac. In contrast, pleural effusion has more irregular borders.

The DH view into the thorax can allow for evaluation of the presence or lack of the 'glide sign' (which will be discussed in more depth with the

TFAST³ below). Lack of the glide sign can increase suspicion for the presence of a pneumothorax. The DH view can also be used to assess for US B-lines (previously called lung rockets or comet tails; see TFAST³ section).

4. Finally, for an advanced DH view assessment, the probe should be fanned dorsocaudally away from the gall bladder toward the great vessels. Here an advanced operator may be able to estimate intravascular fluid volumes. This component to the AFAST³ examination is beyond the scope of this chapter (see Further Reading section).

Splenorenal view

The SR view surveys for free fluid around the spleen, left kidney, and retroperitoneal and peritoneal spaces. Classically, free fluid found in this view is between the spleen and colon; other structures should be evaluated as detailed below.

Obtain the SR view in the following way:

1. With the patient in right lateral recumbency, place the curvilinear US probe longitudinally (US marker placed cranially toward the patient's head), parallel to the spine, just caudal to the last rib (at the costal arch), and fan the probe cranially under the rib. In order to distinguish loops of fluid-filled bowel/colon or a fluid-filled gravid uterus from free fluid, evaluate the structure in both longitudinal and transverse planes. To image in transverse, slowly rotate the US probe 90 degrees so that the notch is facing the patient's right-hand side (i.e. moving to the AFAST³ operator's left).
2. Return the probe to the start position, direct it caudally, and then fan from side to side. While fanning back and forth, the AFAST³ operator can evaluate the retroperitoneal space. Free fluid within the retroperitoneal space should raise concern for differentials such as ongoing hemorrhage, sterile and nonsterile effusions, and uroabdomen.

Cystocolic view

The CC view surveys for free fluid around the urinary bladder and body wall. Despite the colic component of the name, the colon wall is the only thing that can be imaged as the gas present in the colon will create artifact obscuring the remainder of the colon. Therefore, most of the imaging for the CC view is focused around the urinary bladder. In very young puppies and kittens a small amount of free fluid in this view has been described as a normal finding but other fluid accumulations are considered pathologic.

Obtain the CC view the following way:

1. Place the curvilinear US probe longitudinally (US indicator/notch pointed cranially toward the patient's head) just cranial to where the flank meets the body wall.
2. Direct the probe toward the gravity-dependent region – a pocket made up of the urinary bladder, colon, and the body wall. A classic finding with free fluid is an anechoic triangle between the urinary bladder and abdominal body wall. The CC view has multiple chances for artifacts that should be kept in mind. Fluid within the urinary bladder will create an acoustic enhancement artifact, causing soft tissues visible deep to the urinary bladder to appear more hyperechoic than normal. Additionally, a gas-filled colon may create reverberation and shadowing artifacts that may obscure tissues deep to the colon. The operator can sometimes alleviate some of the artifact by manipulating the colon out of view by gentle alterations of pressure and slight position changing of the US probe.

Hepatorenal view

The HR view surveys for free fluid along the most gravity-dependent area of the AFAST³ examination. Despite being named the hepato-renal view, it is not normal to visualize the liver or the right kidney during this component of the AFAST³ assessment. The liver is only seen in this view when there is significant hepatomegaly. The right kidney is not actively imaged unless trauma is suspected to the right kidney. In situations where it is important to view the right kidney, the patient is moved into left lateral or sternal recumbency to facilitate imaging.

Obtain the HR view the following way:

1. Place the probe longitudinally (the notch/indicator facing cranially toward the patient's head) just below/right lateral to the umbilicus with the animal in right lateral recumbency. Often loops of bowel and occasionally the spleen are seen with this view. To help differentiate free fluid from loops of bowel, image the structures in both longitudinal and transverse US planes. To image in transverse, rotate the US probe slowly 90° so that the notch is facing the

patient's ventrum or toward to the AFAST[3] operator's left-hand side.

2. Direct the US probe toward the table into the gravity-dependent area of the scan. Look for fluid accumulation in this region. In some cases, the US probe can be used to gently direct the loops of bowel out of the field of view.

3. If trauma to the right kidney is suspected, roll the patient slightly dorsal (dorsolateral positioning) to allow the probe to be placed under the patient in order to visualize the right kidney and retroperitoneal space. Larger patients may need to be placed in left lateral recumbency to image the right kidney. This view can also be obtained with the patient in sternal recumbency in hemodynamically compromised patients. This view is not obtained in a typical AFAST[3].

Abdominal fluid scoring system

The abdominal fluid score (AFS) has been utilized clinically to survey for development or resolution of a hemoabdomen, ongoing hemorrhage, and worsening volumes of free fluid. The scoring system consists of a numeric grading system (0–4). For each quadrant surveyed during an AFAST[3] examination containing fluid, a score of 1 is added to the AFS. It is recommended to record results on a standardized template to allow continuity of communication of findings between veterinarians and serial screenings. A template also promotes completion of a full examination. See Further Reading section for examples of such templates.

The TFAST[3] examination

The examination is performed starting on the left-hand side and continuing to the right-hand side (Fig. 7.3). The TFAST[3] views consist of the left and right pericardial site (PCS) views, right and left chest tube sites (CTS), and the DH view. These views are outlined in Fig. 7.3.

Chest tube site view

The CTS view has been used predominately to diagnose the presence or absence of a pneumothorax, but can also be used clinically to assess for US B-line artifacts (previously known as lung rockets/comet tails/ring-down) and the step, shred, and node signs (Fig. 7.6).

The CTS is performed via the following steps.

1. The transducer is placed on the chest wall at the highest point of the thorax in right lateral recumbency (approximately the dorsal third of the thorax, at the level of approximately the eight to ninth intercostal spaces in normal chested dogs and cats and seventh to eighth intercostal space in barrel chested or brachycephalic breeds). This point is usually aligned with and dorsal to the xiphoid process. The indicator notch of the transducer should be facing cranially (toward the patient's head). Theoretically, when there is a pneumothorax, this region will accumulate air since this is the highest point (least gravity-dependent) portion of the chest. The operator should ensure that the diaphragm and liver are out of the field of view, as the presence of these structures in the CTS view may interfere with imaging and create a false positive step sign. In brachycephalic patients or those with an intra-abdominal mass that is pushing the diaphragm forward, it may be necessary to move up one intercostal space.

2. Next, the operator should attempt to isolate the 'bat/gator sign.' This sign consists of the two rib heads that appear as hypoechoic shadowing artifact and the interposed intercostal space (Fig. 7.6A).

Once the gator sign is isolated, the observer must look for the presence of the 'glide sign.' The glide sign (also called lung slide in human TFAST[3]) is created by movement of the pulmonary–pleural line cranially and caudally along the thoracic wall as the patient inspires and expires. The PPL appears as a bright hyperechoic line. If the glide sign is present, then a pneumothorax at that chest level is unlikely. Shallow and rapid breathing may make observing the glide sign more difficult and could possibly result in a false diagnosis of a pneumothorax.

There should be visible air reverberation artifact within the lung creating parallel A-lines (Fig. 7.6A). These A-lines do not typically move. The US transducer may need to be moved horizontally and pivoted dorsally or ventrally to achieve an oblique image to more accurately obtain the glide sign.

3. Assess for B-lines. Ultrasound B-lines are also referred to as US lung rockets. They are created when fluid is immediately next to air within the peripheral lung parenchyma, specifically the outer 1-3mm. The B-lines appear as hyperechoic streaks that run parallel to the rib space; they may oscillate back and forth with respiration and will obliterate the perpendicular A-lines (Fig. 7.6B). It is normal to have 1-2 B-lines

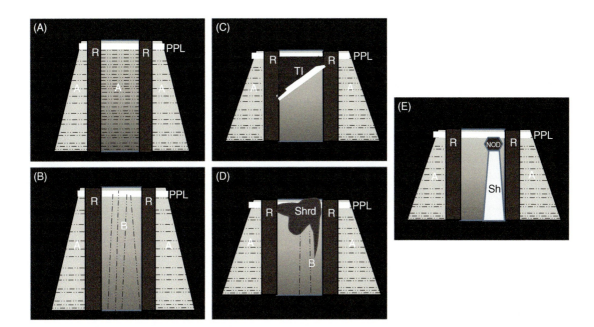

Fig. 7.6. Lung ultrasound findings at the chest tube site. (A) Normal dry lung with the gator and glide sign: The gator/bat sign consists of the two rib heads (R) that appear as hypoechoic shadowing artifacts connected via the intercostal space. The ribs appear as the gator's eyes and the intercostal space is the bridge of the gators nose. Once the gator sign is isolated, the observer must look for the presence of the 'glide sign.' The glide sign is the observation of the pulmonary–pleural line (PPL) moving cranially and caudally along the thoracic wall as the patient inspires and expires. The pulmonary–pleural line on US appears as a bright hyperechoic line. The aeration of normal dry lung air creates reverberation artifact which appears as parallel lines extending beyond the PPL termed A-lines (A). (B) Ultrasound B-lines (wet lung); are also referred to as US lung rockets. They are created when fluid is immediately next to air within the peripheral lung parenchyma, specifically the outer 1–3 mm. The B-lines appear as hyperechoic streaks that run parallel to the rib space shadowing. They may oscillate back and forth with respiration and will obliterate the perpendicular A-lines. It is normal to have one or two B-lines per lung field due to changes in density of aerated lung. More than three B-lines is consistent with interstitial edema or a 'wet' lung. Pattern distribution, additional TFAST view evaluation, clinical picture, and corresponding radiographs can help differentiate between pneumonia, non-cardiogenic pulmonary edema, and cardiogenic pulmonary edema. (C) Step/tissue sign (complete lung consolidation). The step sign is used to describe a discontinuity in the pulmonary–pleural line during TFAST[3] evaluation, usually associated with thoracic wall or pleural space disease and/or lung consolidation without aeration (TI). The tissue sign due to lack of aerated lung has also been described as a 'hepatized' or liver-like appearance. Conditions associated with the step sign include rib fractures, pulmonary masses, pleural effusion, diaphragmatic hernia, mediastinal masses and, at times, severe left-sided cardiomegaly. The tissue sign is similar to the shred sign without aerated lung appreciated; peripheral lung tissue is consolidated making it appear hepatized. (D) Shred sign (dense but not complete lung consolidation). The shred sign occurs when there is a deviation from the expected continuity of the PPL by the presence of hypoechoic, echo-poor tissue (Shrd). This hypoechoic tissue is caused by peripheral lung tissue consolidation. This sign is differentiated from step/tissue sign by the fact that there is not complete consolidation of the peripheral lung tissues. Thus, hyperechoic B-lines (B) consistent with areas of aerated lung adjacent to the consolidated areas still appear. (E) Nodule sign (mass effect). The nodule sign (Nod) appears within the peripheral lung tissue as a focal well marginated hypoechoic structure surrounded by deeper aerated lung. In dry lung with a nodule, attenuation artifact creates a hyperechoic shadow deep to the nodule as depicted by Sh in the image. The nodule sign is only appreciated if the structure is present within peripheral lung. Deeper pulmonary masses may not be appreciated without additional imaging.

per lung field as normal reverberation artifact from changes in density of aerated lung. When multiple B-lines are visualized in the lung (> 3), this is consistent with increased lung density secondary to a loss of aeration in the lung periphery. This typically occurs with interstitial pulmonary infiltrates (contusions, cardiogenic pulmonary edema, non-cardiogenic pulmonary edema, or pneumonia).

4. Assess for the step sign. The step sign is used to describe a discontinuity in the pulmonary–pleural line, usually associated with a thoracic wall or pleural space discontinuity (Fig. 7.6C). Conditions that lead to the step sign include rib fractures, pulmonary masses, pleural effusion, a diaphragmatic hernia, a mediastinal mass, and potentially left-sided cardiomegaly. The presence of a step sign warrants additional imaging such as thoracic radiography. Do not look for the step sign caudal to the CTS as the normal lung-diaphragm-liver interface can create what looks like a step sign.

5. Repeat steps 1-4 on the right hemithorax.

Pericardial sites

The pericardial sites (PCS) are used to look for pericardial effusion and, with training, can be utilized to assess left-sided heart volume status and systolic contractility. Both left and right PCS should be assessed during a TFAST[3] examination.

The PCS exam is performed as follows:

1. The TFAST[3] operator should palpate the heart's point of maximum intensity and place the probe at that site. If the point of maximum intensity cannot be identified, place the transducer probe on the contralateral gravity-dependent side between intercostal spaces three through five (Fig. 7.3). When trying to find the location of the heart quickly, the author moves the elbow to the level of the costochondral junction and puts the transducer probe at this location. Place the US probe with the indicator/notch facing dorsally toward the spine. Slide the transducer slightly dorsally and adjust the depth of the transducer to focus the heart within the distal/bottom third of the US viewing window. Fan the probe slightly to obtain both a four-chamber (Fig. 7.7A) and five-chamber view (right parasternal long-axis view) of the heart while evaluating for pericardial effusion. The chamber sizes can also be subjectively observed in this view. In health, the left ventricle should be approximately three to four times the size of the right ventricle, the atria should be symmetrical, and the interventricular septum should be straight. See Further Reading section for more information on focused echocardiogram assessment.

2. Rotate the transducer until the indicator/notch is perpendicular to the elbow. This should reveal the transverse (right parasternal short axis) view of the heart. When at the level of the mitral valve, this view will reveal the classic 'mushroom view'. At this level the TFAST[3] operator can subjectively assess contractility of the ventricle while also looking for pericardial effusion. With advanced training the operator can also measure ventricular volumes at the end of systole and diastole, measure left ventricular wall thickness, and calculate fractional shortening. The details of measuring and performing these calculations is beyond the scope of this chapter. See Further Reading section for detail regarding focused echocardiogram assessment.

3. The operator can assess the left atrium:aorta (LA:Ao) ratio. The LA:Ao ratio is performed to gauge suspicion for left-sided heart failure in the dyspneic patient. The LA:Ao ratio is performed using the US transducer probe with the indicator/notch facing toward the elbow. Typically, the probe is moved up one intercostal space or lightly fanned cranially to obtain a right parasternal apical transverse (short axis) view of the heart base. In this view the US TFAST[3] operator should be able to see the aorta, left atrium and right ventricular outflow tract/pulmonary artery (Fig. 7.7B). The aorta at the level of the aortic valve will appear as the classic 'Mercedes Benz' view. At this level, the operator can assess the LA:Ao ratio by measuring the diameter of the chambers. An LA:Ao ratio < 1.5 is normal. Typically cats with heart failure have significantly increased LA:Ao ratios of >2.0.

Diaphragmaticohepatic view

The DH view is the final site to assess for pleural and pericardial effusion during a TFAST[3] (see Fig. 7.3). This view allows imaging of the pleural and pericardial sites with less air interference and can evaluate the diaphragm for herniation. See the previous AFAST[3] section of this chapter for a description on how to acquire images in this view. When an animal is in respiratory distress, pressing the US probe into the DH site may be uncomfortable or stressful. Moving the US transducer probe from the subxiphoid location to a location slightly pericostally will allow for easier breathing while still obtaining the same information.

Other information obtained during TFAST[3]

LUNG POINT (PNEUMOTHORAX) If present, the severity of a pneumothorax is gauged by determining the lung point. The lung point is the position along

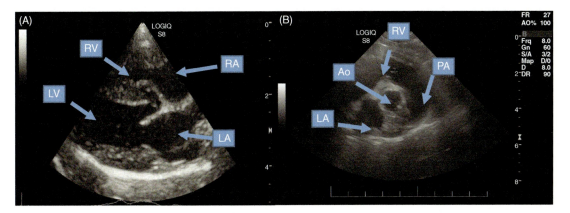

Fig. 7.7. Ultrasound views of the heart. Cranial is toward the left-hand side of the image in both figures. (A) Four-chamber right parasternal long-axis view. The four-chamber view is obtained with the US probe pointed toward the spine within intercostal spaces three to five. Once in focus, the operator can subjectively compare chamber sizes while looking for pericardial effusion. In health, the left ventricle (LV) should be approximately three to four times the size of the right ventricle (RV), the atria (LA and RA) should be symmetrical in size, and the interventricular septum should be straight. In conjunction with a comparison of chamber sizes, physical examination findings and radiographic changes can increase or decrease clinical suspicion for underlying heart disease. (B) LA:Ao ratio. Right parasternal basilar short axis view. In this view, the operator can identify the left atrium (LA), aorta (Ao), pulmonary artery (PA) and right ventricular outflow tract (RV). This view is obtained by pointing the transducer toward the patient's elbow and moving cranially one rib space from the four-chamber right parasternal long-axis view. The operator can assess for the left atrium:aortic (LA:Ao) ratio. The LA:Ao ratio is performed to assist in assessing for suspicion for left-sided heart failure in the dyspneic patient.

the thorax where the glide sign or the presence of B-lines is resumed. The lung point is found by sliding the US transducer ventrally along the thorax; the point at which the lung resumes contact with the chest wall and the glide sign resumes is the lung point (Fig. 7.8).

If the lung point is present in the dorsal one-third of the thorax (point 1 in Fig. 7.8), there is a mild pneumothorax. If the lung point is associated with the middle one-third of the thorax (point 2 in Fig. 7.8), then there is a moderate pneumothorax. If the lung point is present in the ventral one-third of the thorax (point 3 in Fig. 7.8) or is nonexistent, this suggests a massive pneumothorax. The location of the lung point can be used to determine/characterize severity of a pneumothorax at time of triage as well as tracking pneumothorax serially in the hospitalized patient. In addition, determination of the lung point can be used to gage presence or worsening of a pneumothorax after invasive procedures such as thoracocentesis, lung aspirates, or thoracotomy.

CARDIAC TAMPONADE (PERICARDIAL EFFUSION) If pericardial effusion is discovered at either the DH or PCS sites, it is important to evaluate for concurrent cardiac tamponade. Cardiac tamponade occurs when the pericardium is filled with fluid to the point that the intrapericardial pressure exceeds the filling pressure of the right atrium and, in severe cases, the right ventricle. When the filling pressures are exceeded, the heart chambers collapse and cannot fill. This leads to decreased cardiac output and hypovolemic shock. During an US, cardiac tamponade is represented by inward collapse of the right atrium ± the right ventricle with wall fluctuations between systole and diastole. Seeing cardiac tamponade indicates the need for immediate pericardiocentesis in the hemodynamically compromised patient.

VETBLUE The VetBLUE protocol consists of evaluating four different views on each hemithorax (caudodorsal lung lobe region, perihilar lung lobe region, middle lung lobe region, and the cranial lung lobe region; see Fig. 7.5) just as with TFAST[3], and evaluating for the presence of B-lines, glide signs with A-lines, and the presence of shred, tissue, or nodule signs (Fig. 7.6). Interpretation of each finding is the same as with TFAST[3]. It is designed to evaluate only the lungs.

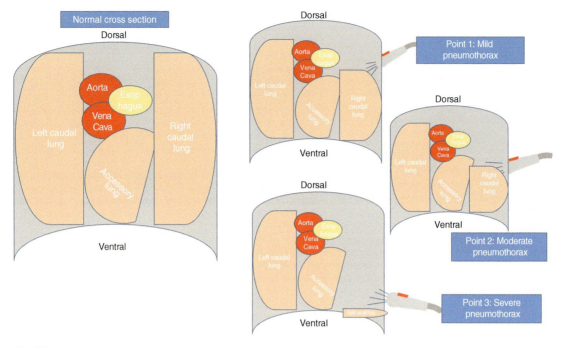

Fig. 7.8. Pneumothorax severity determined through the lung point. This diagram depicts a cross section of a patient at the level of the 8th rib space. In a normal lung, the operator should be able to see the glide sign when imaging the lung from dorsal to ventral. With pneumothorax, we are unable to see the glide sign because the lung is displaced from the chest wall. The severity of the pneumothorax can be determined via determining the lung point. The lung point is the point at which the lung resumes contact with the chest wall and the glide sign resumes. The lung point is located by sliding the US transducer dorsally to ventrally along the thorax while maintaining the gator sign (see Fig. 7.6). The right-hand side of the figure depicts three areas of lung point determination and the associated severity of the pneumothorax (see the text for details).

The VetBLUE examination

1. With the patient in standing or sternal recumbency, the US probe is placed with the probe notch/indicator facing toward the patient's head at the level of approximately the TFAST[3] CTS (directly dorsal to the xiphoid within the upper one-third of the thorax at approximately the eighth to ninth intercostal space). This is the caudodorsal lung lobe region (point 1 in Fig. 7.5). The focus point of the US transducer should be adjusted to the level of the hyperechoic pulmonary–pleural line (approximately 4–6 cm in depth) to allow evaluation for A-lines with a glide sign, B-lines, or changes such as the shred or nodule signs. Pleural effusion can also be identified. If B-lines are seen the operator can semi-quantify them as 1, 2, 3, or >3 before moving onto the next site. The US operator should ensure that the probe is not placed too far caudally as imaging caudal to the diaphragm may result in a false tissue sign by inadvertently imaging the patient's liver.

2. The above assessment is repeated at each of the other sites on both left and right hemithorax. The left perihilar lung lobe region is found within the central one-third of the thorax between intercostal spaces six and seven (point 2 in Fig. 7.5). The left middle lung lobe region is located specifically in the lower one-third of the thorax over the heart at the level of the fourth and fifth intercostal spaces (point 3 in Fig. 7.5). The left cranial lung lobe region is found by placing the probe in the ventral one-third of the thorax cranial to the heart at approximately intercostal spaces two and three (point 4 in Fig. 7.5); often the patient's thoracic limb is extended cranially to achieve this view.

3. After completing the four views on the left hemithorax, the US operator should repeat steps on the right hemithorax.

Findings of the VetBLUE should be recorded in a standard fashion for comparison between operators and serially over time within one animal. The developers of the VetBLUE have a specific recording protocol (see Further Reading section for more information).

Ultrasound-guided vascular access

In the human literature, there have been descriptions of both dynamic real-time and static UST for vascular access. The static technique uses the linear US probe to isolate the area of the vascular structure prior to performing a blind venipuncture. The dynamic technique uses the US to guide the needle into the vessel in real time. Human medicine describes the use of a needle guide, but veterinary reports largely use a freehand technique for both arterial and venous vascular access. For the purpose of this chapter, we will discuss the dynamic real-time freehand approach.

The US-guided vascular access examination

1. The desired vascular access location is aseptically clipped and cleaned as detailed above, the entire technique is performed sterilely.
2. If attempting central venous catheter placement within a large vein, an assistant distends the vein by applying digital pressure proximal to the point of imaging and catheter insertion. If imaging for arterial catheter access (femoral artery), the area of the desired artery is explored with the US without the need for digital occlusion.
3. The US probe should be manipulated with the operator's non-dominant hand while imaging the desired vessel in either the transverse or longitudinal

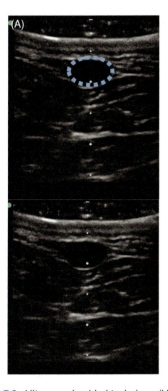
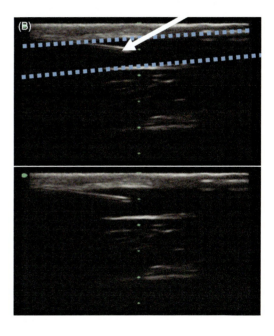

Fig. 7.9. Ultrasound-guided technique (UST) for vascular access (A) transverse and (B) longitudinal approaches. In each image the dot along the left upper edge of the image indicates either left or cranial/distal when the introducer notch is pointed toward the point of insertion. The top images for both (A) and (B) have the hyperechoic vessel walls outlined with blue dotted lines and the images below have no additional markings. In (B) there is an introducer catheter within the anechoic lumen of the vessel (indicated by the white arrow). The introducer catheter is the hyperechoic structure passing through the dorsal vascular wall into the anechoic vessel lumen. When imaged in transverse, the vessels appear as anechoic circles (A). When imaged in a longitudinal plane (B), the vessels are denoted by parallel lines (hyperechoic vessel walls) surrounding the anechoic vascular lumen, similar to an equals sign.

Table 7.2. A comparison of the transverse and longitudinal techniques for ultrasound-guided vascular access.

	Transverse plane	Longitudinal plane
Vessel identification	Easier to identify vessel	Due to limited beam footprint, harder to align US beam with vasculature
	Vessels appear as anechoic circular structures	Vessels appear as anechoic stripes with hyperechoic walls (similar to an equal sign)
	Veins may collapse with pressure	Veins will easily collapse with pressure
	Arteries may have visible pulsation of blood	Arteries may have visible blood pulsation
	Arteries are more difficult to collapse	Arteries are more difficult to collapse
Needle identification	Appears as hyperechoic dot	Appears as hyperechoic tube
	Needle makes a bullseye sign when inside the vessel lumen	Easy to see needle profile within the vessel (hyperechoic tube within the vessel)
	Can be hard to judge depth of needle until inside vessel	Easy to judge depth of needle insertion
	Relatively easy to keep needle and vessel in same plane	Hard to keep needle in plane with vessel
Learning curve	Larger probe footprint	Smaller probe footprint
	Easier to stay in plane with vessel	Harder to stay in plane with vessel
	Considered easier to learn	Considered more technically challenging for novice
Depth of structures	Harder to adjust depth in real time	Easy to adjust depth of approach in real time
	Easier to utilize in deeper structures such as when there is neck pathology (edema, cellulitis, hematomas)	Easier to utilize for superficial structures and use when normal neck anatomy
	Harder to use when neck anatomy normal (structures too superficial)	Easier to use when neck anatomy is normal

US, ultrasound.

plane. To image the desired vessel, the operator should place the US probe with the notch/indicator pointed distally toward the point of catheter insertion. When imaged in transverse the vessels appear as anechoic circles (Fig. 7.9A). When in imaged in a longitudinal plane, the vessels appear as parallel lines (similar to an equal sign) made up of the hyperechoic vessel walls and anechoic vascular lumen (Fig. 7.9B). To differentiate between vein and artery, the operator may look for pulsation of the vessel (consistent with being an artery). The operator may also observe that a vein will more easily collapse with pressure applied to it than an artery.

4. Once the vessel is identified, the operator determines if he would like to catheterize in a transverse or longitudinal plane. See Table 7.2 for the pros and cons of each approach and below for a description.

For *transverse orientation* venipuncture, the operator should alter the image depth and focus so that the vessel is in the center of the US screen and appears as an anechoic circle (Fig. 7.9A). The needle or introducer catheter should be held with the dominant hand and introduced through the skin 1–2 cm rostral to the US probe and perpendicular to the indicator/notch on the linear transducer. The angle that the needle or introducer catheter should be inserted into the skin is dependent upon the depth of the vessel and distance of insertion rostral to the US transducer probe (for arterial catheterizations, the operator may need a steeper angle of approach than a vein).

Once the needle or introducer catheter are inserted into the skin, the US probe can be moved slightly rostrally to see the hyperechoic needle as it inserts into the anechoic vessel. Seeing the hyperechoic tip of the needle within the anechoic vessel has been described as a 'bullseye effect' in the human literature. Once this bullseye effect is appreciated, the operator may cannulate the vessel or collect the blood sample.

For *longitudinal orientation* venipuncture, the operator should start by identifying and focusing on the image of the vessel in transverse orientation. Then, the US probe is rotated 90° so that the vessel appears as an anechoic to hypoechoic tract across the screen with the probe indicator/notch facing rostrally. The needle or introducer catheter should be held within the dominant hand and placed through the skin 1–2 cm rostral to the US probe and perpendicular to the indicator/notice on the transducer. The angle that the needle or introducer catheter should be inserted into the skin is dependent upon the depth of the vessel and distance of insertion rostral to the US probe.

Once the needle or introducer catheter is inserted into the skin, the US probe is moved slightly rostrally to visualize the hyperechoic needle as it inserts into the vessel through the dorsal vessel wall (Fig. 7.9B). The vessel wall may bow inward or roll away from the US view. If this occurs, the operator should slightly withdraw the needle or introducer catheter and optimize the image of the vessel before trying again. When the vessel has been successfully penetrated, the bowing of the vessel should resolve and a flash of blood into the catheter or needle should be seen.

5. If the operator is using the UST for vascular access to achieve a central venous catheter, once vascular penetration has been confirmed, the modified Seldinger technique (guidewire-based technique) can be performed for either approach. The US can be used to identify if a guidewire is feeding into the vessel appropriately during that step of the Seldinger technique. See Further Reading section for a more detailed description of the modified Seldinger technique.

7.3 Indications for Ultrasound Evaluation

AFAST[3]/Abdominal Fluid Score

Since its first description in veterinary medicine in 2004 and validation in 2009, AFAST[3] has multiple applications (Table 7.3). It has been shown to be superior to physical examination alone and more sensitive than abdominal radiographs for small amounts of effusion (up to 24% of patients with normal abdominal radiographs have been shown to have fluid present on AFAST[3] examination).

The abdominal fluid score (AFS) has been developed to predict the severity of anemia in the traumatic hemoabdomen by differentiating between a small and large bleeding event. The same AFS system has also been applied in postoperative hemorrhage serial monitoring. The AFS allows for semi-quantification of the degree of hemorrhage for comparison at different time points and may allow veterinarians to predict the future need for blood products. This scoring system has been validated in cases of trauma in dogs but is not predictive for anemia and transfusion requirements in cats.

An AFS of 1–2 is associated with small amounts of bleeding, and an AFS of 3–4 is associated with larger bleeding events. In dogs, higher AFS scores in trauma cases are associated with development of anemia, a higher need for blood transfusions, and, rarely, a requirement for surgical intervention. In trauma patients, the AFS can also help a practitioner to determine sources of blood loss. For example, if a patient without a pre-existing anemia that has a static traumatic AFS of only 1–2 develops anemia in the hospital, a clinician should look for other sources of ongoing hemorrhage including, but not limited to, the pericardial space, pleural space, pulmonary parenchyma, and fracture sites.

Clinically, the AFS has been also utilized for scoring the accumulation of other non-traumatic abdominal effusions. If the effusion amount is increasing, it indicates a need for further diagnostic or therapeutic interventions. These effusions include non-traumatic bleeding (ruptured masses, coagulopathies, and post interventional hemorrhage), urine, septic effusion, and non-septic effusion. The AFAST[3] can be more sensitive in detecting hemorrhage than serial packed cell volume/total solids (PCV/TS), physical examination findings, and radiographs since there is a great ability to compensate for blood loss. Humans with ongoing blood loss have been noted to compensate with normal vital parameters until nearly 30% total blood loss has occurred.

TFAST[3]/VetBLUE

Use of TFAST[3] in veterinary medicine was first documented in 2008 for detection of pneumothorax (Lisciandro, 2008) in trauma patients. This study found that US by an experienced operator had a sensitivity of 95% for detecting pneumothorax. Since then, the TFAST[3] has been utilized to evaluate the intrathoracic organs and thoracic

Table 7.3. Indications for AFAST[3].

Indication	Comments
Screening for intra-abdominal injury following blunt trauma	Aids in differentiation of small versus large amounts of intra-abdominal bleeding in dogs Has not been validated in cats
Screening tool for patient with acute collapse, unexplained hypotension, ventricular arrhythmias, or mentation changes	Pericardial effusion with tamponade and acute hemoabdomen are common reasons for these clinical signs
Screening tool for suspected peritonitis cases	Finding and sampling even small amounts of abdominal effusion can be diagnostic
Monitoring a critically ill patient for abdominal effusion development (septic or non-septic) following fluid resuscitation	Many animals will present without abdominal effusion but after fluid resuscitation will demonstrate small amounts of effusion Sampling effusion can help with making a diagnosis
Postoperative monitoring for ongoing hemorrhage	Detection of intracavitary fluid, especially in increasing amounts, can be consistent with ongoing bleeding hours after surgical procedures Serial monitoring helps to differentiate this fluid from normal postoperative intrabdominal fluid (the fluid amounts are increasing with hemorrhage)
Postoperative peritonitis monitoring	Patients with surgical dehiscence (especially after gastrointestinal tract surgery) may develop abdominal effusion hours to days after surgery Increasing fluid from postoperative baseline can be detected with US
Evaluation of the integrity of the urinary bladder following trauma	Abdominal radiographs may not reveal small amounts of urine but it may be visible on US Increasing amounts of fluid from baseline may be consistent with tear in the urinary tract
Evaluate for pericardial or pleural effusion	Thoracic radiographs may not reveal small amounts of pleural effusion that is visible with US Smaller amounts of pericardial effusion or a more acute bleed will not show changes to the cardiac silhouette on radiographs but will be visible on US
Evaluate for retroperitoneal effusions	Fluid is difficult to diagnose via radiographs Fluid solely in the retroperitoneal space may not be sampled with a blind 4 quadrant abdominal tap but can be sampled with US
Ancillary screening for possible anaphylaxis	A halo sign consistent with gall bladder wall edema may increase clinical suspicion for anaphylaxis or right-hand sided volume overload

AFAST[3], abdominal focal assessment sonographically for trauma /triage/tracking; US, ultrasound.

cavity in blunt trauma cases, as well as triage assessment, and tracking of conditions in the critically ill. See Table 7.4 for clinical applications of TFAST[3].

The TFAST[3] has also more recently been extended into a more focused lung surveillance known as VetBLUE, designed specifically to evaluate lung parenchyma in concert with thoracic radiographic findings (see Fig. 7.4). It is most important in differentiating primary respiratory from respiratory look-alike illnesses to allow for improved emergent treatment of the unstable patient and more focused future diagnostics. For example, patients that have metabolic disorders such as diabetic ketoacidosis may come in with tachypnea. Without performing imaging of the chest and other diagnostics, the patient could mistakenly receive furosemide during stabilization. Administration of furosemide in this sce-

Table 7.4. Indications for TFAST[3].

Indication	Comments
Surveillance for pleural and pericardial space disease in the bluntly traumatized and dyspneic emergency and critical care patient	Useful in cases not stable enough for standard radiography Thoracic radiographs may not reveal small amounts of pleural effusion that is visible on US; smaller amounts of pericardial effusion or a more acute bleed will not show changes to the cardiac silhouette on radiographs but be visible on US Evaluate thoracic wall and pleural space for evidence of disease (step sign; see Fig. 7.6)
Detect and serially monitor pleural effusion	Small amounts of pleural effusion may not be visible or quantifiable on thoracic radiographs
Survey for pericardial effusion	US is the only way to confirm the presence of pericardial effusion short of tapping fluid from the pericardial sac Smaller amounts of pericardial effusion or a more acute bleed will not show changes to the cardiac silhouette on radiographs but is visible on US
Screening for the presence of a pneumothorax in traumatized veterinary patients ± gage severity/progression of pneumothorax	Potential for high accuracy, sensitivity and specificity to detect pneumothorax dependent upon operator skill Serial examinations and use of the lung point (see Fig. 7.8) can rate severity and progression of disease
Survey peripheral lung parenchyma for pulmonary edema and attempt to predict edema distribution patterns	Interpretation of A-lines, B-lines, shred (see Fig. 7.6) Most useful in patients that are not stable enough for radiographs Cost-effective and radiation sparing way to trend disease progression/resolution in the ICU for conditions like pulmonary contusions, pneumonia, or CHF in combination with radiographic findings
Assess left-sided cardiac status through the LA:Ao ratio	Normally, right and left atrium symmetrical, with flat intraventricular septum Changes in chamber size and bowing of the septum suggest the need for full echocardiographic assessment LA:Ao ratio >2 is suggestive of left-sided CHF

Ao, aorta; CHF, congestive heart failure; LA,. left atrium; TFAST[3], thoracic focal assessment sonographically for trauma /triage/tracking; US, ultrasound.

nario would further exacerbate the patient's renal fluid and electrolyte losses. Use of VetBLUE can also help differentiate between upper airway, lower airway, and congestive heart failure as causes for true respiratory dyspnea without the need for thoracic radiography or computed tomography of the lungs. See Table 7.5 for specific indications for VetBLUE.

US-guided advanced vascular access

The bedside application of UST for vascular access has great potential for those with cellulitis, edema, hematomas, challenging anatomy, small size, or critical illness (i.e. those patients who are difficult to catheterize). The application of US guidance for vascular access is initially challenging but has been documented to have a quick learning curve and thus has good potential for application to the veterinary critically ill. Ultrasound can be used to catheterize or draw blood from any peripheral vessel including veins and arteries. See Table 7.6 for indications for US-guided vascular access.

7.4 Pitfalls of Ultrasound Monitoring

AFAST[3]

While the AFAST[3] is a valuable asset to supplement physical examination findings and serially monitor for effusion accumulation, there are a number of limitations. These limitations include but are not limited to the following:

- Does not allow for characterization of the type of effusion. Ultrasound-guided abdominocentesis and ancillary testing is required to fully characterize the effusion.

Table 7.5. Indications for VetBLUE.

Indication	Comment
Rapid determination of the likelihood of interstitial lung edema (dry versus wet lungs)	Achieved via semi- quantitative assessment of the presence or absence of ultrasound B-lines (see Fig. 7.6). ≥3 B-lines is consistent with a 'wet' lung (interstitial disease) Perform within minutes of triage assessment and either before or after interventional procedures
Presence and distribution of B- lines may help predict early signs of left-sided CHF, fluid overload, and lung injury in at risk patients	Changes potentially identified before clinical signs are appreciated Changes detected with US before pulmonary edema evident on radiographs
Identify lung patterns consistent with pulmonary contusions or acute lung injury in a dyspneic patient too unstable for thoracic radiography	Limited to disease located at the periphery of the lungs B-lines consistent with 'wet' lungs
Increase or decrease clinical suspicion for primary respiratory processes such as asthma, aspiration pneumonia, neoplasia, or pulmonary thromboembolism in dyspneic patients too unstable for thoracic radiography	Lung patterns narrow down likely disease etiologies. For example: Aspiration pneumonia → B-lines likely appreciated in region of right middle lung lobe Asthma → dry lungs in all fields Neoplasia → identify nodule sign or tissue sign in the affected lung (peripheral regions) PTE → peripheral parenchymal consolidations visible (shred or tissue sign)
Semi-quantification of the severity of pulmonary contusions	Number and distribution of B-lines at baseline and serially
Trend in respiratory distress patients' response to therapy	Serial examinations and recording the number and distribution of B-lines can provide tangible evidence of disease progression
Identify lung consolidation and degree of consolidation	Observation of shred and tissue signs (both number and location) allows for semi-quantification of degree of lung consolidation
Identify possible nodules	Quantify and record location of nodule sign in peripheral lung tissue

CHF, congestive heart failure; PTE, pulmonary thromboembolism; US, ultrasound; VetBLUE, veterinary beside lung ultrasound examination.

- In severely dehydrated and hypotensive patients, AFAST[3] may be falsely negative. Serial AFAST[3] examinations are important, especially after fluid resuscitation. Typically, reassessment is recommended within four hours of fluid resuscitation, but fluid can accumulate sooner or later than the initial reassessment.
- An AFAST[3] examination cannot reliably predict the degree of anemia in cats with blunt trauma.
- The AFAST[3] is less sensitive for effusion detection in penetrating trauma as compared to blunt trauma.
- As with any US imaging, there can be artifacts during AFAST[3] which can limited the interpretation of AFAST[3]. See Table 7.1 for the various artifacts related to AFAST[3].

TFAST[3]/VetBLUE

While TFAST[3] and VetBLUE are a valuable asset to supplement physical examination findings and serially monitor pleural and pericardial space disease, there are a number of limitations. These limitations include but are not limited to the following:

- TFAST[3] is unable to characterize the type of effusion present in either pleural or pericardial effusion. Either US-guided thoracentesis or pericardiocentesis is needed to sample the fluid found on TFAST[3]. Samples can be analyzed cytologically and/or submitted for culture and biochemical testing to further characterize the effusion. The reader is referred to the Further Reading section for more information.

Table 7.6. Indications for ultrasound-guided vascular access.

Indication	Comment
Placement of central venous catheters and other peripheral venous catheters	Rapid identification of the desired vasculature for venipuncture Helps to identify vessels in patients with peripheral edema, vascular collapse, obesity, hematomas, or of very small size Confirmation of successful cannulation of a vessel
Arterial catheterization/blood sampling	Identify and guide catheterization of arteries Arterial catheterization allows for hemodynamic monitoring and arterial blood sampling in the critically ill Confirmation of successful cannulation of a vessel Improves the ability to identify and sample blood from peripheral arteries
Surveillance for venous and arterial thrombosis development	Serial imaging of veins and arteries to identify and describe thrombosis

- TFAST[3] is meant to be used in conjunction with, rather than in replacement of, thoracic radiographs because US is limited to the peripheral lung tissues.
- Without the complimentary application of VetBLUE, TFAST[3] is limited in its ability to scan for pleural effusion and pulmonary parenchymal changes throughout the entirety of the lung fields.
- In the dyspneic patient, TFAST[3] is limited in the ability to diagnose respiratory look-alike conditions (examples: diabetic ketoacidosis, hypocalcemia, hypoglycemia, hypovolemic shock, and neurologic disease). Therefore, it is best used in concert with other bedside imaging modalities and biochemical testing.
- Subcutaneous emphysema can limit the ability to achieve a gator sign on TFAST[3] due to interruption of sound waves traveling into the thorax. With sufficient pressure, there is the possibility that the free gas may be moved sufficiently to enable accurate images.

Ultrasound-guided vascular access

As with all the ultrasound techniques discussed in this chapter, using US to guide vascular access also has some limitations. These include but are not limited to:

- Superficially located and very small vasculature is difficult to identify and unable to be catheterized via UST. Even mild pressure by the US probe will collapse the vessel and make it impossible to identify.
- The ability to identify blood vessels and thrombosis within the vessels is highly dependent on the operator's US technique. Training and practice is needed for successful use of the UST for vascular access and thrombus identification.
- Identification of veins is more difficult than arteries due to lack of pulsatile blood flow through the veins. Operator training is required to help with confident identification of especially venous structures.
- Use of ultrasound to guide a catheter or needle into a blood vessel requires training and practice for competence.

7.5 Case Studies

Case study 1: AFAST/TFAST/VetBLUE applications in an acutely collapsed patient

Cash, a 7-year-old castrated male Labrador retriever, was presented to the emergency department for evaluation after acute collapse. He lives in a rural environment and has free access to barns where the family is currently treating for an outbreak of rats. Upon assessment, Cash is tachycardic (heart rate 160 bpm), tachypneic (respiratory rate of 45), pale, and has a capillary refill time (CRT) of 3 seconds. His pulse is weak on palpation and his ventral lungs are difficult to auscultate while his dorsal lung fields have harsh bronchovesicular sounds. While simultaneously attempting to place an intravenous catheter and collecting blood work for lactate, packed cell volume/total solids (PCV/TS), prothrombin/partial thromboplastin times (PT/aPTT), complete blood count (CBC), and serum chemistry (CHEM), the point of care ultrasound is used to perform an AFAST[3], TFAST[3], and VetBLUE examination. The AFAST[3]/TFAST[3]/VetBLUE findings are the following:

AFAST³	
DH view	0/4 within the abdominal cavity Positive race-track sign is seen and there appears to be irregular triangles of anechoic fluid within the pleural space
SR view	0/4
CC view	0/4
HR view	0/4

TFAST³/VetBLUE	Right	Left
CTS	Glide sign + <3 B-lines	Glide sign + <3 B-lines
Pericardial site	Pericardial effusion without diastolic compression of the right atrium	Pericardial effusion Pleural effusion
DH	As above in AFAST	
Caudodorsal lung lobe region	>3 B-lines bilaterally	>3 B-lines bilaterally
Perihilar lung lobe region	Glide sign + <3 B-lines	Glide sign + <3 B-lines
Middle lung lobe region	>3 B-lines	>3 B-lines
Cranial lung lobe region	>3 B-lines Small amount of pleural effusion	>3 B-lines Small amount of pleural effusion

+, positive; AFAST³, abdominal focal assessment sonographically for trauma/triage/tracking; CC, cystocolic; CTS, chest tube sites; DH, diaphragmaticohepatic; HR, hepatorenal; SR, splenorenal; TFAST³, thoracic focal assessment sonographically for trauma/triage/tracking; US, ultrasound.

At completion of the AFAST³/TFAST³/VetBLUE assessment, results of the PCV/TS/lactate and PT/aPTT have arrived. The results are 14% / 3.0 mg/dL / 5.0 mmol/L (normal values 35–45% / 4.5–6 mg/dL / <2.0 mmol/L) for PCV/TS/lactate, respectively. Both the PT and aPTT are prolonged. Cash is showing signs of active hemorrhage due to his low total protein and PCV. His elevated lactate shows that he is currently undergoing anaerobic metabolism. This is likely due to a combination of hypovolemic and hypoxemic shock resulting in inadequate oxygen delivery to his tissues. He is showing evidence of secondary hemostasis abnormalities with his prolonged PT and aPTT values. He has evidence of wet lungs within his caudodorsal and middle lung lobes which could be suggestive of pulmonary bleeding or other pulmonary interstitial disease. Additionally, the irregular hypoechoic changes in the pleural spaces are consistent with pleural effusion and he has evidence of pericardial effusion without evidence of tamponade. Given that he is showing signs of active hemorrhage, is clinical for his anemia, and has altered secondary hemostasis, he is a good candidate for fluids and a whole blood transfusion.

Cash receives a whole blood transfusion. At completion of the transfusion, a US-guided thoracentesis is performed and is consistent with hemorrhage. Based on these findings, Cash likely consumed vitamin K antagonist (anticoagulant) rodenticide and has subsequent pulmonary parenchymal, pleural space and pericardial space hemorrhage. He is started on vitamin K. Cash continues to improve after his transfusion and within 36 hours is discharged to the care of his family.

Case study 2: AFAST/TFAST/VetBLUE applications in an acutely dyspneic patient

Indy, a 5-year-old male domestic shorthair cat, was presented to the emergency department for evaluation of changes in breathing character at home. Indy is an indoor only cat and has 12 housemates that are up to date on vaccines and preventative medications. Over the last month his owner has been diffusing the house with cinnamon essential oils daily and has historically smoked within the home throughout Indy's life. His owner has noted that Indy has had a rapid respiratory rate over the last 24 hours; he became worse acutely this evening when she attempted to nebulize Indy with the cinnamon essential oils.

On examination, Indy is open mouth breathing with a respiratory rate of 90 bpm. He has significant expiratory effort and his breathing is shallow. With exertion a dry cough is seen. His mucous membranes are pale and auscultation is difficult as he is vocalizing and thrashing.

Indy is placed into oxygen with an FiO_2 of 40% and a bit later is able to tolerate a TFAST³/VetBLUE assessment. Below is his TFAST³/VetBLUE assessment:

TFAST³/VetBLUE	Right	Left
CTS	Glide sign + <3 B-lines	Glide sign + <3 B-lines

Pericardial site	No evidence of pericardial effusion Symmetrical atrial sizes. An estimated LA:Ao ratio is 1	No evidence of pericardial effusion
DH	No pericardial, pleural or peritoneal effusion appreciated	
Caudodorsal lung lobe region	Glide sign + <3 B-lines bilaterally	Glide sign + <3 B-lines bilaterally
Perihilar lung lobe region	Glide sign + <3 B-lines	Glide sign + <3 B-lines
Middle lung lobe region	Glide sign + <3 B-lines	Glide sign + <3 B-lines
Cranial lung lobe region	Glide sign + <3 B-lines	Glide sign + <3 B-lines

+, positive; CTS, chest tube sites; TFAST[3], thoracic focal assessment sonographically for trauma/triage/tracking; US, ultrasound; VetBLUE, Veterinary Bedside Lung Ultrasound Exam.

Given that the lack of pathologic numbers of B-lines and subjective lack of evidence of left-sided heart enlargement, you have less suspicion for cardiac disease as an etiology for Indy's signs. However, because TFAST[3] only assesses the peripheral lung parenchyma it is elected to try to stabilize Indy further to be able to perform thoracic radiographs. A single dosage of butorphanol 0.2 mg/kg IM is administered, and two puffs of albuterol are administered via an infuser device. After 20 minutes, Indy is breathing better and thoracic radiographs are acquired. Thoracic radiographs show evidence of a diffuse bronchiolar pattern with no evidence of pulmonary edema. The lungs appear hyperinflated with flattening of the diaphragm. Based on his history, TFAST[3]/VetBLUE and thoracic radiograph findings, Indy is likely having an acute exacerbation of feline asthma. It is recommended to consider additional diagnostics for other etiologies for feline bronchopulmonary disease including a CBC, biochemistry panel, urinalysis, feline heart worm testing, fecal examination for lungworms, and bronchoscopy with broncho-alveolar lavage.

After discussion with Indy's family regarding all options, the owner elects for empirical outpatient therapy. Indy is dismissed with oral prednisolone at an anti-inflammatory dose, an albuterol inhaler, empirical fenbendazole, and client education to decrease inhaled irritants in the home. Indy follows up with his primary care veterinarian in 3 days' time and is acting like his normal self.

Case study 3: AFAST/TFAST/VetBLUE applications in an acute abdomen patient

Brindy, a 12-year-old spayed female Sheltie, is presented to the emergency department for vomiting, diarrhea, lethargy, and hyporexia that has progressed to anorexia for 2 days. On presentation, she is severely dehydrated (~9% dehydration), icteric, has prolonged capillary refill time, and dry mucus membranes. She has a skin tent and her mentation is dull. Her eyes are sunken, icteric, and her corneas appear dry. She is unwilling to ambulate on her own. On abdominal palpation, she has significant cranial abdominal discomfort. Her pules are weak, she is tachycardic (170 beats/minute) and tachypneic (45 breaths/minute) and her core body temperature is low at 98°F (36.66°C). Her feces is an orange color and diarrhea in consistency.

An intravenous catheter is placed, and initial orders are given for blood pressure, CBC, biochemistry panel, PT/aPTT, ammonia, lactate, PCT/TS, glucose, and AFAST$_3$. She is hypotensive with a systolic blood pressure of 60 mmHg (normal 80–120 mg/dL) and has elevated lactate at 7.0 mmol/L (normal < 2.0 mmol/L; see chapter 1). She is hypoglycemic at 60 mg/dL and has elevated lactate at 7.0 g/dL. She is hemoconcentrated with a PCV/TS of 60%/8.0 (normal 35–45%/4.5–6.0; see chapter 1) and her serum is icteric. While awaiting benchtop blood work, an isotonic crystalloid fluid bolus of 22 mL/kg is administered and she is placed on an active external warming device. She is also given a 0.5 mL/kg 50% dextrose bolus diluted 1:4 over 5 minutes. Her blood pressure improves to a systolic pressure of 75 mmHg. A second 22 mL/kg isotonic crystalloid bolus is administered. While this is being delivered, the AFAST[3]/TFAST[3]/VetBLUE examinations are performed. Below are her results:

AFAST[3]

DH view	0/4 fluid within the abdominal cavity Contents of the gall bladder appear to be well organized, echogenic debris consistent with a mucocele and the gall bladder wall appears to be thickened with a hypoechoic and hyperechoic ring consistent with a halo effect

SR view	0/4	
CC view	0/4	
HR	0/4	
TFAST³/ VetBLUE	**Right**	**Left**
CTS	Glide sign + <3 B-lines	Glide sign + <3 B-lines
Pericardial site	No evidence of pericardial effusion Symmetrical atrial sizes. An estimated LA:Ao ratio is 1	No evidence of pericardial effusion
DH	As above in AFAST₃	
Caudodorsal lung lobe region	Glide sign + <3 B-lines	Glide sign + <3 B-lines
Perihilar lung lobe region	Glide sign + <3 B-lines	Glide sign + <3 B-lines
Middle lung lobe region	Glide sign + <3 B-lines	Glide sign + <3 B-lines
Cranial lung lobe region	Glide sign + <3 B-lines	Glide sign + <3 B-lines

+, positive; AFAST³, abdominal focal assessment sonographically for trauma/triage/tracking; CC, cystocolic; CTS, chest tube sites; DH, diaphragmaticohepatic; HR, hepatorenal; SR, splenorenal; TFAST³, thoracic focal assessment sonographically for trauma/triage/tracking; US, ultrasound.

Brindy's blood pressure improves to a systolic pressure of 95 mmHg on Doppler and her temperature improves to 98.7°F (37.06°C). Her blood glucose improves to 90 mg/dL. At that time, her remaining dehydration deficit is corrected over 12 hours with a 2.5% dextrose continuous rate infusion. Her vitals are closely monitored for decline. Blood work returns and Brindy has an inflammatory leukogram with a degenerate left shift, she is hemoconcentrated, and has a thrombocytosis. Her PT/aPTT are within normal limits and the ammonia is normal. She has a severe cholestatic pattern with a total bilirubin of 13, is mildly azotemic, hypoglycemic, and has a 13 mg/dL (normal 0.1–08 mg/dL) mildly elevated albumin. These findings are suggestive for possible peritonitis. At this time there is no free fluid to corroborate this suspicion.

She is admitted to the ICU with serial vital monitoring, frequent weights, and urine collection and quantification. She is started on pain medications, broad spectrum antimicrobials, and anti-emetics. A repeat AFAST³ in 2 hours shows accumulation of fluid within the DH view. An US-guided abdominocentesis yields fluid that is submitted for a fluid analysis, a total bilirubin level, and cytology. The cytology shows biliary crystals and degenerate neutrophils. Abdominal total bilirubin is 35 mg/dL (normal 0.1–0.8 mg/dL). Given the bile crystals and the comparative abdominal:serum total bilirubin ratio of >2, the peritoneal effusion is consistent with bile peritonitis. As her hemodynamic status is stable, Brindy undergoes an abdominal exploratory surgery and cholecystectom. She is treated aggressively within the intensive care unit for three days prior to dismissal to her family.

7.6 Summary

Ultrasound has many applications for veterinary emergency and critical care cases. Through adequate training and consistent applications of AFAST³, TFAST³, and VetBLUE, a non-radiologist clinician can gather information to help diagnose and treat his patients. Clinicians also have the potential to serially track changes that can increase sensitivity for detecting dynamic changes in the critically ill patient.

Abbreviations

AFAST³, abdominal focal assessment sonographically for trauma/triage/tracking; CC, cystocolic view; COAST³, cage-side organ assessments for trauma triage and tracking; CTS, chest tube site; CVC, central venous catheter; DH, diaphragmaticohepatic view; HR, hepatorenal view; PCS, pericardial site; SR, splenorenal view; TFAST³, thoracic focal assessment sonographically for trauma/triage/tracking; US, ultrasound; UST, ultrasound-guided technique; VetBLUE, veterinary beside lung ultrasound examination.

Further Reading

Campbell, M.T., Macintire, DK. (2012) Catheterization of the venous compartment. In: Burkitt Creedon, J.M., Davis, H. (eds) *Advanced Monitoring and Procedures for Small Animal Emergency and Critical Care.* WB Saunders Co, Chichester, UK, pp. 51–68.

DeFrancesco, T. (2014) Focused or COAST-ECHO (Heart). In: Lisciandro, G. (ed.) *Focused Ultrasound Techniques for the Small Animal Practitioner.* Wiley and Sons, Ames, Iowa, USA, pp. 40–164.

Jandrey, K. (2015) Abdominocentesis and diagnostic peritoneal lavage. In: Silverstein, D., Hopper, K. (eds) *Small Animal Critical Care Medicine*, 2nd edn. Elsevier, St Louis, Missouri, USA, pp. 1036–1039.

Lisciandro, G. (2014a) The abdominal FAST[3] (AFAST[3]) exam. In: Lisciandro, G. (ed.) *Focused Ultrasound Techniques for the Small Animal Practitioner*. Wiley and Sons, Ames, Iowa, USA, pp. 17–44.

Lisciandro, G. (2014b), Appendix II: Goal-directed templates for medical records. In: Lisciandro, G. (ed.) *Focused Ultrasound Techniques for the Small Animal Practitioner*. Wiley and Sons, Ames, Iowa, USA, pp. 306–313.

Lisciandro, G. (2014c) The thoracic FAST[3] exam. In: Lisciandro, G. (ed.) *Focused Ultrasound Techniques for the Small Animal Practitioner*. Wiley and Sons, Ames, Iowa, USA, pp. 40–164.

Lisciandro, G. (2014d) The VetBLUE Lung Scan. In: Liscandro G. (ed.). *Focused Ultrasound Techniques for the Small Animal Practitioner*. Wiley and Sons, Ames, Iowa, USA, pp. 166–188.

Williams, K., Linklater, A. (2015) Central venous catheter placement: modified Seldinger technique. *Clinicians Brief* 1, 71–75.

Bibliography

Abbott, J.A., MacLean, H.A. (2006) Two-dimensional echocardiographic assessment of the feline left atrium. *Journal of Veterinary Internal Medicine* 20, 111–119.

Adamantos, S., Brodbelt, D., Moores, A.L. (2010) Prospective evaluation of complications associated with jugular venous catheter use in a veterinary hospital. *Journal of Small Animal Practitioners* 51, 254–257.

Beal, M.W., Hughes, D. (2000) Vascular access: theory and techniques in the small animal emergency patient. *Clinical Techniques in Small Animal Practice* 15, 101–109.

Biffi, R. (2014) Introduction and overview of PICC history. In: Sandrucci, S., Mussa, B., (eds) *Peripherally Inserted Central Venous Catheters*. Springer-Verlag, Mailand, Germany, pp. 31–42.

Boon, J.A. (2011) *Veterinary Echocardiography,* 2nd edn. Wiley Blackwell, Ames, Iowa, USA.

Boysen, S.R., Lisciandro, G.R. (2013) The use of ultrasound for dogs and cats in the emergency room. *Veterinary Clinics of North America Small Animal Practice* 43, 773–797.

Boysen, S.R., Rozanski, E.A., Tidwell, A.S., et al. (2004) Evaluation of a focused assessment with sonography for trauma protocol to detect free abdominal fluid in dogs involved in motor vehicle accidents. *Journal of American Veterinary Medical Association* 225, 1198–1204.

Brass, P., Hellmich, M., Kolodziej, L., et al. (2015) Ultrasound guidance versus anatomical landmarks for internal jugular vein catheterization. *Cochrane Database of Systematic Reviews* 1, CD006962.

Brederlau, J., Muellenbach, R., Kredel, M., et al. (2008) Comparison of arterial and central venous cannulations using ultrasound guidance in pigs. *Veterinary Anesthesia Analgesia* 35, 161–165.

Brusasco, C., Corradi, F., Zattoni, P.L., et al. (2009) Ultrasound-guided central venous cannulation of bariatric patients. *Obstetrics Surgery* 19, 1365.

Campbell, M.T., Macintire, D.K. (2012) Catheterization of the venous compartment. In Burkitt Creedon, J.M., Davis, H. (eds), *Advanced Monitoring and Procedures for Small Animal Emergency and Critical Care*. WB Saunders Co, Chichester, UK, pp. 51–68.

Carovac, A., Smajlovic, F., Junuzovic, D. (2011) Application of ultrasound in medicine. *Acta Informatica Medica* 19, 168–171.

Chamberlin, S., Sullivan, L.A., Morley, P.S., et al. (2013) Evaluation of ultrasound-guided vascular access in dogs. *Journal of Veterinary Emergency and Critical Care* 23, 498–503.

Choi, J., Kim, A., Keh, S., et al. (2013) Comparison between ultrasonographic and clinical findings in 43 dogs with gallbladder mucoceles. *Veterinary Radiology and Ultrasound* 55, 202–207.

Denys, B.G., Uretsky, B.F., Reddy, P.S, et al. (1991) An ultrasound method for safe and rapid central venous access. *New England Journal of Medicine* 324, 566.

Filly, R.A. (1998) Ultrasound: the stethoscope of the future, alas. *Radiology* 167, 400.

Froehlich, C.D., Rigby, M.R., Rosenberg, E.S., et al. (2009) Ultrasound-guided central venous catheter placement decreases complications and decreases placement attempts compared with the landmark technique in patients in a pediatric intensive care unit. *Critical Care Medicine* 37, 1090–1096.

Fulton, R. (2014) Focused-basic ultrasound principles and artifacts. In: Lisciandro, G. (ed.) *Focused Ultrasound Techniques for the Small Animal Practitioner*. Wiley and Sons, Ames, Iowa, USA, pp. 1–15.

Heng, H.G., Widmer, W.R. (2003) Appearance of common ultrasound artifacts in conventional vs spatial compound imaging. *Veterinary Radiology and Ultrasound* 51, 621–627.

Hundley, D., Brooks, A., Thomovsky, E., et al. (2018) Comparison of ultrasound guided versus landmark based technique for jugular central venous catheterization in healthy, anesthetized dogs. *American Journal of Veterinary Research* 79, 628–636.

Ianniello, S., Di Giacomo, V., Sessa, B., Miele, V. (2014) First-line sonographic diagnosis of pneumothorax in major trauma: accuracy of e-FAST and comparison with multidetector computed tomography. *Radiology Medicine* 119, 674–680.

Kirpatrick, A.W., Sirois, M., Ball, C.G., et al. (2004) The hand-held ultrasound for penetrating abdominal trauma. *American Journal of Surgery* 187, 978–982.

Lamperti, M. (2014) The choice of a vein in critically ill patients: cost-effectiveness. In: Sandrucci, S., Mussa, B., (eds) *Peripherally Inserted Central Venous Catheters.* Springer-Verlag, Mailand, Germany, pp. 31–42.

Langstron, C.E., Eatroff, A.E. (2018) Hemodialysis catheter associated fibrin sheath in a dog. *Journal of Veterinary Emergency and Critical Care* 28, 366–371.

Legler, D., Nugent, M.K. (1984) Doppler localization of the internal jugular vein facilitates central venous cannulation. *Anesthesiology* 60, 481–482.

Lichenstein, D.A. (2007) Ultrasound in the management of thoracic disease. *Critical Care Medicine* 35, S250–S261.

Lisciandro, G.R. (2011) Abdominal and thoracic focused assessment with sonography for trauma, triage, and monitoring in small animals. *Journal of Veterinary Emergency and Critical Care* 21, 104–122.

Lisciandro, G. (2014a) The abdominal FAST[3] (AFAST[3]) exam. In: Lisciandro, G. (ed.) *Focused Ultrasound Techniques for the Small Animal Practitioner*. Wiley and Sons, Ames, Iowa, USA, pp. 17–44.

Lisciandro, G. (2014b), Appendix II Goal-directed templates for medical records. In: Lisciandro, G. (ed.) *Focused Ultrasound Techniques for the Small Animal Practitioner*. Wiley and Sons, Ames, Iowa, USA, pp. 306–313.

Lisciandro, G. (2014c) The thoracic FAST[3] exam. In: Lisciandro, G. (ed.) *Focused Ultrasound Techniques for the Small Animal Practitioner*. Wiley and Sons, Ames, Iowa, USA, pp. 40–164.

Lisciandro G. (2014d) The VetBLUE Lung Scan. In: Lisciandro, G. (ed.) *Focused Ultrasound Techniques for the Small Animal Practitioner*. Wiley and Sons, Ames, Iowa, USA, pp. 166–188.

Lisciandro, G.R., Lagutchik, M.S., Mann, K.A., et al. (2008) Evaluation of a thoracic focused assessment with sonography for trauma (TFAST) protocol to detect pneumothorax and concurrent thoracic injury in 145 traumatized dogs. *Journal of Veterinary Emergency and Critical Care* 8, 258–269.

Lisciandro, G.R., Fosgate, G.T., Fulton, R.M. (2014) The frequency and number of ultrasound lung rockets (B-lines) using a regionally-based lung ultrasound examination named VetBLUE (Veterinary Bedside Lung Ultrasound Exam) in dogs with radiographically normal lung findings. *Veterinary Radiology and Ultrasound* 55, 315–322.

Mandell, D.C., Drobatz, K. (1995) Feline hemoperitoneum: 16 cases (1986–1993). *Journal of Veterinary Emergency and Critical Care* 5, 93–97.

Matisushima, K., Frankel, H.L. (2011) Beyond focused assessment with sonography for trauma: ultrasound creep in the trauma resuscitation area and beyond. *Current Opinions in Critical Care* 17, 606-612.

McGee, D.C., Gould, M.K. (2003) Preventing complications of central venous catheterization. *New England Journal of Medicine* 348, 1123–1133.

McMurray, J., Boysen, S., Chalhoub, S. (2016) Focused assessment with sonography in nontraumatized dogs and cats in the emergency and critical care setting. *Journal of Veterinary Emergency and Critical Care* 26, 64–73.

Miller, A.H., Roth, B., Mills, T., et al. (2002) Ultrasound guidance versus the landmark technique for the placement of central venous catheters in the emergency department. *Academy of Emergency Medicine* 9, 800–805.

Milling, T.J. Jr, Rose, J., Briggs, W.M., et al. (2005) Randomized, controlled clinical trial of point-of-care limited ultrasonography assistance of central venous cannulation: The third sonography outcomes assessment program (SOAP-3) trial. *Critical Care Medicine* 33, 1764.

Mohammadi, A., Ghasemi-Rad, M. (2012) Evaluation of gastrointestinal injury in blunt abdominal trauma FAST is not reliable: the role of repeated ultrasonography. *World Journal of Emergency Surgery* 20, 2.

Muhm, M. (2002) Ultrasound guided central venous access: is useful for beginners, in children, and when blind cannulation fails. *British Medical Journal* 325, 1373–1374.

Muir, W. (2001) Trauma physiology, pathophysiology, and complication implications. *Journal of Veterinary Emergency and Critical Care* 16, 253–263.

Mussa, B. (2014) Advantages, disadvantages, and indications of PICCs in inpatients and outpatients. In: Sandrucci, S., Mussa, B., (eds.) *Peripherally Inserted Central Venous Catheters*. Springer-Verlag, Mailand, Germany, pp. 43–51.

Nguyen, B., Prat, G., Nowak, E., et al. (2014) Determination of the learning curve for ultrasound-guided jugular central venous catheter placement. *Intensive Care Medicine* 40, 66–73.

Portillo, E., Mackin, A., Hendrix, P.K., et al. (2005) Comparision of modified Seldinger and through the-needle jugular catheter placement techniques in the dog. *Journal of Veterinary Emergency and Critical Care* 16, 88–95.

Reminga, C.L., Silverstein, D.C., Drobatz, K.J., et al. (2018) Evaluation of the placement and maintenance of central venous catheters in critically ill dogs and cats. *Journal of Veterinary Emergency and Critical Care* 28, 232–243.

Ringold, S.A., Kelmer, E. (2008) Freehand ultrasound-guided femoral arterial catheterization in dogs. *Journal of Veterinary Emergency and Critical Care* 18, 306–311.

Rishniw, M., Erb, H.N. (2000) Evaluation of four 2-dimensional echocardiographic methods of assessing left atrial size in dogs. *Journal of Veterinary Internal Medicine* 14, 429–435.

Rozycki, G.S. (1998) Surgeon performed US: its use in clinical practice. *Annals of Surgery* 228, 16–28.

Rozycki, G.S., Ochsner, M.G., Schmidt, J.A., *et al.* (1995) A prospective study of surgeon-performed ultrasound as the primary adjuvant modality for injured patient assessment. *Journal of Trauma* 39, 492–498.

Sargsyan, A.E., Hamilton, D.R., Nicolau, S., *et al.* (2001) Ultrasound evaluation of the magnitude of pneumothorax: a new concept. *American Journal of Surgery* 21, 232–235.

Soldati, G., Sher, S., Testa, A. (2011) Lung and ultrasound: time to reflect. *European Review for Medical and Pharmacological Sciences* 15, 223–227.

Scoppettuolo, G., Mussa, B. (2014) Clinical problems associated with the use of peripheral venous approaches: infections. In: Sandrucci, S., Mussa, B., (eds.) *Peripherally Inserted Central Venous Catheters.* Springer-Verlag, Mailand, Germany, pp. 95–109.

Udobie, K.F., Rodriguez, A., Chiu, W.C., *et al.* (2001) Role of ultrasonography in penetrating abdominal trauma: a prospective study. *Journal of Trauma* 50, 475–479.

Viscasillas, J., Sanchis, S., Sneddon, C. (2014) Ultrasound guided epidural catheter placement in a dog. *Veterinary Anesthesia Analgesia* 41, 330–331.

Ward, J., Lisciandro, G., Ware, W., *et al.* (2018) Evaluation of point of care thoracic ultrasound and NT-proBNP for the diagnosis of congestive heart failure in cats with respiratory distress. *Journal of Veterinary Internal Medicine* 32, 1530–1540.

Williams, K., Linklater, A.. (2015) Central venous catheter placement: Modified Seldinger technique. *Clinicians Brief* 1, 71–75.

Yonei, A., Nonoue, T., Sari, A. (1986) Real-time ultrasonic guidance for percutaneous puncture of the internal jugular vein. *Anesthesiology* 64, 830–831.

8 Electrolyte Monitoring

ELIZABETH J. THOMOVSKY*

Purdue University College of Veterinary Medicine, West Lafayette, Indiana, USA

This chapter will review electrolytes of immediate concern (sodium, calcium, phosphorus, and potassium) that often need to be monitored and treated in the emergent patient, their basic function in the body, and the most common situations that warrant monitoring of each electrolyte. It is important to recognize when electrolytes need persistent and continual monitoring and when electrolytes require less intense monitoring. The methods of measurement of each electrolyte as well as possible pitfalls in measurement will also be presented in addition to several clinical examples of electrolyte monitoring in action.

8.1 Basic Physiology and Anatomy

Sodium

Sodium (Na) is ubiquitous in the body and is intimately involved in control of osmolality in the blood, cells, and interstitial tissues. The location of sodium particles (intracellular versus extracellular) is determined by the action of sodium transporters and Na/K (potassium) ATPase pumps. In many locations in the body such as the brain, heart, kidneys, and skeletal muscle, sodium is preferentially moved into one location in order to set up a concentration gradient across cell membranes; maintenance of this gradient is crucial for appropriate cellular and organ function. Because sodium is so abundant in the body, changes in sodium concentrations can be related to multiple different systems. In addition, the animal's sodium level is a *concentration*, usually measured in mmol or mEq of sodium/dL of water on blood work. This means that the amount of body water can have profound effects on the sodium reported in a blood panel.

Therefore, when interpreting changes in sodium, it is important to remember that in most cases, the hyper- or hyponatremia is actually due to changes in the *water* levels in the bloodstream, rather than actual alterations in the amount of sodium. This is why terminology that is often used in the literature to describe changes in sodium refers to the free water deficit. Essentially when there is a *free water deficit* and water levels are low in the blood, then the *sodium is high* (i.e. the decrease in water concentrates the sodium particles, resulting in hypernatremia). Conversely, when there is a *free water excess* and water levels are relatively high in the blood, the *sodium is low* (i.e. the increased water dilutes the sodium particles in solution, resulting in hyponatremia).

See Fig. 8.1 for the basic mechanisms underlying the development of hypernatremia and hyponatremia. Interested readers can obtain more detail regarding sodium regulation in the Further Reading section. While not the focus of this chapter, changes in serum sodium concentration should also be associated with similar changes in serum chloride (Cl) levels, as alterations in overall water content of the blood should dilute or concentrate both ions concurrently. In order to know if the increase or decrease of chloride relative to sodium/water is proportional, mathematical corrections (see Chapter 5) can be applied to 'correct' the chloride relative to the free water gain or loss. Gains or losses of chloride in excess of what can be explained by changes in sodium/water levels have their greatest impact on regulation of the acid–base status of the body, as further discussed in Chapter 5.

In general, large alterations in sodium (either high or low) can lead to clinical signs in the patient. However, relatively small changes in sodium that

---

* Corresponding author: ethomovs@purdue.edu

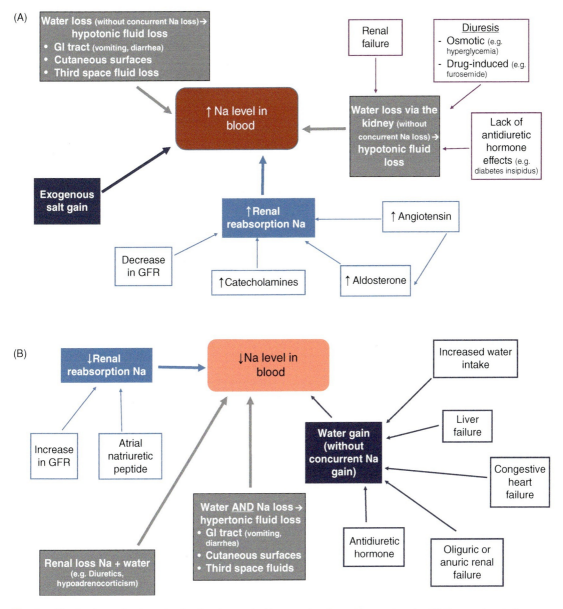

Fig. 8.1. The basic mechanisms for the development of hypernatremia and hyponatremia. (A) Hypernatremia is a result of either a gain of sodium (ingestion of salt without water, infusion of hypertonic fluids with a high sodium content), a loss of free water in excess of sodium loss (hypotonic fluid or pure water losses), or retaining sodium in excess of water at the level of the kidney. (B) Conversely, hyponatremia results from losing sodium in excess of water, gaining pure water that dilutes blood sodium, or retaining less sodium at the level of the kidney. GFR, glomerular filtration rate; GI, gastrointestinal; Na, sodium.

occur very *rapidly* can also result in clinical signs. Clinical signs are most commonly neurologic since the effects of changes in blood osmolality are most evident in cells of the nervous system. Neurologic signs can include changes in behavior/mentation, ataxia, and seizures or seizure-like events. In some cases (especially in more chronic conditions), clinical signs can be non-specific such as anorexia or weakness and lethargy. In general, the more chronic the change in sodium, the less severe the clinical signs directly attributable to the sodium abnormality since the brain has more time to adapt.

Sodium loss or a gain in water leads to hyponatremia and in turn a hypo-osmolar plasma. If this happens acutely, the cells in the brain are relatively hyperosmolar compared to the plasma, and the excess water will shift from the plasma into the cytoplasm. This in turn can lead to cellular swelling, causing cerebral edema and signs ranging from lethargy and vomiting to changes in mentation, seizures, and even death. If the hyponatremia is more chronic, the brain cells have a chance to adapt and will reduce their own osmolality through the loss of intracellular potassium and other intracellular organic osmoles such as amino acids. This reduces the difference in osmolality between the brain cells and the hypo-osmolar plasma, leading to less movement of water from the plasma into the brain cells, less cerebral edema, and blunting of clinical signs.

Conversely, hypernatremia – whether from gain of sodium particles or loss of plasma water – leads to a hyperosmolar plasma. Acutely, plasma that is hyperosmolar compared to cellular fluid will draw water out of the cells of the brain, leading to shrinkage of those cells. This can lead to an overall decrease in brain volume that, in the most severe cases, can cause rupture of blood vessels in the brain and sudden intracerebral hemorrhage. Less acutely, the dehydrated nerves can become demyelinated. Signs of demyelination can take up to 72 hours or more to become clinically apparent. If the hypernatremia is more chronic, the cells of the central nervous system will have a chance to adapt, accumulating and producing 'idiogenic osmoles' (intracellular solutes such as amino acids and electrolytes) to raise their own osmolality closer to that of the plasma. This will reduce the movement of water out of the cells, ensuring that the cells are protected and resulting in fewer or less obvious clinical signs.

Calcium

Calcium volumes in the body are relatively small, especially as compared to sodium. However, like sodium, calcium is found in many locations in the body and is integral to many cellular functions. Calcium is incorporated and stored in body tissues (bones, teeth) and plays a crucial role in electrophysiology (nerve conduction, cardiac conduction, and muscular tone) and intracellular signaling, and is a cofactor for many enzyme systems including the coagulation system.

The largest proportion of calcium is stored in the skeleton (99% of all calcium) with the remaining 1% (i.e. the extracellular calcium) free and able to exchange between the blood and the extracellular bony matrix. This extracellular calcium is found in three forms – ionized (iCa), complexed (i.e. bound to phosphate, bicarbonate, sulfate, citrate, and lactate), and protein bound (primarily to albumin). Typically, since iCa is the fraction of calcium that is the most important in cellular functions, it is the calcium that should be monitored clinically rather than total calcium. See Fig. 8.2 for basic calcium metabolism and regulation by the body.

In general, extremes of calcium will be clinically important. Ionized hypercalcemia (usually accompanied by total hypercalcemia) can lead to cell death secondary to the toxic effects of excessive calcium. While all cells can be affected, central nervous system, renal, cardiac, and gastrointestinal (GI) tract cell death lead to the most obvious clinical signs. Clinical signs include polyuria and polydipsia as the body tries to reduce the higher calcium concentration by diluting the calcium, as well as increasing urinary excretion. Some animals become lethargic and weak, and concurrent anorexia and vomiting often occur. The latter clinical signs are likely due to impaired muscle contraction of smooth muscle in the GI tract leading to ileus, in addition to death of gastrointestinal tract cells. As with sodium, the faster the hypercalcemia develops, the more severe the clinical signs. However, the more chronic the hypercalcemia, the more likely that mineralization of soft tissues will occur due to a high phosphorus × calcium product (greater than 60–70 predisposes to mineralization), resulting in organ dysfunction. While mineralization can occur in any tissue, clinical signs usually manifest first in the kidneys as progressive renal failure.

Ionized hypocalcemia (usually accompanied by total hypocalcemia) causes a variety of clinical signs including muscle tremors that often appear seizure-like, facial/muzzle pruritus resulting in facial rubbing, a stiff gait, or even behavioral changes including restlessness, disorientation, or hypersensitivity to stimuli. Changes in electrical activity of the heart (arrhythmias) can also occur and rarely these animals display polyuria or polydipsia. Both extremes – hypocalcemia and hypercalcemia – can potentially be fatal if untreated.

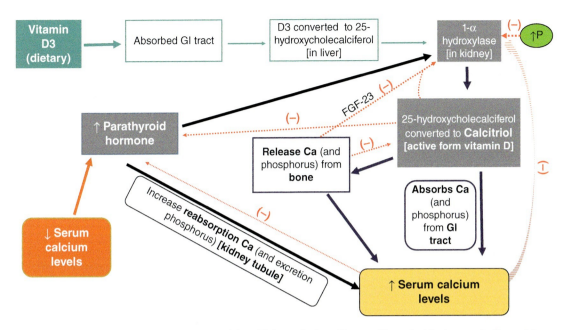

Fig. 8.2. The basic mechanisms involved in calcium (Ca) metabolism. The most important factors controlling calcium levels are calcitriol (the active form of vitamin D; 1,25-dihydroxyvitamin D) and parathyroid hormone. Calcitriol primarily works to increase calcium absorption from the gastrointestinal (GI) tract and releases calcium from the bony matrix via increased osteoclast activity. Parathyroid hormone production is stimulated by hypocalcemia and can similarly increase osteoclast activity to release calcium from bony stores. It also acts directly on the kidneys to increase calcium reabsorption in the renal tubules and indirectly stimulates calcitriol production in order to increase gastrointestinal tract reabsorption of calcium. Negative feedback occurs to maintain calcium levels in the normal range (*as indicated by dotted/hatched lines with parenthetical minus signs*). Specifically, high serum calcium levels decrease parathyroid hormone release and have an inhibitory effect on calcitriol activation by inhibiting 1-α hydroxylase (and therefore the conversion of inactive vitamin D into calcitriol). In addition, production of fibroblast growth factor 23 (FGF-23) from the bone in response to high levels of serum phosphorus and calcitriol also inhibits 1-α hydroxylase. This collectively leads to less renal reabsorption, less gastrointestinal absorption, and decreased bone mobilization of calcium. High levels of calcitriol will also decrease parathyroid hormone release. Additionally, hyperphosphatemia (↑P) will decrease calcitriol activation, decreasing calcium levels.

Phosphorus

Phosphorus is an electrolyte that is often overlooked when treating emergency and critically ill patients as it rarely requires urgent intervention to treat. Phosphorus is the primary negatively charged ion (anion) within the cytoplasm of cells similar to potassium which is the primary intracellular cation (positively charged ion) in cells. Phosphorus is extremely important in maintaining cell membranes in all tissues of the body (as part of the phospholipid cell membrane) as well as being an integral part of adenosine triphosphate (ATP), the energy currency of the body. Phosphorus is found in an organic form (e.g. phospholipids, found within soft tissues) and an inorganic form (e.g. serum phosphorus or bound in bones) with the ability to shift back and forth between the various forms. Approximately 15% of phosphorus is organic while the remaining 80–85% of phosphorus is inorganic. The phosphorus measured on a blood panel is the inorganic phosphorus; this inorganic phosphorus can be protein bound (10–20%), free (the negatively charged ion, PO_4^-), or complexed to other molecules (e.g. sodium, magnesium, or calcium). See Fig. 8.3 for an overview of phosphorus metabolism.

Clinical signs of phosphorus alterations are not readily apparent, affecting 'unseen' functions in the body. When hypophosphatemia occurs (typically when phosphorus levels are ≤1.0 mg/dL), cell membranes become fragile leading to hemolysis of red blood cells, impaired phagocytic effects of

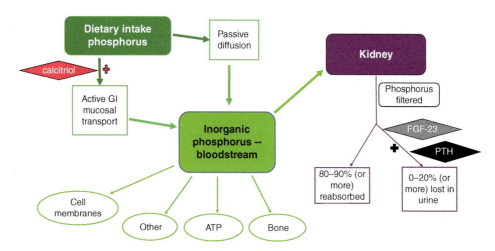

Fig. 8.3. Basic phosphorus (P) metabolism. Inorganic phosphorus is ingested in the diet and then either diffuses into the bloodstream or is actively transported across gastrointestinal (GI) mucosal cells into the bloodstream from the gastrointestinal lumen. Active transport of phosphorus from the GI lumen is upregulated in the presence of calcitriol. Once in the bloodstream, the inorganic phosphorus can be incorporated into multiple structures including cell membranes, ATP, and the bony matrix, in addition to playing a role in the coagulation system and white blood cell function. Phosphorus in turn is filtered at the level of the kidney where it is either reabsorbed or lost in the urine. Phosphorus loss in the kidney is increased in the presence of parathyroid hormone. Osteocyte production of fibroblast growth factor 23 (FGF-23) in response to hyperphosphatemia also increases renal excretion of phosphorus. See Fig. 8.2 for more information about regulation of PTH and calcitriol. ATP, adenosine triphosphate; GFR, glomerular filtration rate; PTH, parathyroid hormone.

leukocytes, and compromised platelet functionality/lysis of platelets. Red blood cells also have less 2,3 diphosphoglycerate (2,3 DPG – see Chapter 4) and cannot release oxygen as readily to the tissues. If muscle cells lyse due to hypophosphatemia (rhabdomyolysis), patients can be weak or in pain, and eventually decreases in cellular energy (ATP) will alter brain functions and lead to encephalopathies and mentation changes. Changes in heart muscle functions and/or arrhythmias can also occur in severe hypophosphatemia, as can GI signs including ileus, vomiting, and diarrhea.

In contrast, hyperphosphatemia leads to a decrease in the serum calcium concentration by reducing the activity of 1-α hydroxylase (and therefore reducing calcitriol production; see Fig. 8.2) as the body attempts to prevent the phosphorus × calcium product from exceeding 60–70 which will place the animal at risk for calcification of tissues. Therefore, the clinical signs seen with hyperphosphatemia are typically related to hypocalcemia (see the Calcium section). Since hyperphosphatemia is often associated with calcification of tissues and resulting disruption of tissue function, especially in the kidneys, patients may also display signs of vomiting, lethargy, or polyuria/polydipsia attributable to kidney failure.

Potassium

Potassium is the primary cation found within cells. Its concentration is similar to the extracellular concentration of sodium, helping to maintain the electrochemical balance. The majority of potassium (66–75%) is contained within muscle cells. The primary role of potassium is maintaining the resting membrane potential of the cell, specifically playing an important role in repolarization of muscle and nerve cells during each action potential. Therefore, alterations in potassium (especially hyperkalemia) can lead to arrhythmias which can potentially be life threatening. See Fig. 8.4 for an overview of potassium metabolism.

It is important to understand that the potassium concentration in the bloodstream is in proportion to the potassium levels in the intracellular compartment. Therefore, when blood potassium levels are low, it means the intracellular compartment is also depleted of potassium. Similarly, if a patient is hyperkalemic, the intracellular compartment is

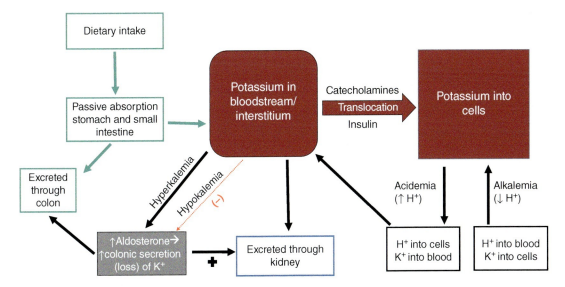

Fig. 8.4. Basic potassium (K$^+$) metabolism. Potassium originates in the diet and is absorbed from the stomach and small intestine and enters the bloodstream. Excess potassium will remain in the intestinal tract and be excreted through the colon. In addition, potassium can be secreted back into the colon for excretion, a process that increases in response to aldosterone. Once in the bloodstream, potassium can translocate into cells and become intracellular potassium; the translocation process is increased by the presence of insulin and catecholamines. Intracellular potassium levels are also influenced by the pH of the bloodstream. Acidemia (increased levels of hydrogen ions, H$^+$) will cause the exchange of hydrogen ions for potassium, increasing the concentration of potassium in the blood as the hydrogen ions are moved into cells. In contrast, alkalemia will lead to the movement of potassium ions into cells in exchange for the outward movement of hydrogen ions into the bloodstream. When a patient is hypokalemic, aldosterone release is suppressed leading to potassium retention in the kidney (dotted line).

replete with potassium. However, since potassium will translocate into and out of cells in response to changes in factors such as the patient's acid–base status, the measured blood potassium levels can be deceiving. For example, in conditions marked by acidemia such as diabetic ketoacidosis, potassium will shift out of cells in exchange for hydrogen ions. This can lead to a measured normal blood potassium level even though the cells are globally potassium depleted (see Fig. 8.4).

Clinical signs of potassium depletion are associated with the relative lack of potassium within muscle cells. The lack of potassium leads to an inability to contract properly or as strongly causing muscle dysfunction and weakness. The classic sign of hypokalemia in cats is weak cervical musculature leading to a ventroflexed neck and plantigrade stance, but generalized lethargy, gait changes, and weakness can also be seen with hypokalemia. Some hypokalemic patients also display polyuria and polydipsia. This is largely due to the effects of aldosterone, specifically the suppression of this hormone in cases of hypokalemia (Fig. 8.4). Lower levels of aldosterone will cause loss of sodium in the kidney (while retaining potassium), leading to polyuria. Hypokalemia can also reduce insulin release, causing hyperglycemia, that might contribute to the polyuria and polydipsia noted. In extreme cases, difficulty breathing (weak diaphragm), muscle cell death leading to rhabdomyolysis, and even electrocardiogram (ECG) changes can occur. These electrical changes can make hypokalemic patients with arrhythmias more refractory to treatment, especially with class I antiarrhythmics (e.g. lidocaine). Hypokalemia does not usually cause observed clinical signs until K$^+$ levels are significantly less than 3.0 mEq/L.

Hyperkalemia also causes muscle weakness (usually K$^+$ levels >7.5–8.0 mEq/L). When an animal is hyperkalemic, its cell membranes are initially more excitable than in a normal setting since the resting membrane potential of the cells is higher (more positive) than at normal potassium levels. In cardiac muscle cells, this initial hyperexcitability is followed by an *inability* to depolarize, leading to bradycardia and/or other bradyarrhythmias (although rarely tachyarrhythmias may occur). Hyperkalemic animals may also be acidemic. Often hyperkalemia occurs concurrently with decreased renal excretion of acids, but acidemia may also occur when hydrogen ions translocate out of the cells into the bloodstream in exchange for potassium ions shifting into the cells to improve the hyperkalemia (see Fig. 8.4).

8.2 How the Monitor Works

When measuring electrolytes, clinicians are limited to either measuring them on a bench-top analyzer as part of a full chemistry panel (either in-house or sent out to a laboratory) or via a point-of-care analyzer. There are two main ways that laboratory machines measure electrolytes – flame photometry (flame atomic emission spectrometry) or ion-selective electrodes (ISE). Flame photometry is an older technology where the sample is heated via a flame or burner until the liquid portion of the sample evaporates, leaving the ions. These ions are excited when they absorb energy from the flame and, after the heat is removed, they return to their normal (non-excited state) while giving off a characteristic wavelength of radiation. This radiation signature and its magnitude is measured by the analyzer and in turn is proportional to the concentration of the electrolyte in the blood.

The downside of flame photometry is that for electrolytes other than sodium and potassium, the absorption and resulting release of radiation from the electrolytes is too variable to be reliable and/or the analyzers cannot detect electrolytes at a low enough level to be clinically useful. In addition, some electrolytes can alter the flame temperature or react with the flame or environment to make new compounds (e.g. calcium combines with oxygen from the flame to form CaO), nullifying their ability to be measured. Therefore, if flame atomic emission spectrometry is used, it is limited to determining potassium and sodium levels.

The other major technology used in laboratory machines is ISE to measure electrolyte concentrations. This technology is used for sodium, chloride, ionized calcium, and potassium. With ISE, one electrode is in contact with or contains a reference solution with a known concentration of an electrolyte to be measured and the other electrode is in contact with the blood sample. The two solutions then 'meet' in the center portion of the testing slide, forming a concentration cell. The resulting electrical potential of this junction between reference solution and sample solution is measured (i.e. the 'junction cell') and correlated to the ionic concentrations and types. Specifically, a volt meter is used to determine the electrical potential and a microprocessor mathematically converts this voltage into the concentration of the ion in the blood sample. Typically, there is either an ion-specific membrane through the test electrode so that only the electrolyte of interest can move into the junction cell and be measured or separate ISE for each electrolyte to be measured.

Direct and indirect ISE techniques exist. With direct ISE, the blood sample is presented to the electrode and the electrolyte levels are directly measured. With indirect ISE, the blood sample is first diluted in a buffer by the machine before being presented to the electrode; this allows for measurement of the electrolyte activity versus the concentration of the buffer solution. This yields values most closely correlated to flame photometry which is the historic gold standard. Most laboratories and point-of-care instrumentation use indirect ISE. Most bedside point-of-care analyzers use a miniaturized version of ion-specific electrode technology to determine electrolyte concentrations which may be direct or indirect ISE.

Laboratory machines also use colorimetry to measure total calcium and phosphorus in laboratory analyzers. The complexed and ionized calcium in the blood reacts with a dye such as orthocresolphthalein to form a colored complex; this complex is measured spectrophotometrically and the amount (density) of the color is indicative of the volume of calcium. A similar technique is used for free or complexed inorganic phosphorus, except a different dye (molybdate) is used.

8.3 Indications

Sodium

When handling emergency or critical care patients, sodium is generally a marker of the volume of water in the plasma relative to the amount of sodium ions. Monitoring sodium is most important in animals with kidney disease (or other non-renal causes of diuresis such as hyperglycemia or mannitol administration), polyuria/polydipsia, vomiting, and/or diarrhea. Clinicians can alter sodium values with the administration of either hypertonic fluids (hypertonic saline) or hypotonic fluids (5% dextrose in water or 0.45% sodium chloride) in large quantities or over long periods of time. See Table 8.1 for common diseases leading to sodium alterations. Box 8.1 provides broad suggestions as to how often to measure serum sodium values in different hospitalized cases and case study 1 details a case in which aberrant sodium values were treated. An in-depth discussion of the treatment of sodium disorders is beyond the focus of this chapter (see Further Reading section for more information).

Calcium

When working up an emergency patient, altered calcium levels are differentials for clinical signs such as polyuria or polydipsia, vomiting, tremors, arrhythmias, or weakness. Patients with conditions such as dystocia that may receive calcium therapy should also have baseline levels measured prior to treatment. See Table 8.2 for a list of common diseases for which hypercalcemia or hypocalcemia are differentials, leading to the need to measure calcium levels. Since iCa is the most clinically important fraction of calcium, when there is concern that hypocalcemia or hypercalcemia is contributing to the animal's clinical condition, iCa should be measured.

There are no hard and fast rules as to when treatment must occur for hypocalcemia or hypercalcemia. However, the author typically treats hypocalcemia when iCa levels are less than 1.0 mmol/L and/or the patient is showing clinical signs suggestive of hypocalcemia despite higher iCa levels. Similarly, the author typically instigates treatment for hypercalcemia when iCa levels are higher than 1.4 mmol/L. The exception to these rules is extremely debilitated critically ill patients who often have ionized hypocalcemia. The etiology of hypocalcemia of critical illness is multifactorial, including downregulation of vitamin D during inflammatory states, causing decreased levels of iCa. This is usually a transient change and resolution of the underlying disease and inflammation should normalize iCa levels. Therefore, critically ill patients typically do not require treatment for their hypocalcemia unless the iCa is less than 0.70–0.80 mmol/L and/or they are showing clinical signs compatible with hypocalcemia.

Phosphorus

Measurement of phosphorus levels by themselves are not that important in most emergency or critically ill patients since the phosphorus levels will usually normalize with treatment of the underlying disease (Table 8.3). The exception is when the underlying disease process directly causes extremes

Table 8.1. Diseases commonly associated with hyper- or hyponatremia.

Hypernatremia	Hyponatremia
Loss of water in excess of sodium (free water loss): • Vomiting • Diarrhea • Renal failure • Diuresis • Third space fluid accumulation (peritoneal or pleural effusion) • Deficiency of or lack of response to antidiuretic hormone (e.g. central or nephrogenic diabetes insipidus) • Drugs (e.g. glucocorticoids, diuretics) • Fever • Prolonged inadequate access to water Sodium gain: • Ingest in diet (e.g. salt toxicity, paint ball intoxication) • Hypertonic saline administration • Sodium bicarbonate administration • Excess aldosterone (e.g. hyperaldosteronism) • Hyperadrenocorticism	Gain of water in excess of sodium (free water gain): • Hyperglycemia • Liver failure • Congestive heart failure • Renal failure • Excess antidiuretic hormone (e.g. syndrome inappropriate antidiuretic hormone) Loss of sodium in excess of water: • Vomiting • Diarrhea • Third space fluid accumulation (peritoneal or pleural effusion) • Cutaneous loss (e.g. burns, wounds) • Hypoadrenocorticism • Drugs (e.g. diuretics)

> **Box 8.1. Suggested monitoring in hospitalized patients with sodium disorders.**
>
> *Measure sodium concentrations at least every 4-6 hours:*
>
> - Documented hypernatremia (typically >160–170 mEq/L) that is being treated
> - Documented hyponatremia (typically < 90–100 mEq/L) that is being treated
>
> The goal is to ensure that the sodium does not normalize at a rate faster than 0.5–1.0 mEq/L/h to avoid significant changes in osmolality in the plasma that can affect the cells of the brain.
>
> Correct CHRONIC hypernatremia (present more than 48–72 hours) relatively slowly with frequent monitoring of sodium levels (sometimes more frequently than every 4–6 hours if levels are changing rapidly) during treatment to allow for adjustment of fluid rates.
>
> Correct ACUTE hypernatremia more quickly (i.e. if you know the abnormality occurred within the last 8 hours, you can correct it within the next 8 hours) with more or less frequent monitoring depending on the situation.
>
> *Measure sodium concentration at least every 12-24 hours:*
>
> - Persistent vomiting or diarrhea while hospitalized, especially large volumes
> - Diuresis
>   - Renal failure (e.g. polyuric renal failure)
>   - Non-renal diuresis (e.g hyperglycemia, mannitol administration, furosemide administration)
>   - Post-obstructive diuresis
> - Regurgitation, especially large volumes
> - Effusion in thorax or abdomen, especially when being removed via active or passive drainage
>
> *Measure sodium concentration at presentation (frequency of rechecking depends on the patient's clinical condition and response to treatment):*
>
> - Historical vomiting or diarrhea
> - Clinical dehydration on examination
> - Suspicion of hypoadrenocorticism (along with serum potassium)
> - Thoracic or abdominal effusions
> - Heart failure
> - Renal failure
> - Liver failure
> - Diuretic administration
> - History of sodium gain (e.g. salt toxicity)
> - Cutaneous wounds or burns, especially when covering more than 20% of the body and/or damaging the dermis and epidermis (i.e. 2nd degree burns or more severe)
> - Any critically ill animal receiving fluid therapy

of phosphorus that can lead to clinical complications. The most common emergency and intensive care unit cases with significant alterations in their phosphorus levels that will not normalize without direct treatment of the phosphorus are those with diabetic ketoacidosis and kidney failure. In diabetic ketoacidosis (and any other disease leading to a significant osmotic diuresis in the kidney), excessive water and phosphorus loss occur through the kidney, leading to hypophosphatemia. Complicating matters in diabetic ketoacidosis, treatment with insulin will worsen hypophosphatemia by shifting phosphorus into cells. In contrast, patients with renal failure (leading to a decreased glomerular filtration rate) are unable to excrete phosphorus appropriately, leading to retention of phosphorus and hyperphosphatemia. See Table 8.3 for a list of the most common causes of hypophosphatemia and hyperphosphatemia. However, regardless of the etiology of the alterations in phosphorus, phosphorus values are rarely checked more often than every 6–12 hours (and usually every 24 hours or longer) since most alterations in phosphorus occur slowly and/or parallel improvements in other disease parameters are monitored more regularly (i.e. as the azotemia improves in a renal failure patient, so does the phosphorus).

Table 8.2. Diseases associated with hypercalcemia or hypocalcemia.

Hypercalcemia[a]	Hypocalcemia
Hyperparathyroidism **A**ddison's disease (hypoadrenocorticism) **R**enal disease **D** – Hypervitaminosis **D** **I**diopathic hypercalcemia **O**steomyelitis (caused by bacterial or fungal disease of the bone) **N**eoplastic disease (especially lymphoma, anal sac apocrine gland adenocarcinoma)	Hypoparathyroidism Hypoalbuminemia Chronic renal failure Hypovitaminosis D Pancreatitis Eclampsia Starvation Ethylene glycol intoxication Administration Ca binders such as phosphate enemas or bicarbonate Intestinal malabsorption Cellular breakdown (e.g. rhabdomyolysis, tumor lysis syndrome)

[a]Mnemonic for differentials for hypercalcemia: HARD ION.

Table 8.3. Common diseases causing hypophosphatemia or hyperphosphatemia.

Hyperphosphatemia	Hypophosphatemia
Renal failure Hypoparathyroidism Hyperthyroidism Increased intake of dietary phosphorus Vitamin D intoxication (e.g. rodenticide) Phosphate enema Release of phosphorus from other cells: • Tumor lysis syndrome • Rhabdomyolysis • Hemolysis Metabolic acidosis (shifting out of cells to follow hydrogen ions)	Renal diuresis (e.g. furosemide) Hyperparathyroidism Eclampsia Decreased dietary intake Vitamin D deficiency Malabsorption Phosphate binders Translocation into cells • Treatment diabetic ketoacidosis • Insulin administration • Respiratory alkalosis • Hypothermia

Potassium

Potassium levels are commonly altered in sick animals. Low potassium results from gastrointestinal losses (vomiting and diarrhea) or (rarely) chronically decreased potassium intake (anorexia). In addition, diseases affecting the kidney and its ability to reabsorb potassium can lead to hypokalemia including renal failure as well as any other diuresis-inducing disorder such as post-obstructive diuresis or diabetes mellitus. On the other hand, high potassium most commonly results from renal failure or an inability to excrete potassium in the urine as seen with urethral obstruction. See Table 8.4 for a list of the most common diseases that lead to hyperkalemia and hypokalemia.

If potassium levels are mildly to moderately elevated (<7.5 mEq/L) or mildly to moderately decreased (>2.5 mEq/L), potassium levels can be monitored every 12–24 hours while treating the underlying disease and/or supplementing potassium. However, if potassium levels are less than 2.5 mEq/L, the author will test potassium levels every 4–6 hours during supplementation until the potassium levels are close to 3.0 mEq/L or above. This is both to ensure that supplementation of potassium is improving the levels as well as to be able to identify when to lessen the degree of supplementation. If potassium levels are greater than 7 or 7.5 mEq/L, actions are typically taken to reduce the potassium levels, and potassium is rechecked until it is consistently dropping toward normal or is at least below 6 mEq/L. See Section 8.4 for general information on how to supplement low potassium or decrease high potassium levels and case study 2 for an example of managing hyperkalemia; the interested reader is urged to consult additional resources related to treating electrolyte abnormalities

Table 8.4. Common diseases leading to potassium abnormalities.

Hyperkalemia	Hypokalemia
Renal failure Decreased urinary excretion • Urethral obstruction • Ureteral obstruction • Uroabdomen • Poor renal perfusion/reduced GFR Hypoadrenocorticism (decreased aldosterone) Release from damaged/destroyed cells • Rhabdomyolysis • Tumor lysis syndrome • Hemolysis Metabolic acidosis (shifting out of cells) Insulin deficiency Drug therapy • Beta blockers • ACE-inhibitors • Potassium-sparing diuretics (e.g. spironolactone) • Excessive potassium supplementation	Renal diuresis Renal failure Gastrointestinal losses (vomiting or diarrhea) Decreased intake (chronic) Translocation into cells • Treatment diabetic ketoacidosis • Insulin • Respiratory alkalosis • Hypothermia Metabolic alkalosis (shifting into cells) Catecholamines (exogenous or endogenous) Drug therapy • Loop diuretics (e.g. furosemide) • Albuterol overdose • Thiazide diuretics (e.g. hydrochlorothiazide)

ACE, acetylcholine esterase; GFR, glomerular filtration rate.

for more information on treatment of potassium disorders (see Further Reading section).

8.4 Interpretation of the Findings

The reader is referred to multiple other sources in the Further Reading section regarding detailed approaches to treating electrolytes. As with any clinical situation, ensure that the patient is not hypovolemic and displaying clinical signs of shock before focusing on treating measured electrolyte abnormalities. Table 8.5 presents some very broad and general approaches to treating abnormalities in the electrolytes discussed in this chapter.

Table 8.5. Generalized approach to treating electrolyte abnormalities.[a]

Electrolyte	Approach when hyper-	Approach when hypo-
Sodium	*Typically ≥160–170 mEq/L* Administer fluid therapy to replace free water deficit (and dilute the sodium) 1. Calculate water deficit Water deficit = weight (kg) × ($[Na]_{current}/[Na]_{normal} - 1$) Assume $[Na]_{normal}$ = 140–145 mEq/L *Some sources will multiply the above number by 0.6 to represent the proportion of the body's weight that is water, making the equation:* Water deficit = Weight (kg) × 0.6 × ($[Na]_{current}/[Na]_{normal} - 1$) 2. Select hypotonic fluid (5% dextrose in water or 0.45% saline) 3. Fluid rate = water deficit to patient over time[b] + maintenance fluids + replacement of any ongoing losses	*Typically when <130 mEq/L* As long as a patient is not hypervolemic on examination (e.g. liver failure, congestive heart failure, oliguric or anuric renal failure), administer fluid therapy rich in sodium to increase [Na][c] Calculated as: maintenance + dehydration replacement + replacement of any ongoing losses Treat the underlying cause leading to water retention (and dilution of Na).

Continued

Table 8.5. Continued.

Electrolyte	Approach when hyper-	Approach when hypo-
Calcium	*Typically when iCa >1.4 mmol/L* Techniques to lower calcium levels while treating the underlying cause: 1. Administer 0.9% saline fluid (Na in fluid induces calciuresis in the renal tubules) 2. Furosemide (induces renal calciuresis) 3. Glucocorticoids (various mechanisms) 4. Calcitonin (reduces osteoclast formation/activity) 5. Bisphosphonates (e.g. pamidronate; decrease osteoclast function/activity)	*Typically when iCa <0.8–1.0 mmol/L* 1. Treat the underlying cause 2. If significant clinical signs (e.g. tetany/seizures/cardiac arrhythmias): • Administer calcium (typically in the form of 10% calcium gluconate) IV slowly (over 5-10 min) or SQ • A continuous IV infusion of calcium gluconate may be needed • Start oral vitamin D therapy if the cause of hypocalcemia will be persistent • Start oral calcium carbonate therapy chronically, usually in concert with oral vitamin D therapy 3. If minimal to no clinical signs: • Consider starting oral vitamin D and oral calcium therapy without IV or SQ calcium gluconate • It may take a long period of time to normalize calcium unless the underlying disorder is rapidly corrected
Phosphorus	*Typically when $[PO_4^{3-}] > 7.0$ mg/dL* In most cases, no specific therapy is required to reduce phosphorus concentrations emergently 1. Treat the underlying disease 2. Administer fluid therapy to increase the glomerular filtration rate and filter phosphorus in the kidney 3. Administer oral phosphate binders (e.g. aluminum hydroxide) to reduce dietary intake of phosphorus once patient is eating	*Typically when $[PO_4^{3-}] < 1.5$ mg/dL* 1. Treat the underlying disease 2. Supplement phosphorus intake intravenously with phosphorus solution (often potassium phosphate solutions) 3. Recheck serum phosphorus levels every 6–12 hours 4. Monitor hematocrit tubing for signs of hemolysis/decreasing PCV
Potassium	*Typically when $[K^+] > 7.5$ mEq/L* Techniques to rapidly reduce potassium levels (while treating the underlying cause): 1. Administer crystalloid fluids with low to no K^+ content (increase GFR and wasting of K^+ by the kidneys) 2. Furosemide therapy (stimulates potassium wasting in the kidney) 3. Calcium gluconate (protects myocardium from effects of hyperkalemia; does not reduce potassium levels) 4. Insulin and dextrose (insulin pushes potassium into cells, dextrose prevents reflex hypoglycemia) 5. Sodium bicarbonate (moves potassium into cells in exchange for hydrogen ions)	*Typically when $[K^+] < 2.5$ mEq/L* 1. Supplement potassium (usually potassium chloride solutions) intravenously. Usually added to intravenous crystalloid fluid bag for administration. Concentrations $[K^+] > 80$ mEq/L should be given via central line to avoid phlebitis. In order to avoid negative cardiac side effects from potassium, the maximum rate of potassium supplementation is 0.5 mEq/kg/h 2. Chronically, oral potassium supplements are available (potassium gluconate)

iCa, ionized calcium; GFR, glomerular filtration rate; IV; intravenous; K^+, potassium, $[K^+]$, concentration of potassium in (mEq/L); Na, sodium; [Na], concentration of sodium (mEq/L); $[PO_4^{3-}]$, concentration of phosphorus (mg/dL); SQ, subcutaneous.
[a]Doses for specific medications are not included as the reader should reference other sources dedicated to treatment when faced with a clinical case (see Further Readings for treatment-related references).
[b]When replacing water losses for CHRONIC hypernatremia (>24–48 hours), remember that sodium levels should not decrease at a rate faster than 0.5–1.0 mEq/L/h to avoid rapid shifts of water into the brain cells causing cerebral edema. Therefore, chronic hypernatremia should be corrected relatively slowly with frequent monitoring of sodium levels (usually every 4–6 hours) during treatment to allow for adjustment of fluid rates. If the sodium levels are dropping too quickly with hypotonic fluids, fluids with a greater

Continued

Table 8.5. Continued.

concentration of sodium can be administered instead (lactated Ringer's solution, Plasmalyte, 0.9% saline) to slow the rate of sodium decline.
With ACUTE hypernatremia, sodium levels can be corrected quickly with high fluid rates (i.e. if you know the abnormality occurred within the last 8 hours, you can correct it within the next 8 hours).
^{c}When replacing sodium levels in CHRONIC hyponatremia (>24–48 hours), sodium levels should not increase at a rate faster than 0.5–1.0 mEq/L/h to avoid dehydrating the cells of the brain by increasing the osmolality of the blood too quickly (and drawing water out of the brain cells into the bloodstream). As with hypernatremia, sodium levels are typically checked every 4-6 hours to monitor the rate of the sodium increase and adjust the fluid rates accordingly.
With ACUTE hyponatremia, the sodium levels can be corrected as quickly as they occurred without concern.

8.5 Pitfalls of the Monitor

In general, electrolyte monitoring (whether done on a point-of-care instrument or a laboratory-based machine) is widely performed and time tested. Many publications have compared a variety of point-of-care instruments versus laboratory-based instrumentation in humans and various animal species. Electrolyte testing (Na, K, iCa) has high agreement between the two types of instrumentation in dogs and cats.

As with any laboratory machine, quality control and calibration should be performed per the instructions included with that instrument. Many of the point-of-care instruments do internal calibration and quality control. For example, an i-STAT system performs internal electronic simulation several times daily on its own to ensure viability of the ion-specific electrodes and notifies the operator with a warning message if the internal electronic simulation fails. Most point-of-care instruments still recommend periodic intermittent operator calibration. When point-of-care instruments use cartridges to effect electrolyte measurement, calibration is done automatically when the cartridges are inserted into the machine. In most cases, the manufacturer does not suggest that cartridges in a lot or box be checked against controls as long as cartridges are stored within the temperature limits, used within the expiration dates, and otherwise handled according to the manufacturer's recommendations. Some laboratories will independently test the cartridges according to protocols dictated by individual institutions.

Sodium

The biggest interference with *flame photometric* testing of sodium occurs when there is excessive lipemia or hyperproteinemia. Sodium is present in the aqueous portion of a blood sample (usually about 93% of the sample in health), but is not present in the approximately 7% of the blood occupied by proteins and lipids. However, flame photometric techniques report the amount of sodium per *total* volume of sample. Because the lipid and protein component is usually fairly small, for most samples this does not significantly affect the measured value. However, if the protein or lipid content of the blood is significantly greater than 7%, there will be a much smaller proportion of the sample which is aqueous from which to derive the sodium content. Therefore, when the sodium value is compared to the total sample volume (which is higher because of the lipemia and/or hyperproteinemia), the sodium concentration will be falsely lowered. This is termed pseudohyponatremia.

Typically, if lipid is causing pseuohyponatremia, the lipid is visible to the naked eye in the blood sample. Generally, 1 mg/dL of serum triglyceride reduces the sodium by 0.002 mEq/L so large amounts of triglyceride are required to significantly alter sodium concentrations. Similarly, patients with dramatic enough hyperproteinemia to affect laboratory results usually have viscous plasma. For hyperproteinemic cases, each 1 g/dL of protein above the level of 8 g/dL reduces the sodium concentration by 0.25 mEq/L.

When using ISE testing (whether it be a point-of-care analyzer or a laboratory machine), hyperlipidemia and hyperproteinemia generally do not alter sodium measurements unless there are large changes in lipid levels (typically triglyceride levels greater than 650 mg/dL), since the concentration of sodium is measured directly rather than versus the volume of the plasma. However, inappropriate dilution of the sample with anticoagulant or intravenous (IV) fluid contamination can alter results. Anticoagulant dilution occurs when too little blood is added to a tube containing sodium heparin anticoagulant. The 'extra' sodium heparin that is unbound to blood will falsely elevate the sodium. Similarly, if a patient is receiving sodium bromide as an anti-epileptic, the extra sodium can elevate the measured sodium levels. Potassium bromide (a cation with a single positive charge similar to sodium) may also be interpreted by the machine as sodium and falsely elevate blood sodium levels. If a blood sample is drawn from a sampling IV line that has not had an appropriate waste sample drawn first, there may be significant hemodilution of the sample with excessive lactated Ringer's solution or 0.9% saline or there can be *in vitro* dilution of a blood sample with isotonic crystalloid fluids. In both situations, the sodium in the isotonic crystalloid solutions can falsely increase sodium levels.

In contrast, any molecule that increases serum osmolality (β-hydroxybutyrate, glucose, mannitol, lactate) can decrease sodium concentrations by drawing more water into the plasma compartment where the sample is measured, even though the total body content of sodium may be normal. See Further Reading section readings for more information about mathematical correction factors for sodium in states of hyperosmolality.

Potassium

When using flame photometric methods to measure potassium, both lipemia and hyperproteinemia can potentially increase the non-aqueous proportion of the blood, leading to a false decrease in the serum potassium concentrations similar to that seen with sodium (see above for mechanism).

Potassium levels have also been shown to falsely decrease with ion-specific electrodes when triglyceride levels are higher than 650 mg/dL due to dilution of the sample with the potassium-free triglyceride component. Ion-selective electrode measurement of potassium can also be decreased when there is contamination of the sample with fluids that contain little to no potassium (0.9% sodium chloride, lactated Ringer's solution) or when osmotically active particles such as mannitol draw water into the intravascular compartment.

Potassium can be falsely elevated when using ISE or flame photometric testing. Anything that leads to cellular rupture and release of potassium into the sample can falsely elevate the potassium. This would include hemolysis due to placing samples on ice for prolonged periods and significant delays in testing after sample collection. Similarly, hemolysis induced by blood collection could increase potassium levels. In general, the potassium content of red blood cells in most veterinary species is low enough to not cause clinically significant changes in potassium levels, but widespread hemolysis or hemolysis of red blood cells from dog breeds such as the Akita which contain higher than normal amounts of potassium might cause clinically significant alterations in potassium levels.

Platelets and white blood cells can also leak potassium into plasma with prolonged storage; this is generally not an issue unless there are excessively large numbers of cells as in thrombocytosis (typically >500,000 cells/hpf) and leukocytosis (>70,000 cells/hpf). In addition, potassium release from both white blood cells and platelets during activation and coagulation in prolonged storage conditions can lead to hyperkalemia in states of leukocytosis and thrombocytosis. Normally platelet activation leads to increases in serum potassium that are generally 0.3–0.5 mmol/L greater than plasma, but these differences can be significantly increased with profound thrombocytosis. Conversely, leukocytes can also absorb potassium, which may falsely lower levels if the patient has a profound leukocytosis or leukemia.

Calcium

Total calcium

Total calcium is measured via colorimetric methods where a dye (orthocresolphthalein complexone or Arsenazo III) complexes with calcium and causes a color change. Therefore, anything that falsely alters the degree of color change by binding to the dye can falsely elevate total calcium levels. This would include lipemia and hemolysis. However, hyperbilirubinemia will falsely decrease calcium levels by binding to the calcium and not allowing calcium to complex with the dye. Use of anticoagulants such as EDTA, citrate, or oxalate can bind calcium, lowering the total calcium measurements. Thrombocytosis can also falsely increase total calcium levels in serum due to release of calcium during clotting.

In addition, since total calcium levels include the calcium that is protein bound, changes in protein concentration (primarily albumin) will alter measured total calcium levels. Therefore, hypoalbuminemia will cause a decreased total calcium level. Similarly, if levels of albumin are elevated, measured total calcium levels will be (falsely) increased.

iCa

Ionized calcium is only measured by ion-selective electrodes. Historically, other positively charged electrolytes such as magnesium, lithium, and potassium would interfere with the measurement of iCa, causing falsely increased iCa levels. However, newer ion-selective electrodes are less likely to have interference and present more reliable measures of iCa, minimizing the chances that magnesium, sodium, or administration of sodium or potassium bromide will falsely increase iCa concentrations. Another reason for falsely increased iCa levels is release of calcium from the silicone separator in blood tubes. Follow your analyzer's instructions for the appropriate tube type to minimize such changes but often lithium heparin tubes are used.

Other medications may decrease iCa levels by binding calcium that would normally be in the ionized (free) form. These medications include acetaminophen, salicylates (i.e. aspirin), and acetylcysteine. Heparin mixed with whole blood (as opposed to serum) can lower iCa levels by 0.05–0.26 mmol/L in dogs and 0.05–0.14 mmol/L in cats. This occurs exclusively in inappropriately heparinized samples when too much heparin is combined with too little blood. Common situations would include not putting enough blood in a pre-heparinized blood gas syringes or adding unmeasured amounts of heparin to a syringe. The appropriate amount of liquid heparin to add to a syringe when testing for iCa is 10 IU/mL.

Changes in blood sample pH can also affect measured iCa levels. Acidemia causes dissociation of calcium from proteins and falsely elevates iCa levels. In contrast, alkalemia can lead to increased Ca binding to proteins, falsely lowering iCa levels. The most common cause of erroneous alkalemia occurs when blood samples are stored exposed to air for long periods of time. Long-term exposure to air will cause a decrease in carbon dioxide levels as it is lost to the environment, resulting in alkalemia.

Phosphorus

Phosphorus is measured by a colorimetric test and is therefore affected by factors that alter the color of the serum. Therefore, icterus, lipemia, and hemolysis will alter colorimetric testing and falsely increase phosphorus levels. Similarly, hyperproteinemia (especially when due to increased serum globulins) will lead to opaque precipitates in the serum that falsely elevate serum phosphorus levels detected by colorimetric testing. In addition, glassware contaminated with detergents and even medications can lead to color changes or precipitates in the serum that alter colorimetric testing and falsely increase phosphorus levels.

Hemolysis of the blood sample will also release phosphorus into the serum from the hemolyzed cells, increasing the amount of serum phosphorus measured. Long-term storage of blood samples can also falsely increase phosphorus levels as phosphorus leaches out of red and white blood cells and thrombocytes into the sample. This is especially common in situations with larger than normal numbers of cells in the blood (e.g. thrombocytosis or leukocytosis).

Conversely, mannitol will draw water into the serum and dilute phosphorus levels (true decreases in serum phosphorus) or it can interfere with phosphorus binding to molydate (the dye used in colorimetric testing) and falsely decrease the measured phosphorus levels. Recent carbohydrate-rich food intake will also decrease circulating serum phosphorus because the resulting insulin release in response to the carbohydrates will push phosphorus transiently into cells, creating a falsely low serum phosphorus at the time of measurement. Actual circulating phosphorus levels can be measured after a fasting period to remove the effect of insulin release on phosphorus.

8.6 Case Studies

Case study 1: The hypernatremic cat

An approximately 10-year-old female spayed domestic long-haired cat named Norah was presented to the hospital for evaluation. She had been adopted and spayed approximately 5 weeks prior to presentation by her current owners. Since her spay, she had lost three pounds and had never eaten or drunk well. She also had a spay site infection immediately after the surgery that resolved with antibiotic therapy administered 1 and 4 weeks postoperatively. For the 4 days prior to presentation, Norah had been receiving meloxicam orally once daily and she had also been receiving triple antibiotic eye lubricant three times daily in both eyes for 2 weeks to treat ocular discharge.

At presentation, she was hypothermic (98.4°F; 36.9°C), mildly tachycardic (heart rate 212 beats per minute) and was very thin (2.0 kg; body condition score 2/9). She had mucopurulent ocular discharge and blepharospasm in both eyes with a fractured right maxillary canine tooth. There was evidence of dehydration on examination (prolonged skin tenting, tacky mucous membranes). She appeared to be weak and was obtunded. She also had a grade I–II/VI left-sided systolic heart murmur with normal lung sounds and was estimated to be approximately 8% dehydrated.

Bloodwork was performed which revealed evidence of hemoconcentration: total protein 10.8 g/dL (normal 6.0–8.0 g/dL) and hematocrit 62% (normal 30–45%). She also had azotemia characterized by a blood urea nitrogen (BUN) of 294 mg/dL (normal 15–25 mg/dL) and creatinine 12.60 mg/dL (normal 0.9–2.3 mg/dL). She was severely hypernatremic with a *sodium concentration of 207 mEq/L (normal 148–157 mEq/L)*. Her urine specific gravity was 1.024 suggesting an inappropriate concentrating ability given her clinical dehydration.

Norah was diagnosed with renal failure and dehydration with concurrent chronic hypernatremia (based on the duration of her clinical signs). During the first night of hospitalization, the initial goal was to correct her dehydration and observe for changes in her sodium during that correction period. She was given an isotonic crystalloid that was comparatively high in total sodium content to slow the overall decrease in sodium as she was rehydrated and attempt to keep her rate of sodium decrease no more than 1 mEq/L/h.

Therefore, she was initially placed on 0.9% saline fluids to correct an estimated 8% dehydration over 12 hours plus administer maintenance fluids. Her estimated dehydration deficit was 160 mL (13.3 mL/h given over 12 hours) and her maintenance fluid rate was calculated at 3.3 mL/h (40 mL/kg/day). The total fluid rate was 17 mL/h or 215 mL/kg/day. She was also given famotidine and maropitant to treat uremia-associated gastrointestinal disease from her renal failure and started on ofloxacin and cidofovir topically to treat the corneal ulcer. She almost immediately started eating in the hospital and her mentation improved during the initial overnight period with fluid therapy.

Since her renal failure and hypernatremia were likely chronic, the goal was to reduce her sodium levels by no more than 0.5–1.0 mEq/L/h to prevent cerebral edema formation. Please see Table 8.6 for the serial BUN, creatinine, and Na levels in Norah. Her fluid rates and fluid types are included on the chart for reference as well as the frequency at which her sodium levels were checked. Footnotes to the table provide rationale for the various fluid rates selected. The chart is not meant as a guide for treatment but simply to illustrate the fluctuations in Na levels in a real clinical case.

Norah was discharged on the day 6 of hospitalization and was reportedly doing well at home.

Case study 2: The hyperkalemic cat

A 6-year-old male neutered domestic shorthaired cat named Stormy was presented to the hospital for evaluation of vocalizing and vomiting. The owners also felt that he had been more lethargic than usual overnight. He had a history of a prior urethral obstruction, was indoor–outdoor, and had no other pre-existing health problems.

On presentation, Stormy was quiet, alert and responsive with normal heart and lung sounds. His heart rate was 180 beats per minute. He was hypothermic (temperature 96.5°F; 35.8°C). A large firm bladder was palpated in the abdomen that could not be expressed. He was diagnosed with a urethral obstruction.

Bloodwork was performed which revealed a BUN >140 mg/dL, creatinine 14.6 mg/dL, and *potassium of >9.0 mEq/L*. Stormy was given a bolus of intravenous crystalloids (plasmalyte, 20 mL/kg), calcium gluconate (100 mg/kg of 10% calcium gluconate), and insulin/dextrose (0.5 U/kg regular insulin + 2 g of 25% dextrose/unit of insulin) to treat his hyperkalemia. General anesthesia was induced with hydromorphone and propofol to allow placement of a urinary catheter to relieve the obstruction. After the fluid bolus and relief of the obstruction, his potassium was 7.9 mEq/L, creatinine was 12.2 mg/dL, and BUN was >140 mg/dL.

Please see Table 8.7 for the subsequent interventions and values for Stormy's potassium over the next few days of his hospitalization. Each time Stormy received a fluid bolus as indicated below, it

Table 8.6. Serial sodium, blood urea nitrogen, and creatinine values and the fluid interventions taken in response to blood values in an elderly cat with renal failure. Footnotes to the table provide further rationale for the various fluid rates selected.

Time (hours)	BUN (mg/dL) Normal: 15–35	Creatinine (mg/dL) Normal: 0.9–2.3	Na (mEq/L) Normal: 148–157	Rate of Na change (mEq/L/h)	Fluid type and rate
0	294	12.6	207	–	0.9% NaCl at 215 mL/kg/day
12			198	−0.7	0.9% NaCl at 165 mL/kg/day[a]
19	236	9.7	196	−0.28	0.9% NaCl at 165 mL/kg/day
22			193	−1	0.9% NaCl at 165 mL/kg/day
26			186	−1.75	0.9% NaCl at 165 mL/kg/day
37	125	5.5	188	+0.18	0.9% NaCl at 120 mL/kg/day[b]
43			186	−0.33	0.9% NaCl at 120 mL/kg/day
49			183	−0.5	0.9% NaCl at 120 mL/kg/day
61	83	4.1	180	−0.25	0.9% NaCl at 100 mL/kg/day[b]
72			173	−0.63	0.9% NaCl at 100 mL/kg/day
84	67	2.6	165	−0.66	0.9% NaCl at 100 mL/kg/day
92	66	2.6	163	−0.25	0.9% NaCl at 60 mL/kg/day[c]
101	63	2.6	161	−0.22	0.9% NaCl at 60 mL/kg/day
108	59	2.4	160	−0.14	0.9% NaCl at 40 mL/kg/day
113	60	2.4	156	−0.8	0.9% NaCl at 40 mL/kg/day Discharged later that day to owner

BUN, blood urea nitrogen; 0.9% NaCl (also known as 'normal saline') is an isotonic crystalloid fluid with a sodium content of 154 mEq/L.
[a]At approximately 12 hours of hospitalization, Norah's dehydration was improved based on her physical examination findings (weight was 1.9 kg). Her water deficit was calculated as shown in Table 8.5. In Norah's case, we did not multiply by the 0.6 factor.

Water deficit = Weight (kg) × ($[Na]_{current}/[Na]_{normal} - 1$)

= 1.9 kg × (198/145 −1) = 694mL

Since it was likely a chronic hypernatremia (and Norah had a heart murmur), we wanted to replace this sodium deficit over 72 at the fastest. This would equate to ~10 mL/h in addition to her maintenance fluid rate (40 mL/kg/day= 3 mL/h) or 13 mL/h (165 mL/kg/day) total.
[b]At approximately 36 hours of hospitalization, Norah's Na, BUN, and creatinine values were dropping consistently and her dehydration seemed to be completely resolved. Her heart murmur was persistent but unchanged. She was eating and drinking water readily. Due to concerns about fluid overload with continued high IV fluid rates and the fact that she was definitely taking in large amounts of water per day in her canned food intake and water intake in addition to her fluids, her IV fluid rate was decreased. Reducing her fluid rate to first 120 mL/kg/day and then to 100 mL/kg/day at 61 hours of hospitalization were somewhat arbitrary decisions to reduce her fluid therapy ~20–25% each day but were supported by the fact that her sodium continued to decrease. She was also kept on 0.9% NaCl since her sodium was continuing to decrease on that fluid type at a reasonable rate (overall 0.5-1 mEq/h). If her sodium values had not continued to decrease, her fluid type would have been changed to lactated Ringer's solution or plasmalyte, both of which contain less sodium per mL than 0.9% NaCl or potentially even a hypotonic fluid such as 0.45% NaCl or 5% dextrose in water. In addition, if she had displayed any hyperchloremia from the 0.9% NaCl, her fluid type would have been changed to a fluid with less chloride content.
[c]Between 84 and 92 hours of hospitalization, Norah's Na, BUN, and creatinine had reached a plateau. Therefore, fluid weaning was continued by first reducing the fluid rate by approximately one-third and then, when Na, BUN, and creatinine remained at a plateau, reducing her to maintenance fluids (40 mL/kg/day) at 108 hours of hospitalization prior to discharge.

Table 8.7. Serial potassium values in an obstructed cat.

Time	K+ (mEq/L) Normal: 2.9–4.2	Intervention
Presentation	>9.0	Bolus 20 mL/kg plasmalyte 100 mg/kg of 10% calcium gluconate bolus 0.5 U/kg regular insulin + 2 g of 25% dextrose/unit of insulin 120 mL/kg/day plasmalyte + 2.5% dextrose infusion[a] Pass urethral catheter under general anesthesia
Post-unblocking	7.9	Bolus 10 mL/kg plasmalyte 120 mL/kg/day plasmalyte + 2.5% dextrose solution Administer additional plasmalyte to match urine production above and beyond the fluid rate above
3 h post-unblocking	5.9	Bolus 10 mL/kg plasmalyte 120 mL/kg/day plasmalyte + 2.5% dextrose solution[b] Administer additional plasmalyte to match urine production above and beyond the fluid rate above
12 h post-unblocking	5.8	Bolus 10 mL/kg plasmalyte 0.25 U/kg regular insulin + 2 g of 25% dextrose/unit of insulin 120 mL/kg/day plasmalyte + 2.5% dextrose solution Administer additional plasmalyte to match urine production above and beyond the fluid rate above
16 h post-unblocking	5.9	120 mL/kg/day plasmalyte + 2.5% dextrose solution Administer additional plasmalyte to match urine production above and beyond the fluid rate above
19 h post-unblocking	6.0	120 mL/kg/day plasmalyte + 2.5% dextrose solution Administer additional plasmalyte to match urine production above and beyond the fluid rate above
23 h post-unblocking	5.3	120 mL/kg/day plasmalyte[c] Administer additional plasmalyte to match urine production above and beyond the fluid rate above
31 h post-unblocking	4.1	120 mL/kg/day plasmalyte Administer additional plasmalyte to match urine production above and beyond the fluid rate above
43 h post-unblocking	3.6	60 mL/kg/day plasmalyte + 0.1 mEq/kg/h KCl[d] Administer additional plasmalyte to match urine production above and beyond the fluid rate above
51 h post-unblocking	3.4	60 mL/kg/day plasmalyte + 0.1 mEq/kg/h KCl Administer additional plasmalyte to match urine production above and beyond the fluid rate above
67 h post-unblocking	3.9	60 mL/kg/day plasmalyte + 0.1 mEq/kg/h KCl Administer additional plasmalyte to match urine production above and beyond the fluid rate above
75 h post-unblocking	3.7	60 mL/kg/day plasmalyte + 0.1 mEq/kg/h KCl Administer additional plasmalyte to match urine production above and beyond the fluid rate above
91 h post-unblocking	4.2	60 mL/kg/day plasmalyte Discharged to owner later that day

IV, intravenous; K+, potassium; plasmalyte is an isotonic crystalloid fluid with 10 mEq/L of potassium present in the solution.
[a]Stormy was given a 2.5% dextrose infusion with his IV fluids to ensure that his blood glucose did not drop due to the residual effects of the insulin he had been given.
[b]His blood glucose had decreased to <20 mg/dL so an additional bolus of 10 mL of 25% dextrose was given to correct blood glucose.
[c]Dextrose supplementation was discontinued due to several normal blood glucose measurements after last dose of insulin 12 hours prior.
[d]KCl supplementation was added to ensure that the potassium levels did not fall significantly lower than this with prolonged fluid therapy and the continuing post-obstructive diuresis Stormy was experiencing.

was to improve kidney perfusion and increase renal excretion of potassium. Stormy was discharged on the day 4 of hospitalization and did not return with an additional urethral obstruction. Table 8.7 is not meant as a guide to treatment but simply to illustrate the changes in potassium in response to various interventions in a real clinical case.

Case study 3: The chronically hypocalcemic dog

Queenie, an 8-year-old female spayed Pit Bull Terrier was presented to the hospital for evaluation of abnormal behavior. For at least 24 hours prior to presentation, the owners reported that she was squinting her eyes, shaking her head and pawing at her face. She seemed to be restless and they also noted muscle tremors as well as rhythmic teeth clicking. The owners felt that she was becoming progressively weaker and having more and more trouble getting up on the couch. She had been eating well until the day of presentation when she did not have an appetite. Her water consumption was unchanged. She received no medications other than monthly heartworm preventative. There was no history of toxin exposure.

While at her primary care veterinarian's office being examined prior to presentation at the hospital, she became laterally recumbent with worsening muscle tremors and blood was noted in her mouth. Bloodwork at her primary veterinarian's office revealed hypocalcemia and hypernatremia (exact values unknown).

On presentation to our hospital, Queenie was ambulatory but severely obtunded. Her temperature was 100.6°F (38.1°C), heart rate 90 beats per minute, and respiratory rate 44 breaths/min. Her level of awareness waxed and waned, ranging from being almost stuporous to mild obtundation. She had multiple erythematous regions on her skin with scattered crusts and superficial abrasions. There was a scab on her tail and a 3 cm rounded pedunculated mass on the right lateral phalanx of her front leg. Ophthalmologic examination revealed

Table 8.8. Serial ionized calcium levels in a dog with hypoparathyroidism presenting for neurologic signs and cardiac arrhythmias.

Time (hours)	iCa levels (normal 1.2–1.3 mmol/L)	Intervention
Presentation (time 0)	0.48	1 mL/kg 10% calcium gluconate IV over 30 minutes 1.0 g/kg IV mannitol over 30 minutes
1	1.22[a]	120 mL/kg/day plasmalyte
8	0.72	90 mL/kg/day plasmalyte
21	0.69	60 mL/kg/day plasmalyte
27	0.66[b]	60 mL/kg/day lactated Ringer's solution 1 mL/kg 10% calcium gluconate IV over 30 minutes *Calcium carbonate tablets started at 50 mg/kg by mouth every 12 hours* *Calcitriol started at 0.02 mg/kg by mouth every 12 hours*
33	0.79	60 mL/kg/day lactated Ringer's solution
41	0.79	60 mL/kg/day lactated Ringer's solution
65	0.53[c]	60 mL/kg/day lactated Ringer's solution Sent home later that day

iCa, ionized calcium; plasmalyte is an isotonic crystalloid with 5 mEq/L of calcium; lactated Ringer's solution is an isotonic crystalloid with 3 mEq/L of calcium.
[a]Due to the initial improvement in iCa values (and clinical condition) with calcium gluconate treatment and the fact that Queenie had not been worked up at all for her clinical signs, the iCa levels were initially just observed and not treated again.
[b]After about 24 hours of hospitalization when hypoparathyroidism became the top differential, Queenie was started on oral vitamin D (calcitriol) and oral calcium carbonate. She was given one more bolus of calcium gluconate since any increase in iCa due to calcitriol can take hours to days to become apparent.
[c]Even though Queenie's iCa levels had actually dropped while in the hospital when she was receiving calcium carbonate and calcitriol orally, she was not displaying any cardiac signs and her mentation had improved from presentation. The owners requested that she be discharged for continued care at home.

small punctate lesions on her lenses bilaterally that were consistent with chronic hypocalcemia.

Her total calcium was low (5.8 mg/dL, normal 9.7–12.3 mg/dL). An ionized calcium (iCa) on a bedside monitor revealed 0.48 mmol/L (normal 1.2–1.3 mmol/L) with all other electrolytes normal or near normal including the sodium reported by her primary care veterinarian (Na= 131 mEq/L; normal 139-150 mEq/L). An electrocardiogram (ECG) placed at the time of presentation revealed a variety of heart rates and rhythms ranging from sinus bradycardia (heart rate 50–60 bpm) to an idioventricular rhythm (heart rate 90–100 bpm) and then an escape rhythm (heart rate <40 bpm). During the period when she was displaying various bradyarrhythmias, her measured blood pressure was 240 mmHg. She was given 1 mL/kg of 10% calcium gluconate IV slowly over 30 minutes to address her hypocalcemia while observing the ECG for worsening bradycardia. She was also given mannitol (1 g/kg IV over 30 minutes) to treat a possible Cushing's reflex (obtunded mentation with bradycardia and hypertension). These signs seemed to resolve with treatment but it was unclear if the calcium gluconate or the mannitol had a greater effect.

Table 8.8 shows Queenie's serial iCa measurements and the intervention taken in response to each one. This table is not meant as a guide to treatment but simply to illustrate alterations in calcium in response to various interventions in a real clinical case.

Queenie was worked up for her hypocalcemia and diagnosed with primary hypoparathyroidism on the basis of an inappropriately low parathyroid hormone level (0.6 pmol/L; normal 0.5–5.8 pmol/L) in the face of a low iCa (0.86 mmol/L; normal 1.25–1.45 mmol/L). She was discharged 3 days after presentation on oral calcium carbonate tablets and vitamin D to manage her hypoparathyroidism. Follow-up 4 months after discharge revealed that Queenie was doing well aside from intermittent episodes once or twice a week wherein she would run in circles chasing her tail and then freeze, but was responsive to her name during those events. Her mentation was back to normal and she was otherwise doing well.

Further Reading

Matthews, K.M. (2017) *Veterinary Emergency and Critical Care Manual*, 3rd edn. Lifelearn, Guelph, Ontario, Canada.

Plunkett, S.J. (2013) *Emergency Procedures for the Small Animal Practitioner*, 3rd edn. Saunders Elsevier, Philadelphia, Pennsylvania, USA.

Bibliography

Bleul, U., Gotz, E. (2014) Evaluation of the i-STAT portable point-of-care analyzer for determination of blood gases and acid-base status in newborn calves. *Journal of Veterinary Emergency and Critical Care* 24, 519–528.

Burnett, R.W., Covington, A.K., Fogh-Andersen, N., et al. (2000) Use of ion-selective electrodes for blood-electrolyte analysis. Recommendations for nomenclature, definitions, and conventions. International Federation of Clinical Chemistry and Laboratory Medicine (IFCC). Scientific Division Working Group on Selective Electrodes. *Clinical Chemistry and Laboratory Medicine* 38, 363–70.

Dalal, B.I., Brigden, M.L. (2009) Factitious biochemical measurements resulting from hematologic conditions. *American Journal of Clinical Pathology* 131, 195–204.

DiBartola, S.P. (2012) Disorders of sodium and water: hypernatremia and hyponatremia. In: Dibartola, S.P. (ed.) *Fluid, Electrolyte and Acid-Base Disorders in Small Animal Practice*, 4th edn. Elsevier, St. Louis, Missouri, USA, pp. 45–79.

DiBartola, S.P., de Morais, H.A. (2012) Disorders of potassium: hypokalemia and hyperkalemia. In: Dibartola, S.P. (ed.) *Fluid, Electrolyte and Acid-Base Disorders in Small Animal Practice*, 4th edn. Elsevier, St. Louis, Missouri, USA, pp. 92–119.

DiBartola, S.P., Willard, M.D. (2012) Disorders of phosphorus: hypophosphatemia and hyperphosphatemia. In: Dibartola, S.P. (ed.) *Fluid, Electrolyte and Acid-Base Disorders in Small Animal Practice*, 4th edn. Elsevier, St. Louis, Missouri, USA, pp. 195–211.

Estridge, B.H., Reynolds, A.P. (2012) Principles of chemistry instrumentation. In: Estridge, B.H., Reynolds, A.P. (eds) *Basic Clinical Laboratory Techniques*, 6th edn. Delmar Cengage Learning, Clifton Park, New York, USA, pp. 622–629.

Higgins, C. (2007) Pseudohyponatremia. Available at: https://acutecaretesting.org/en/articles/pseudohyponatremia (accessed 1 March, 2019).

Learn more about flame photometry (2019) Available at: www.sciencedirect.com/topics/medicine-and-dentistry/flame-photometry (accessed 15 February 2019).

Liamis, G., Liberopoulos, E., Barkasa, F., et al. (2013) Spurious electrolyte disorders: a diagnostic challenge for clinicians. *American Journal of Nephrology* 38, 50–57.

Nikolac, N. (2014) Lipemia: causes, interference mechanisms, detection, and management. *Biochemia Medica (Zagreb)* 24, 57–67.

Schenk, P.A., Chew, D.J., Nagode, L.A., *et al*. (2012) Disorders of calcium: hypercalcemia and hypocalcemia. In: Dibartola, S.P. (ed.) *Fluid, Electrolyte and Acid-Base Disorders in Small Animal Practice*, 4th edn. Elsevier, St. Louis, Missouri, USA, pp. 120–194.

Stockham, S.L., Scott, M.A. (2008) Monovalent electrolytes and osmolality. In: *Fundamentals of Veterinary Clinical Pathology*, 2nd edn. Blackwell Publishing, Ames, Iowa, USA, pp. 495–558.

Tappin, S., Rizzo, F., Dodkin, S., *et al*. (2008) Measurement of ionized calcium in canine blood samples collected in prefilled and self-filled heparinized syringes using the i-STAT point-of-care analyzer. *Veterinary Clinical Pathology* 37, 66–72.

Verwaerde, P., Malet, C., Lagente, M., *et al*. (2002) The accuracy of the i-STAT portable analyser for measuring blood gases and pH in whole blood samples from dogs. *Research in Veterinary Science* 73, 71–75.

Walker, H.K., Hall, W.D., Hurst, J.W. (eds) (1990) *Clinical Methods: The History, Physical and Laboratory Examinations*, 3rd edn. Butterworth, Boston, Massachusetts, USA.

West, E., Bardell, D., Senior, J.M. (2014) Comparison of EPOC and i-STAT analyzers for canine blood gas and electrolyte analysis. *Journal of Small Animal Practice*, 55, 139–144.

Coagulation

ELIZABETH J. THOMOVSKY* AND AIMEE C. BROOKS

Purdue University College of Veterinary Medicine, West Lafayette, Indiana, USA

9.1 Basic Physiology and Anatomy

Coagulation is a complex process that involves the interaction of the body (typically the vascular endothelium), the platelets, and a host of coagulation factors with the goal to prevent the patient from bleeding excessively after injury. There are two parts to the coagulation system – primary (platelet-based) and secondary (coagulation factor-based) hemostasis. The historic belief was that primary coagulation occurs first with platelets coming to an area, creating a platelet plug, and then activating the secondary coagulation system (clotting factors). This standard 'cascade' for secondary coagulation was described as a linear flow of coagulation factors (Fig. 9.1) that occurs after the platelet becomes activated. Since this does not adequately describe the actual interactions of the various cells involved in coagulation, an 'advanced' model of coagulation was introduced in 1992 (see below).

Primary hemostasis

Platelets are typically thought of as the first responders for coagulation. The platelet itself is an anuclear cell created in the bone marrow by megakaryocytes. Its main function is to provide a surface for coagulation and to store various factors that are important in the events related to coagulation and inflammation. It is covered with a variety of glycoproteins that mediate adhesion to the endothelium and to other platelets, as well as mediating signaling between the platelets and other cells. This 'crosstalk' is critical in activating platelets and calling other cells to the area. The two most important storage organelles in the platelet are the alpha and dense granules (see Table 9.1). Each contain various cytokines and other proteins such as platelet factor 4, factors V and XIII, fibrinogen, von Willebrand's factor (vWF), serotonin, adenosine diphosphate (ADP) and calcium. The latter three items are in the dense granules and the other listed factors are in the alpha granules. Some of these items are involved in clot formation (factors V and XIII, vWF, fibrinogen, Ca), others are involved in mediating vascular tone to vasodilate locally to allow for ease of clot formation (serotonin), and still others aid in platelet activation (ADP).

Platelet plug formation is divided into three phases: initiation, activation, and adhesion (also known as aggregation) (Fig. 9.2). *Initiation* occurs when a platelet that is rolling through the blood vessel detects disruption or damage to the endothelium. Damage to the endothelium leads to exposure of collagen and vWF. Exposed vWF interacts with GPIb/V/IX (a platelet glycoprotein receptor) causing adhesion of platelets to the damaged site on the endothelium. In addition, the glycoprotein receptor GPVI on the platelet surface binds to exposed collagen, and both collagen and the remaining exposed subendothelial materials bind to GPIIb/IIIa (another platelet surface glycoprotein receptor; also known as integrin α_{IIb}/β_3) and other platelet surface receptors. This initial binding to damaged endothelial surfaces constitutes the initiation phase of platelet plug formation.

The *activation* phase occurs as these platelets that are bound to vWF and/or collagen are stimulated to change shape from a disk to a sphere. As they change shape, the platelets both create pseudopods that can 'grab' more platelets, and are stimulated to release the contents of their alpha and dense granules. These granule contents work to further enhance platelet adhesion and activation (see Table 9.1). Additionally, the activated platelets have various enzymes including flippases, floppases, and scramblases, which work to change the charge of the cell surface as well as change the population of lipid-based cell surface markers to make the platelet

---

* Corresponding author: ethomovs@purdue.edu

© CAB International, 2020. *Basic Monitoring in Canine and Feline Emergency Patients*
(eds E.J. Thomovsky, P.A. Johnson and A.C. Brooks)

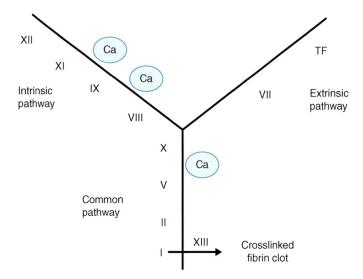

Fig. 9.1. Traditional ('waterfall') model of secondary hemostasis. The extrinsic 'arm' of the coagulation cascade begins with exposed tissue factor (TF or factor III) that cleaves factor VII to factor VIIa (activated factor VII). The activated factor VII then triggers the common pathway of coagulation by cleaving factor X to Xa that, in the presence of calcium (Ca), will activate factor V. Factor Va then cleaves prothrombin (factor II) to thrombin (factor IIa) which in turn causes fibrinogen (factor I) to activate to fibrin (factor Ia). The resulting fibrin is then crosslinked into the final 'hard' clot by the action of factor XIII. The intrinsic 'arm' of the coagulation cascade is also able to activate the common pathway to make fibrin and a crosslinked clot. The intrinsic arm classically begins with factor XII becoming activated to XIIa which then cleaves factor XI to XIa in the presence of Ca. The activated factor XI will stimulate conversion of factor IX to IXa in the presence of Ca which then activates VIII to VIIIa. The activated factor VIII will subsequently trigger the common pathway.

Table 9.1. Summary of the most common contents of platelet granules and their most common function in coagulation.

Platelet granules	Function
vWF (α granules)	Platelet–platelet and platelet–endothelium binding
Fibrinogen (α granules)	Platelet–platelet and platelet–endothelium binding
Factor V (α granules)	Secondary hemostasis, forms part of prothrombinase complex
Factor XIII (α granules)	Secondary hemostasis, crosslinks fibrin strands
Antithrombin (α granules)	Inhibits secondary hemostasis, inhibits thrombin and factor X
TFPI (α granules)	Inhibits secondary hemostasis, inhibits extrinsic factor tenase complex
Protein S (α granules)	Inhibits secondary hemostasis, inhibits factors VIII and V
Plasmin/plasminogen (α granules)	Initiates fibrinolysis
Prothrombin (α granules)	Activates platelets, involved in secondary hemostasis
Calcium (dense granules)	Important cofactor for all stages of secondary hemostasis
ADP (dense granules)	Binds to ADP receptor on the platelet cell surface causing platelet activation
Serotonin (dense granules)	Causes platelet aggregation, platelet activation, local blood vessel dilation
Thromboxane A_2 (created in platelet)	Manufactured via the arachidonic acid cascade within the platelet. Binds to the TXA_2 receptor on the platelet surface to activate platelets

ADP, adenosine diphosphate; TFPI, tissue factor pathway inhibitor; TXA_2, thromboxane A2; vWF, von Willebrand factor.

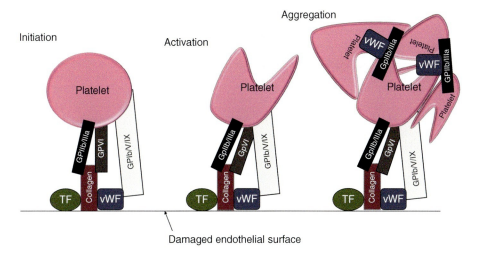

Fig. 9.2. The stages of platelet plug formation. Initiation occurs when exposed collagen/subendothelial factors and von Willebrand's factor (vWF) on the endothelial surface interacts with platelet surface glycoprotein receptors GPIIb/IIIa, GPIb/V/IX, and GPVI on the cell surface. Activation then involves a change in platelet shape from discoid to round with pseudopods. Additionally, the activity of various enzymes and mediators released from the platelet granules (see the text for more information) leads to a change in the signaling milieu on the platelet's surface. Finally, aggregation describes the connection of various activated platelets with each other to form a platelet plug. Typically, aggregation is facilitated by GPIIb/IIIa expressed on the surface of each activated platelet with vWF released from the alpha granules of the activated platelets. TF = tissue factor; GP = glycoprotein; vWF = von Willebrand's factor.

membrane a procoagulant surface and provide various types of cellular signaling. Activation of platelets also causes the expression of various glycoproteins including p-selectin and CD40 ligand on the cell surface and activates the GPIIb/IIIa integrin. The GPIIb/IIIa integrin is the primary surface glycoprotein that attaches to other platelets in the presence of vWF and causes *adhesion (aggregation)* of platelets. Typically, aggregation also occurs in the presence of fibrinogen either released from alpha granules or created by the secondary coagulation cascade.

In summary, damaged endothelium has the ability to grab and hold onto platelets that are passing by (adhesion). These platelets in turn become activated: changing shape, altering the charge on the cell surface, and releasing their granule contents to allow them to aggregate with other platelets and create the platelet plug. However, this does not occur by itself but in tandem and simultaneously with the secondary coagulation cascade.

Secondary hemostasis

The secondary coagulation cascade is mediated by clotting factors. These clotting factors are produced by the liver and certain factors (II, VII, IX, and X) require carboxylation by vitamin K to become fully activated. Secondary coagulation is triggered by the same tissue damage that causes platelet adhesion. Damaged endothelial walls expose tissue factor (TF) as well as collagen, subendothelial factors, and vWF. While TF is expressed in endothelial tissues constitutively, increased amounts of TF are found in inflammatory conditions. Additionally, TF is found on monocytes and platelets, especially under pro-inflammatory conditions, providing a more mobile surface upon which secondary coagulation can occur. In more recent literature, microparticles have been described which are blebs of cell membranes from platelets, monocytes, or other (especially inflammatory) cells. These microparticles are essentially small traveling pieces of cell membrane that express TF on their surfaces. Microparticles are significant because they provide a possible mechanism for the formation of thrombi in tissues distant from sites of endothelial damage and are likely a large player in systemic inflammatory illnesses like sepsis.

The initial phase of the secondary coagulation cascade is known as the *initiation phase* (see Fig. 9.3). The goal of the initiation phase is to make a very small amount of thrombin (factor II) through two steps. The first step of initiation is to take exposed TF on some sort of cell surface (vascular endothelium, platelet, or microparticle) and bind it to factor VII and Ca. Factor VII is the only coagulation factor that circulates in the bloodstream, and it has the shortest half-life of all the coagulation factors (approximately 6 hours). The calcium used in this reaction is often released from dense granules in activated platelets. This complex of factors (conveniently the same factors listed in the extrinsic arm of the coagulation cascade; see Fig. 9.1) is known as the *extrinsic factor tenase complex*. And as predicted by the traditional coagulation cascade, this extrinsic factor tenase complex cleaves factor X to form activated factor X (Xa). It also concurrently cleaves factor IX to activated factor IX (IXa). All these reactions occur on the cell surface.

In the second step of initiation (see Fig. 9.3B), the activated factor X binds to factor V and Ca (both typically released from activated platelet dense granules) on the same cell surface to form the prothrombinase complex. The prothrombinase complex works to cleave prothrombin (II) to activated thrombin (IIa). Initiation yields a relatively small amount of thrombin that is needed to fulfill several functions:

- Thrombin is a potent platelet agonist which activates platelets and facilitates ongoing platelet-to-platelet aggregation (see Fig. 9.2).
- Thrombin activates scramblase to move phosphatidylserine to the platelet surface (in order to make platelet surfaces negatively charged and friendly to further procoagulant reactions).
- Thrombin generates more activated factor VIII.
- Thrombin activates factor XI to generate further amplification of coagulation (see text below and Fig. 9.4).
- Thrombin can activate fibrinogen to fibrin in order to form the clot (see text below and Fig. 9.4).
- Thrombin activates factor XIII to crosslink the fibrin (see text below and Fig. 9.4).
- Thrombin activates various anticoagulant and anti-fibrinolytic systems (see text below and Figs 9.5 to 9.7).

The *amplification phase* of coagulation is the second stage of secondary coagulation (see Fig. 9.4). As explained in the updated model of hemostasis, amplification occurs CONCURRENTLY with the prothrombinase complex activation in initiation because factor IX activated by the extrinsic factor tenase complex (see Fig. 9.3A) binds to factor VIII and Ca (usually released from alpha granules in activated platelets) on the cell surface to form the *intrinsic factor tenase complex*. This complex cleaves inactive factor X to active factor X. This creates more factor Xa that can bind to Ca and

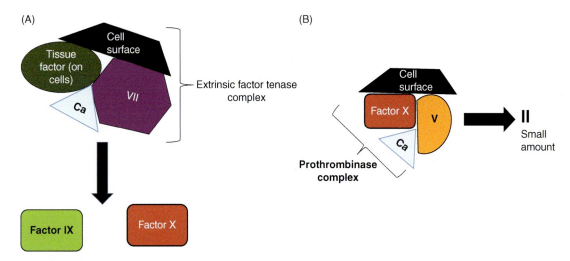

Fig. 9.3. Initiation of secondary hemostasis. (A) Tissue factor (TF), exposed on damaged endothelium or another cell surface, binds to circulating factor VII and activates it in the presence of calcium (Ca). This complex (endothelial cell surface + Ca + VIIa + TF) is called the extrinsic factor tenase complex. The extrinsic factor tenase complex then activates factor X and IX. (B) Continuing with the initiation phase, the activated factor X binds to Ca and factor V on the endothelial surface to create the prothrombinase complex that cleaves a relatively small amount of prothrombin to thrombin.

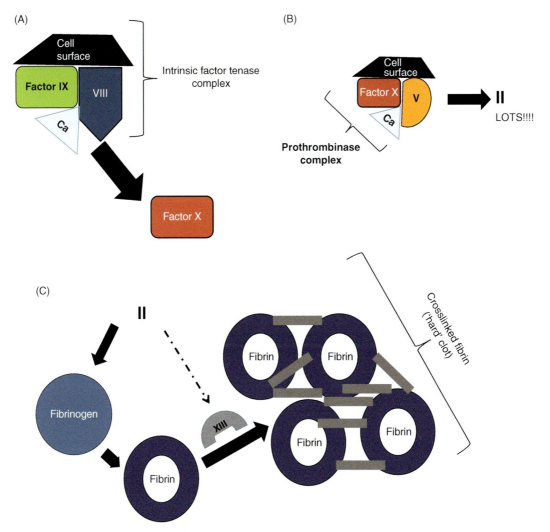

Fig. 9.4. Amplification and propagation of secondary coagulation. (A) The activated factor IX generated during initiation binds to factor VIII and calcium (Ca) on a cell surface to form the intrinsic factor tenase complex. This complex activates factor X. (B) The activated factor X combines with factor V and Ca to form the prothrombinase complex. The prothrombinase complex causes the conversion of prothrombin to thrombin. Since this reaction is occurring on many cell surfaces (including platelets) during amplification and propagation, large amounts of thrombin are created, also known as the 'thrombin burst.' (C) Thrombin will in turn cause activation of fibrinogen to fibrin that, in the presence of factor XIII (also activated by thrombin), will cause crosslinking of the fibrin to form the clot.

factor V on the cell surface (both usually released from dense and alpha granules respectively) to form more *prothrombinase complexes* and cleave a *large* volume of prothrombin to thrombin.

The final stage of secondary coagulation is termed *propagation* and describes the recruitment of activated platelets to the area to further coagulation (see Fig. 9.4). The recruited activated platelets release fac-

tors from their granules including V, VIII, vWF, and Ca which are involved in the various stages of secondary coagulation. Also (and arguably most importantly), the activated platelets provide more negatively charged phospholipid surfaces upon which coagulation can occur. This leads to further amplification and more and more thrombin production (i.e. the 'thrombin burst'). A large quantity of thrombin means a large amount of fibrinogen can be cleaved to fibrin. The fibrin is stimulated by factor XIII to cross-link the platelets and create the firm 'final' clot.

Fibrinolysis

One of the most interesting things about coagulation is that while it is ramping up to form a clot, negative feedback processes are almost immediately activated that cause fibrinolysis (Fig. 9.5). The goal of fibrinolysis is to break down the fibrin that is formed to: (i) control the size of the clot; and (ii) break down any unnecessary clots. Fibrinolysis is mediated by plasmin, an enzyme that cleaves fibrin and fibrinogen to fibrin degradation products (FDPs). Tissue plasminogen activator (tPA) and urokinase plasminogen activator (uPA) cleave plasminogen to plasmin to activate fibrinolysis. Thrombin and venous occlusion activate tPA and fibrinolysis in an attempt to ensure that the clot does not get too large. Factor XIII and plasmin itself activate uPA, acting as negative feedback so that clot formation does not become too exuberant.

While FDP production may simply indicate cleavage of fibrin or fibrinogen in general, crosslinking of fibrin only occurs in clots. Fibrin degradation products that are made from breakdown of *crosslinked fibrin* are called D-dimers and indicate breakdown of an actual clot (not just fibrin/fibrinogen) is occurring. Therefore, measurement of elevated D-dimers can sometimes be used to indicate the presence of a thrombotic event.

However, since clot stability is also needed to control bleeding, there are also fibrinolysis inhibitors whose goal is to ensure that all fibrin is not broken down as quickly as it is formed (Fig. 9.6). The end result is that a *properly* sized clot is created but no extra clots are formed. There are three main fibrinolysis inhibitors: (i) thrombin activatable fibrinolysis inhibitor (TAFI); (ii) α-2 antiplasmin; and (iii) plasminogen activator inhibitor (PAI-1). As indicated by its name, as thrombin is being produced, it activates TAFI which in turn removes lysine residues from the clot so that plasmin cannot bind to the clot and break it down. Similarly, α-2 antiplasmin directly inhibits the activity of plasmin so that it cannot break down the fibrin/fibrinogen. The role of PAI-1 is to inhibit the activators of plasmin (tPA and uPA) so that no plasmin can be formed and therefore no fibrinolysis can occur.

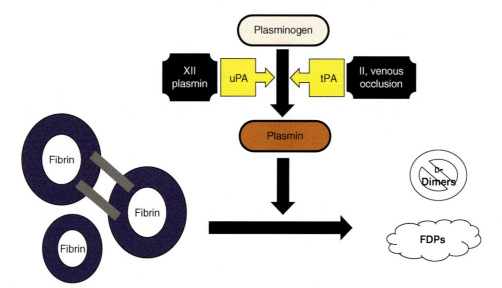

Fig. 9.5. Fibrinolysis. Plasminogen is cleaved to plasmin by the action of tissue plasminogen activator (tPA) and urokinase plasminogen activator (uPA). The presence of thrombin (II) and venous stasis from vascular dilation in the area of the clot activate tPA which is typically circulating in the plasma. Plasmin itself and factor XII both activate uPA found within cells in the area of tissue damage. Plasmin breaks down fibrinogen, fibrin, and crosslinked fibrin to fibrin degradation products (FDPs). The specific FDP created when crosslinked fibrin (present only in clots) is broken down is known as a D-dimer.

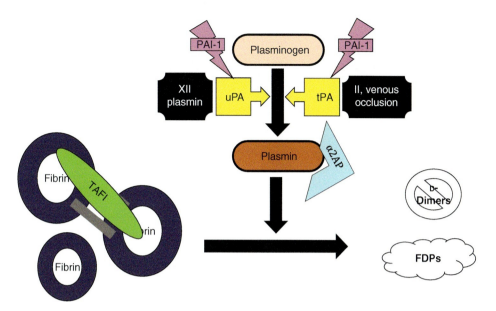

Fig. 9.6. Fibrinolysis with endogenous inhibitors. The same fibrinolysis process as shown in Fig. 9.5 is shown here. The three major fibrinolysis inhibitors found within the body have been added to the figure to show their sites of activity. Thrombin activatable fibrinolysis inhibitor (TAFI) is produced in response to thrombin (II) and blocks the ability of plasmin to recognize a clot by removing signature lysine residues from the surface of the clot. Plasmin activator inhibitor (PAI-1) will inhibit tissue plasminogen activator (tPA) and urokinase plasminogen activator (uPA) so that less plasmin is formed. Finally, α-2 antiplasmin (α2AP) directly binds to plasmin to inhibit its activity. FDPs, fibrin degradation products.

Taken together, fibrinolysis and fibrinolysis inhibitors exquisitely balance the need for a clot with making the clot too large.

Anticoagulation

The body also has a host of endogenous anticoagulants which work to control the formation of the clot itself (rather than simply breaking down the clot once it forms via fibrinolysis; Fig. 9.7). Tissue factor pathway inhibitor will inhibit the initiation phase of secondary hemostasis by blocking the activation of Factor X, specifically by inhibiting the extrinsic factor tenase complex. Tissue factor pathway inhibitor is stored in platelets and endothelial cells so as to be close to the site of action and is released in response to heparin or is bound to lipoproteins and circulates through the body.

Additionally, protein C and protein S are endogenous anticoagulants affecting mainly the amplification and propagation phases. When thrombin is formed, some of it binds to thrombomodulin (which is found on the same endothelial cell surface where coagulation is occurring). When thrombin and thrombomodulin bind together, proteins C/S are activated and they in turn inactivate factors V and VIII so that the intrinsic factor tenase complex and the prothrombinase complexes cannot be formed.

Heparan sulfate (the endogenous form of heparin) is also bound to the endothelial cell wall and will work in concert with circulating antithrombin to inactivate factor X and thrombin. Other endogenous anticoagulants work to directly inhibit factor X (α-1 protease inhibitor) and thrombin (α-2 macroglobulin). Any inhibition of factor X and/or thrombin will inactivate the prothrombinase complex and/or cleavage of fibrinogen to fibrin.

Coagulation is a complex interplay of processes. It is important to remember that: (i) all processes (coagulation, fibrinolysis, anticoagulation, and antifibrinolysis) are occurring simultaneously; (ii) everything occurs on a phospholipid bilayer rather than in space; and (iii) thrombin is the only molecule that is procoagulant, anticoagulant, pro-fibrinolytic, and anti-fibrinolytic all at the same time.

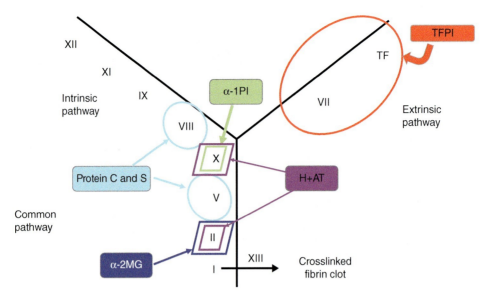

Fig. 9.7. Sites of action of the endogenous anticoagulants. Tissue factor pathway inhibitor (TFPI) essentially blocks the initiation of coagulation (i.e. the entire extrinsic arm of the traditional coagulation cascade) by inhibiting the extrinsic factor tenase complex (see Fig. 9.3A). Inhibition of the prothrombinase complex (i.e. the common pathway of the traditional coagulation cascade) occurs in the form of heparan (H) and antithrombin (AT) which inhibit factor X and II, as well as α-1 protease inhibitor (α-1PI) which inhibits factor X and α-2 macroglobulin (α-2MG) which inhibits factor II. Proteins C and S inhibit factors V and VIII, impeding amplification and propagation as well as formation of factor II (i.e. the intrinsic and common pathways of the traditional coagulation cascade).

9.2 How the Coagulation Tests Work

Analysis of primary hemostasis (platelets)

Obtaining a platelet count should always be the first diagnostic test in patients presenting with evidence of a primary hemostatic disorder. If clinical signs of a primary hemostatic disorder are present (petechia, ecchymosis, epistaxis, etc.; see Section 9.3), but platelet counts are determined to be within normal limits, the clinician may suspect a defect of platelet function, also known as a thrombocytopathia. All of the tests for platelet function will be abnormal if the patient has thrombocytopenia, so it is *imperative* that a low platelet count be ruled out *first* before performing platelet function testing.

Platelet count

Blood should be collected into anticoagulant tubes, most commonly EDTA. The platelet count can then be assessed either by an automated analyzer as part of a complete blood count (CBC), or manually by visual assessment of a stained blood smear. While it is generally good practice to always perform a manual blood smear review on every CBC, it is *essential* to perform visual examination of a blood smear if a thrombocytopenia is diagnosed via an automated analyzer to rule out a spuriously low platelet count due to platelet clumping. While readers should use the reference ranges specific to their analyzer/institution, normal platelet counts in dogs and cats are generally between 200–500 K/μL.

The automated analyzer uses changes in impedance or laser light scatter to assess the size and granular contents of each cell in a blood sample to differentiate between platelets, erythrocytes, and leukocytes (including the different white blood cell types). If platelets are clumped together into larger units, they may not be counted or be counted accidentally as other cell types (especially leukocytes). Many newer CBC analyzers will report when platelet clumping is suspected, but it is good practice to always perform a manual slide review and confirm the presence of platelet clumps. When clumping is present, it is safe to assume that the analyzer count is likely lower than the patient's actual platelet count; how much higher the actual platelet count is above that number is unknown.

BLOOD SMEAR EVALUATION Blood smear evaluation allows for detection of platelet clumps, manual estimation of platelet numbers, and evaluation of platelet morphology. The feathered edge and body of the smear are first scanned for frequent platelet clumps. If clumping is present, all manual and automated estimates should be viewed as minimums that will underestimate the true value.

A manual platelet estimate is taken by counting individual platelets within the monolayer of the smear per high powered field (HPF; 100× oil objective). The number of platelets per field is counted over ten fields and averaged. Each platelet per HPF represents approximately 15,000–20,000 platelets/μL. For example, if there was an average of four platelets/HPF, then 4 × 15 or 4 × 20 = a platelet estimate between 60,000–80,000/μL. See Figs 9.8 and 9.9 for examples of the typical appearance of canine and feline platelets.

Platelet function tests

BUCCAL MUCOSAL BLEEDING TIME The most commonly available 'cage-side' test for platelet function is a buccal mucosal bleeding time or BMBT. In the absence of thrombocytopenia, an abnormal BMBT is interpreted as a defect in platelet or vessel wall function, including things like vWF release from the platelets or endothelial cells. To perform a BMBT, the patient's upper lip is tied back to expose the inner mucosal surface; mild sedation may be required to facilitate the procedure depending on patient temperament. Using a commercially available spring loaded lancet, a small standardized incision is made on the inside of the lip at the level of the maxillary canine tooth. Filter paper is used to dab away flowing blood ventral to the incision, with care taken not to touch the incision itself and disturb any forming clots. The time from creation of the incision until a cease in blood flow is recorded, with normal in dogs between 1.7–4.2 minutes, and cats 1–2.4 minutes. While this test is insensitive to mild conditions, it should be prolonged with moderate to marked platelet function defects.

VON WILLEBRAND'S DISEASE TESTING Von Willebrand's disease (vWd) is the most common inherited thrombocytopathia in dogs. The function of vWF is to allow platelet aggregation (see Fig. 9.2). Specific testing for vWF is done by looking directly for the antigen associated with vWF (vWF:Ag assay). This testing is most commonly performed as an enzyme-linked immunoassay (ELISA) or latex-enhanced immunoassay (LIA) wherein antibodies specific to the vWF

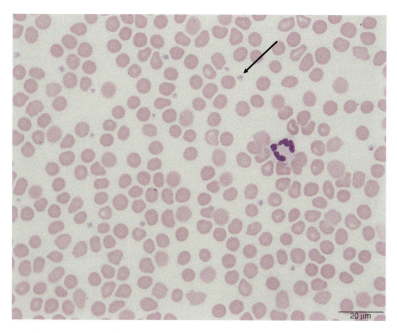

Fig. 9.8. Canine blood smear. A typical platelet is indicated by the arrow. There is one mature neutrophil present in the monolayer depicted in the figure.

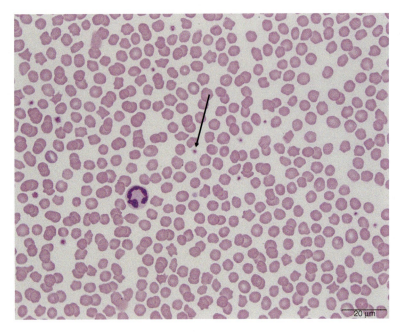

Fig. 9.9. Feline blood smear. A typical platelet is indicated by the arrow. There is one mature neutrophil present in the monolayer depicted in the figure.

antigen bind to vWF and trigger a colorimetric change or change in turbidity that correlates with the amount of vWF present in the sample. The results are reported as a percentage compared to a 'normal' vWF level from the pooled serum of several unaffected dogs. Normal activity is 70–80%. Levels between 50–69% are borderline, and levels <50% are considered abnormal.

OTHER PLATELET FUNCTION TESTING The gold standard analysis of platelet function is *aggregometry*. The basic principle is that addition of a platelet activator to the sample in vitro should cause aggregation of functional platelets. This aggregation can be detected generally by either increasing light passing through the sample (as the heavier aggregated platelets fall out of solution), or an increase in electrical impedance as the aggregating platelets adhere to electrodes within the sample. Depending on the sample and methodology used, aggregometry generally requires advanced training and sample handling. Thus it is usually performed at referral laboratories or research institutions.

Another benchtop analyzer available for commercial use that can evaluate platelet function is the Platelet Function Analyzer (PFA)-100® (Siemens Healthcare Diagnostics, Inc., Tarrytown, New York, USA). This machine aspirates blood through a small opening in a disposable single-use cartridge that is coated with platelet agonist (collagen or ADP). The amount of time it takes for the activated platelets to plug the opening is called the closure time. If the closure time is prolonged (>180 seconds) then thrombocytopathy should be suspected.

Additional tests of platelet function (e.g. viscoelastic methodologies, flow cytometry) are limited in availability to referral laboratories or research institutions, but are additional options for work-up of more complex or uncommon cases. See Further Reading section for more information on these additional platelet function testing methodologies and their interpretation.

Analysis of secondary hemostasis: Coagulation factors

Red-top tube test (Lee-White method)

The most commonly utilized coagulation tests in clinical practice are those that assess coagulation factor activity in plasma. The simplest test is the Lee-White method, also called the 'red-top tube' test. Whole blood placed in a red-top tube should form a clot as the negative charge on the glass tube activates the intrinsic and common pathways (see Fig. 9.1). Cats generally clot in < 8 minutes and dogs within 3–13 minutes, although times up to 21 minutes have been reported in healthy dogs. As this method is highly subjective and prone to significant variation, additional methods to standardize surface activation have been developed.

Activated clotting time (ACT)

The ACT test uses a tube containing diatomaceous earth (gray top tube) to more consistently activate coagulation than in the Lee-White method. Similar to glass, diatomaceous earth is negatively charged and can activate factor XII to initiate coagulation via the intrinsic pathway, but the larger surface area activates coagulation more effectively than glass alone. Two milliliters of whole blood is added to the gray top tube, mixed by inversion, and then incubated at 37°C (body temperature) for 60 seconds. After 60 seconds, the tube is checked by inversion every 5 to 10 seconds for visual evidence of development of a clot. The time from initial contact of blood with the tube until visual development of a clot is the ACT; in dogs, reported normal values range from 60–110 seconds, and in cats 50–75 seconds.

The ACT is not a very sensitive test and is only abnormal in patients that have severe (<10% factor activity) hemostatic deficits. Also, because it depends on the platelets present in the blood sample to provide procoagulant phospholipid surfaces for amplification and propagation, it can be prolonged in cases of severe (<10,000/μL) thrombocytopenia.

Activated partial thromboplastin time (aPTT) and prothrombin time (PT)

More sensitive tests of secondary hemostasis include the aPTT and PT. For these tests, blood anticoagulated with 3.2% citrate (blue-top tube) is used. The sample in the blue-top tube is combined with standardized quantities of calcium, phospholipids, and an activator, and all testing is performed at 37°C.

The aPTT tests the *intrinsic* and common pathway (see Fig. 9.1), because a surface activator (kaolin, ellagic acid, or silica) is used, similar to the diatomaceous earth of the ACT. However, because the various components of the aPTT (phospholipids, calcium, activator) are more standardized and the optical detection method for fibrin formation in plasma is more sensitive than a visual exam, the aPTT can detect when factor activity drops to <35%. The PT is similar, but since the activator used is TF, the PT test looks for deficiencies in the *extrinsic* and common pathway of the cascade. It has a similar sensitivity to the aPTT, detecting when factors in the extrinsic and common pathways drop below approximately 35% activity.

For both tests, the time from addition of the activator to the first formation of fibrin within the sample is the result. The formation of fibrin can be detected by changes in optic density or electrical impedance of the samples. The PT and aPTT are not affected by primary hemostatic disorders. However, because the test result is reported once a small amount of fibrin is created, they do not reflect disorders of hemostasis that may occur after this point (e.g. abnormalities in the amplification or propagation of coagulation that lead to the thrombin burst [see Fig. 9.4B] or alterations in fibrinolysis [see Fig. 9.5]).

The reference ranges specific to the individual laboratory or analyzer should be used for interpretation of these tests as the duration to form fibrin is specific to the strength of the activator used. The standardization of the PT to the strength of activator used is the basis of the 'international normalized ratio' or INR. To calculate an INR, the PT value generated at the laboratory is divided by the mean PT value in that lab's reference range. This allows comparison of the degree of PT elevation versus normal between laboratories. While the INR is commonly used in human medicine to monitor warfarin-type anticoagulant therapy, it is rarely used in veterinary medicine.

Specific factor testing

While tests such as the PT and aPTT test the functionality of larger pathways of the coagulation system, it is possible to measure amounts or activity of certain individual factors as well. Unfortunately, these tests are often performed at reference laboratories or only available at research or referral institutions. This limits their clinical utility if the patient's status is time sensitive. As an example, fibrinogen quantities (factor I) are most commonly directly measured by the Clauss assay. In this test, a high level of thrombin is added to diluted plasma and the change in optical density caused by the precipitation of fibrin is compared to samples of known concentration.

For cases of suspected individual factor deficiencies, such as hemophilia, the *activity levels* of specific coagulation factors can also be measured. This is done by mixing the patient's plasma with test plasma that is known to be deficient in the specific clotting factor of interest. A PT or aPTT (depending on location of the factor of interest in the intrinsic or extrinsic cascade) is performed on the pooled plasma sample. The degree of prolongation of either PT or aPTT is used to extrapolate the activity of the coagulation factor of interest. While these tests may not be readily available for the acutely bleeding animal who is likely emergently receiving fresh frozen plasma or whole blood (see Section 9.4), sample collection prior to administration of blood products can be analyzed at a later time for a definitive diagnosis. For stable patients, screening for specific factor activities can help presurgical planning for elective procedures and inform breeding decisions.

Fibrin degradation products

Measurement of elevations of components such as FDPs may indicate pro-thrombotic and procoagulant states such as disseminated intravascular coagulation. Fibrin degradation products are formed from the breakdown of fibrinogen, fibrin, or crosslinked fibrin. Elevated D-dimers, which are a subtype of FDPs created only by breakdown of actual thrombi (i.e. crosslinked fibrin formed in the amplification and propagation phases, see Fig. 9.4), are more sensitive and specific for the diagnosis of thrombosis. Both FDP and D-dimer assays are typically performed by semi-quantitative latex agglutination. In each of these tests, antibodies against the product of interest are bound to latex beads suspended in solution. When the product is present, the beads clump and fall out of solution, which is detected as decreasing turbidity of the sample.

Viscoelastic testing

As blood clots, it goes from a liquid state to a more solid 'gel-like' consistency. This physical change is the basis of viscoelastic testing methodologies such as thromboelastography (TEG) or rotational thromboelastometry (ROTEM). Rather than measuring specific cell or protein activities as in previous tests, these assays examine how the mechanical properties of the sample change over time as a way to assess overall clot kinetics and strength. This 'global' overview of hemostasis combined with graphical outputs that allow for quick visual assessment of results has made this form of testing grow in popularity in recent years. Viscoelastic testing is becoming more widely available in both human medicine and veterinary referral institutions.

In general, when performing viscoelastic testing, citrated whole blood is incubated in a chamber with calcium plus some form of activator (ellagic acid, TF, etc.). As the blood clots, the chamber will be physically affected in some way depending on the methodology of the specific analyzer. For example, in the TEG, the changes in rotational force applied to a pin within the chamber by the clotting blood is measured (e.g. initially the pin moves freely but its movement slows and changes as the blood clots). The signal from the chamber is translated into a characteristic tracing. Several variables can be measured from this tracing which represent various aspects of clot formation speed, clot strength, and rate of clot breakdown. While the entire viscoelastic assay may run for 60–90 minutes, the early physical appearance of the tracing as well as many of the variables are often apparent within 10–20 minutes of initiation of the test. Please see Further Reading section for more information on viscoelastic testing and interpretation of the various parameters.

9.3 Indications

In general, coagulation testing is pursued in response to the clinical presentation of the animal. Clinical clues can guide the clinician to a suspicion of either a primary or a secondary hemostatic disorder.

Primary hemostatic disorders

Primary hemostatic disorders involve the platelets. With primary hemostatic disorders, animals will bleed at gingival surfaces in the mouth or other mucosal surfaces such as the nose. They will also display petechia or ecchymosis which is essentially pinpoint or larger areas of bleeding under the skin (Fig. 9.10). Other common areas to find bleeding are in the bladder leading to hematuria, within the anterior chamber of the eye causing hyphema (Fig. 9.11), or in the gastrointestinal (GI) tract causing melena.

Primary hemostatic disorders can be divided into two large categories – thrombocytopenia or

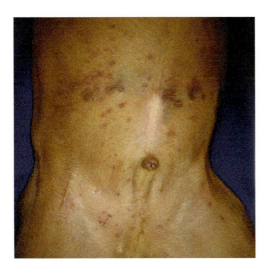

Fig. 9.10. Petechia and ecchymoses on the ventral abdomen of a dog. Note the smaller pinpoint petechiations and the larger areas of ecchymoses in this dog with thrombocytopenia.

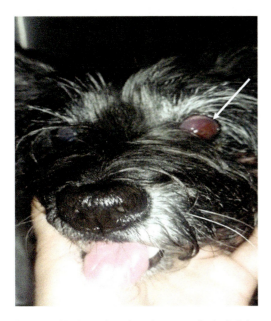

Fig. 9.11. Hyphema in a thrombocytopenic dog's left eye. The white arrow indicates the visible hyphema.

thrombocytopathy. Thrombocytopenic conditions occur when platelet counts drop to such low levels that bleeding occurs. Typically, to have spontaneous hemorrhage related to a lack of platelets, the platelet count must be <50,0000 platelets/hpf but usually this number is *much* less than this (usually less than 10,000 platelets/hpf) before clinical bleeding is noted. In general, the lack of platelets means that there are not enough cell surfaces for propagation of coagulation as well as a lack of platelet granule contents to help in clot formation (see Section 9.1 for more information).

The most common reasons for thrombocytopenia are lack of production of platelets within the bone marrow, destruction of platelets, or consumption of platelets. Theoretically, any disorder affecting the megakaryocytes can lead to a lack of production of platelets including neoplastic disorders, immune-mediated destruction of bone marrow cells, or other infiltrative disease affecting the bone marrow. Side effects of various drugs including chemotherapeutic agents can also damage the bone marrow. Destruction of mature platelets is almost always secondary to immune-mediated destruction of the platelets (i.e. immune-mediated thrombocytopenia; ITP). Immune-mediated destruction can be idiopathic (primary ITP) or secondary to another underlying disease process ranging from tick-borne disease to neoplasia. Platelets are most commonly consumed during persistent hemorrhage. For example, a chronically bleeding gastric ulcer could lead to mild thrombocytopenia secondary to hemorrhage, or blood loss from trauma could result in a low platelet count. Please see Further Reading section for resources elaborating on the various causes of thrombocytopenia.

Thrombocytopathic conditions occur when there are normal numbers of platelets but the platelets are not functioning normally. The most common inherited platelet disorder is vWd. This disease is most commonly reported in Dobermans but can occur in many other breeds. There is some variability in the disease, but in general vWd results from varying degrees of vWF deficiency. This negatively affects platelet adhesion to the endothelium as well as platelet aggregation (see Fig. 9.2). There are many examples of other less common inherited thrombocytopathies in various breeds of dogs and cats ranging from Basset Hound thrombopathia to Glanzman's thrombasthenia in Otterhounds and Great Pyrenees. Disorders affecting the contents of platelet granules or the granules themselves (e.g. Chediak–Higashi syndrome) have also been described in dogs and cats. The reader is referred to other resources for a more comprehensive list of breed-related platelet disorders.

The other common thrombocytopathies encountered are drug induced, occurring after receiving non-steroidal anti-inflammatory drugs (NSAIDS) or anti-platelet medications such as clopidogrel. In the case of these drugs, platelet activation is blocked either by inhibiting endogenous platelet activator production such as thromboxane A_2 (NSAIDS) or blocking receptors that lead to platelet activation (ADP receptors; clopidogrel). There is some research in human medicine indicating that colloid administration can also affect platelet function through a variety of mechanisms although this has not been definitively proven in animals. Please see Further Reading section for a more comprehensive listing of thrombocytopathies.

Secondary hemostatic disorders

Secondary hemostatic disorders affect the clotting factors and range from inherited deficiencies of specific factors (e.g. hemophilia A with a lack of factor VIII) to widespread deficiencies of multiple clotting factors. The most common example of the latter is a lack of functional vitamin K-dependent clotting factors (i.e. factors II, VII, IX, and X) due to anticoagulant rodenticide intoxication or liver disease. However, diseases such as disseminated intravascular coagulation will also affect multiple coagulation factors simultaneously. See Further Reading section for a more comprehensive listing of the various secondary hemostatic disorders found in dogs and cats.

Clinical signs associated with secondary hemostatic disorders are generally associated with bleeding into larger cavities. This is attributed to the fact that although the platelets are present, there is an inability to form fibrin crosslinking of the platelets, resulting in a lack of a 'hard clot.' Larger quantities of bleeding than are typically seen with platelet disorders ensue. Common locations for bleeding from secondary hemostatic disorders include pleural effusion, abdominal effusion, joint effusion, or bleeding into the lung parenchyma itself, although bleeding can theoretically occur anywhere. The clinical signs noted in a patient are consistent with where the blood accumulates. For example, respiratory distress occurs with pleural effusion or bleeding into the pulmonary parenchyma. Hemoptysis is also common with intrapulmonary hemorrhage. Lameness may be present with hemorrhage into joints. No matter the location of the bleeding, if the animal loses a large enough blood volume, it can present with signs of hypovolemia including poor pulses, tachycardia, pale mucous membranes, and obtundation.

9.4 Interpretation of the Findings

Primary hemostasis

With primary hemostatic disorders, treatment options are limited and highly dependent upon the animal's clinical condition as well as the underlying cause of the platelet-related disorder. The approach to these cases can be divided into the emergent, urgent, and stable categories. See Fig. 9.12 for an overview of the approach to these cases.

Emergent primary hemostatic disorders

Emergent cases typically are those animals that are either unstable due to anemia from blood loss and/or actively hemorrhaging with documented development of anemia over time. In cases of thrombocytopenia, these are classically patients with platelet counts less than 10,000 cells/hpf. A good example is an animal with persistent epistaxis resulting in anemia or persistent GI hemorrhage that leads to anemia over the course of several days. In these situations, it is important to stop the bleeding so that red blood cells can either be transfused to improve the anemia or the patient is able to replace red blood cells on its own.

The only option available to emergently stop hemorrhage due to platelet-related bleeding is to transfuse platelets to the patient. There are several options that can provide platelets: fresh whole blood or platelet-rich plasma. Other products touted to provide platelets such as frozen platelet concentrates or lyophilized platelet products are controversial as to the efficacy of the platelets available in the product and the authors suggest doing research into their efficacy prior to using them.

Urgent primary hemostatic disorders

Urgent cases are those cases with known thrombocytopenia or thrombocytopathia which are not currently bleeding but which require a procedure known to induce bleeding. In thrombocytopenic patients, these animals typically have platelet counts of 10,000–50,000 platelets/hpf. An example of such a procedure would be surgery to obtain diagnostic biopsy samples or a bone marrow aspirate to

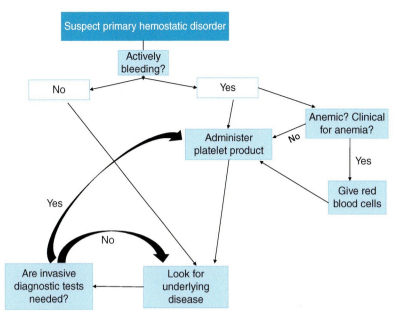

Fig. 9.12. The general approach to the initial clinical management of suspected primary platelet disorders. The single most important initial decision is whether or not the patient requires emergent treatment to stop active bleeding. Otherwise, in all cases a diagnostic workup to look for underlying disease is required prior to definitive treatment.

further diagnose the underlying reason for the hemostatic disorder. These cases should be prophylactically transfused with either fresh whole blood or platelet-rich plasma to provide functional platelets *prior* to the procedure. The exact timing of the transfusion is variable but transfusions are typically given anywhere from 1–4 hours before the procedure (or the blood product can be given during the procedure if necessary). If the animal has a drug-induced thrombocytopathia, ideally the invasive procedure is delayed until the effects of the drug have worn off and the platelets are functional again. In inherited disorders such as vWd, the animal can be given vWF in the blood/plasma products listed above, or by transfusing fresh frozen plasma or cryoprecipitate. Drugs like desmopressin can be given which induce release of vWF from the endothelial cells prior to the procedure.

Stable primary hemostatic disorders

Stable cases are those animals which are thrombocytopenic or have thrombocytopathia but are not actively hemorrhaging. They may or may not have clinical signs such as petechia or ecchymoses. Often in these cases, low platelet counts are discovered incidentally on bloodwork. Other stable cases are those where the animal is known to have a historical thrombocytopathic disease like vWd. It is important to remember when interpreting bloodwork that certain breeds of dogs (Cavalier King Charles Spaniels, Greyhounds) have naturally lower platelet counts that are not pathologic. Stable thrombocytopenic/thrombocytopathic animals do not require emergent transfusion; efforts should instead be directed toward diagnosing their underlying condition and treating it if indicated/possible.

Regardless of the categorization of the animal, once a primary hemostatic disorder is diagnosed, long term treatment involves addressing the underlying disorder (if possible). Most of the inherited thrombocytopathias do not have specific treatment options aside from avoiding situations that might induce hemorrhage, and being aware of the condition when the animal does require procedures that might induce hemorrhage, such as surgery or dental extractions.

Typically, when animals have immune-mediated destruction, platelet counts are extremely low (<5,000–10,000/hpf; normal 200,000–500,000/hpf) with many animals having no platelets present. When platelets are being consumed or lost during hemorrhage, platelet counts are typically higher than immune-mediated cases (often 50,000–150,000/hpf). Regardless if immune-mediated destruction or consumption of platelets secondary to another disease is suspected, it is important to try to diagnose the underlying condition to stop the destruction. This usually involves a systemic workup including testing for tick-borne (Rickettsial) diseases, imaging of the thorax and abdomen looking for underlying neoplasia or other disease, and potentially performing a bone marrow biopsy to evaluate the megakaryocytes and other platelet precursors. While attempting to look for the underlying disease, both primary and secondary immune-mediated destruction is controlled by administration of immunosuppressive drugs including steroids, cyclosporine, mycophenolate mofetil, and azathioprine. Further treatments to apprehend the immune system (intravenous immunoglobulin) or stimulate megakaryocyte platelet release (vincristine) can also be attempted. In many cases, while test results for Rickettsial disease are pending, animals are also prophylactically treated with doxycycline. The reader is referred to the Further Reading section for more information on the specific treatments for ITP. If another underlying disease is diagnosed that is causing platelet consumption, platelet counts should improve once that disease is addressed.

Secondary hemostatic disorders

Secondary hemostatic disorders have only limited treatment options, which are again somewhat dependent upon the cause of the clotting factor disorder. As with platelet disorders, the first clinical decision is whether or not the animal requires emergent treatment to stop bleeding. This is arguably more important in secondary coagulation disorders than primary disorders since secondary disorders often involve larger volumes of hemorrhage than primary disorders.

If an animal is clinical for either anemia (typically packed cell volume <12–15%) or hypovolemia (tachycardia, weak peripheral pulses, obtundation, pale mucous membranes), it requires emergent transfusion of plasma with functional clotting factors as well as red blood cells. Typically, whole blood or multicomponent therapy (packed red blood cells AND fresh frozen plasma) is indicated in these cases. Otherwise, if the animal has prolongations of coagulation tests (e.g. prolonged PT, aPTT, or ACT) without severe anemia or hypovolemia, transfusion with clotting factors alone (i.e. a plasma-containing product without red blood cells) is indicated. Typically, fresh frozen plasma (plasma frozen for <1 year) or frozen plasma (plasma frozen for >1–3 years) can be used in these cases. Note that neither of these products have functional platelets. Also, frozen plasma may contain lesser amounts of factors V and VIII than fresh frozen plasma depending on duration of storage, and therefore may be more limited in its efficacy.

Once hemorrhage is controlled and any anemia is corrected, more diagnostic tests can be conducted to look for the underlying cause of the disorder. The first step is often to look critically at the degree of PT prolongation versus aPTT prolongation to try to narrow down the possible etiologies. See Table 9.2 for an approach to evaluating the PT and aPTT. Subsequently, further diagnostics might include testing for specific clotting factors, investigation into possible anticoagulant rodenticide exposure, or evaluation of liver function. The reader is referred to the Further Reading section for more information on evaluating specific clotting factors and liver function. Longer term treatment and outcomes for these cases are dependent upon the underlying cause. For example, a case of anticoagulant rodenticide intoxication can be treated with vitamin K supplementation until the toxin is cleared from the body (1–6 weeks depending on the product ingested). In contrast, liver functional failure needs to be managed long term and may not be reversible.

9.5 Pitfalls of the Monitor

All laboratory testing is subject to various causes for error. Please see Box 9.1 for a summary of the most common reasons for alterations in the typical coagulation tests. Further detail related to each of the reasons listed in Box 9.1 is found in the text within this section.

Primary hemostasis

Platelet counts

When interpreting platelet counts, the most common spurious finding is a pseudothrombocytopenia that occurs secondary to platelet clumping. Attention to atraumatic venipuncture, gentle sample handling, and reducing the delay in placing the blood in an anticoagulant may help reduce clumping. Despite

Table 9.2. Interpretation of the relative degrees of PT and PTT prolongation.

PT	aPTT	Interpretation
Prolonged >2–2.5 times the high end of the normal range	Normal or prolongation <2 times the high end of the normal range	Suggests extrinsic arm of the coagulation cascade (see Fig. 9.1) primarily affected • Anticoagulant rodenticide intoxication, relatively early in course of disease[a] • Liver failure, relatively early in course of disease[a] Factor VII deficiency
Normal or prolongation <2 times the high end of the normal range	Prolonged >2–2.5 times the high end of the normal range	Suggests intrinsic arm of the coagulation cascade (see Fig. 9.1) primarily affected • Factor XII deficiency • Factor XI deficiency • Factor IX deficiency • Factor VIII deficiency Disseminated intravascular coagulation (multiple factors)
Prolonged >2–2.5 times the high end of the normal range	Prolonged >2–2.5 times the high end of the normal range	Suggests intrinsic and extrinsic arms of the coagulation cascade (see Fig. 9.1) both affected[b] • Anticoagulant rodenticide intoxication (usually PT prolongation is still a greater magnitude than aPTT due to short half-life of factor VII) • Liver failure (usually PT prolongation greater magnitude than aPTT due to short half-life of factor VII) Disseminated intravascular coagulation (usually aPTT prolongation greater magnitude than PT due to consumption of clotting factors involved in amplication/propagation [VIII, IX] more than those involved in initiation [factor VII and TF])

aPTT, activated partial thromboplastin time; PT, prothrombin time; TF, tissue factor.
[a]Factor VII has the shortest half-life of all the coagulation factors and is found in the extrinsic arm of the coagulation cascade. Therefore, early in the course of disease, PT prolongations occur first.
[b]When both values are *greatly* prolonged, especially when PT alone or both PT/aPTT are off the analyzer's scale, the animal has anticoagulant rodenticide intoxication until proven otherwise.

these precautions, platelets (especially in cats) may clump regardless, making a manual review of all blood smears in all species necessary to assess for this artifact. Rough manual estimates made during slide review can be interpreted as a minimum platelet count (see Section 9.2), although the actual platelet count may exceed that range.

Large platelets (such as those commonly seen in Cavalier King Charles Spaniels) may exceed the upper size threshold for platelets on some impedance analyzers and therefore may be miscounted as other cells. Similarly, excessive platelet clumping may be misinterpreted by automated analyzers; the platelet clumps may be counted as neutrophils, basophils, or eosinophils. The misinterpretation of platelet clumps is less of an issue in most modern analyzers which recognize suspected clumping and flag the results for the operator to review.

While most blood samples for platelet/CBC analysis are collected into EDTA anticoagulant, citrated samples can also be used. However, the larger liquid volume of the citrate will cause minor dilution of the blood compared to the reference intervals calculated from EDTA samples. Multiplying the platelet concentration measured on the CBC by 1.1 will correct for the dilution. Heparinized samples are not recommended for platelet counts as platelet clumping is expected with this anticoagulant.

Some breeds of dogs such as Greyhounds and Cavalier King Charles Spaniels have a lower platelet count naturally. Unless these patients also have clinical signs of a primary hemostatic disorder (see Section 9.3) or significantly low platelet counts (<50,000/µL), clinicians should make sure they are using breed-specific cutoffs for thrombocytopenia before initiating a significant diagnostic workup.

> **Box 9.1. Preanalytical variables that may result in erroneous results of commonly used coagulation tests.**
>
> *Falsely lowered platelet count:*
>   Platelet clumping
>   Breed-specific differences in platelet count
>   Citrate tube for CBC analysis
> *Falsely prolonged BMBT:*
>   Anemia
>   Low serum fibrinogen concentration
>   Thrombocytopenia
> *Falsely prolonged PT/aPTT:*
>   Inappropriate tube volume
>   Elevated hematocrit (hemoconcentration)
>   Hemolysis
>   Lipemia
>   Prolonged (unfrozen) storage of plasma
>   Contamination with anticoagulants
>   Clotting in sample
> *Falsely shortened PT/aPTT:*
>   Severe anemia
>   Contamination with Ca
>
> aPTT, activated partial thromboplastin time; BMBT, buccal mucosal bleeding time; Ca, calcium; CBC, complete blood count; PT, prothrombin time.

Platelet function tests

While the BMBT is used as a screening test for thrombocytopathias, it is neither sensitive nor specific. While it will obviously be prolonged in thrombocytopenic patients regardless of platelet function, low fibrinogen levels and significant anemia can also prolong bleeding times.

Platelet aggregation testing can be influenced by many pre-analytical factors. In humans (and likely in animals), things like the time of day, diet, exercise, and supplements have all been shown to affect platelet aggregation. In addition, interpretation of platelet aggregation results as normal or abnormal is difficult. A study by Blois et al. (2015) found high variation in platelet function testing for healthy dogs, implying that interpreting trends within one individual is likely more appropriate than comparing a patient's results to 'normal' reference intervals.

Samples anticoagulated with EDTA cannot be used for platelet aggregation testing as EDTA irreversibly disassociates the GPIIb/IIIa receptor from platelets and prevents fibrinogen binding, making platelets unable to aggregate. In addition, light transmission aggregometry can only be performed on platelet-rich plasma because all red cells must be removed from the sample so as to not interfere with the light transmission methodology. The need to create platelet-rich plasma in turn leads to increased processing of samples before testing, which increases the risk of activating platelets simply by sample handling, potentially also influencing the results of aggregation testing.

Secondary hemostasis

Appropriate filling of the 3.2% citrate tube is very important as the 1:9 citrate to blood ratio is crucial for accuracy of tests that require the addition of calcium to the sample to initiate clotting (PT, aPTT, viscoelastic testing). Underfilling of tubes will result in a higher concentration of citrate in the plasma. In this situation, the standardized amount of calcium added to the sample may not be enough and clotting times may be erroneously prolonged. A tube filled to <90% of the recommended volume should be considered underfilled. Samples with elevated hematocrits have less plasma per unit volume, and therefore result in a decreased plasma:citrate ratio in the tube. This results in an artificial prolongation of clotting times that increases exponentially as hematocrit rises above 55%. In humans, these artifacts have been shown to be clinically relevant and adjustment of citrate levels in samples with hematocrit (Hct) >55% is recommended (see Marlar et al., 2006). A simplified method in humans is to remove 0.1 mL of sodium citrate from a 5 mL 3.2% tube prior to sample collection if the Hct is >55%. To the author's knowledge, this has not been validated in veterinary species.

Conversely, overfilling of tubes or severe anemia (greater amount of plasma present per same volume of whole blood) will result in a lower concentration of citrate in the plasma, which may falsely shorten clotting times. However, one study in humans (Siegel et al., 1998) did not find clinically relevant shortening of clotting times in patients with hematocrits as low as 14%. Contamination of the sample with additional calcium may also falsely shorten clotting times, and contamination with other anticoagulants (such as EDTA or heparin) may falsely prolong clotting times. Therefore, blue-top tubes should be filled first or only after non-additive (red-top) tubes to prevent cross-contamination.

If tubes are filled too slowly or are inappropriately mixed, the blood sample may clot despite the presence of citrate. Samples should be assessed visually or by insertion of wooden applicator sticks into the sample, for presence of clots prior to analysis. Samples containing clots have consumed coagulation factors and fibrinogen that will be removed when centrifuged, and so 'plasma' from these samples (i.e. serum) will lead to a false prolongation of PT and aPTT.

If samples cannot be assessed for secondary hemostasis on whole blood within 1 hour, they should be spun and the plasma separated. Fresh plasma can be tested within 4 hours or it can be tested after freezing. Freezing is most useful when prolonged storage or shipping is necessary for advanced testing such as specific factor testing. Delays in sample analysis without freezing may lead to factor degradation and a false prolongation of clotting times.

Tests that rely on optical methodologies for sample analysis (including some PT, aPTT, fibrinogen, FDP, D-dimer, and aggregometry techniques) may give erroneous results if samples contain significant amounts of other pigments (bilirubin, lipids, free hemoglobin) as these will affect passage of light through the sample. Tests of secondary hemostasis also only detect >90% (ACT) or > 65% (PT, aPTT) loss of coagulation factors. As a result, milder or early phase disease states may go undetected. When assessing hypercoagulability, the PT and aPTT are not reliably shortened in hypercoagulable states and *cannot* be used to assess risk of thrombosis. Finally, although aPTT testing is used primarily to screen for secondary hemostatic conditions, it may be mildly prolonged in vWF deficiencies as the decreased amount of vWF can also result in less factor VIII activity.

Multiple preanalytical and analytical factors may influence viscoelastic testing; for more information on this topic, readers are referred to the PROVETS guidelines (see Further Reading section).

9.6 Case Studies

Case study 1: Intoxication

A 3-month-old male intact Golden Retriever named Teddy was presented to the emergency room for evaluation of coughing on day one. The owners had taken him to a pet store a few days prior to presentation and noted that he had started coughing subsequent to that visit. On day 1 he seemed to have a normal energy level and was eating normally at home despite the cough. The owners had noted that sometimes when he coughed there was a terminal retch with some bloody sputum. At that time, exposure to canine infectious disease complex (CIRDC) at the pet store was suspected and he was treated with over-the-counter cough suppressant.

On day 2, Teddy was re-presented to the hospital for decreased appetite, lethargy, and intermittent continued cough. During his physical examination he was extremely lethargic and noted to have very pale mucous membranes. His respiratory rate was elevated at 96 breaths/min. A packed cell volume/total protein (PCV/TP) was taken which was 12%/5.5 g/dL (normal 40–45%/6–7 g/dL). His CBC showed a mildly decreased platelet count of 100,000/hpf (normal 200,000–500,000/hpf) with normal morphology. A PT/aPTT revealed values too high to read.

Teddy was suspected to have been exposed to anticoagulant rodenticide leading to pulmonary hemorrhage based on the hemoptysis and severe elevations in both his PT and aPTT (see Table 9.2 for rationale). Thoracic radiographs were considered to corroborate this theory but he was too unstable to undergo radiography. Instead, Teddy was immediately administered 120 mL of whole blood and placed in oxygen. He was given vitamin K orally. Two hours after transfusion, his PCV/TP was 22%/6.2 g/dL.

Teddy continued to have tachypnea and displayed respiratory distress when handled for the next 12 hours and he was left in the oxygen cage with minimal handling. Approximately 24 hours after admission to the hospital, he was greatly improved. He was acting more normally with a normal respiratory rate and effort even when handled. He was still anemic (PCV/TP = 26%/6.5 g/dL), which led to a reduced energy level versus a normal puppy. However, his PT/aPTT had normalized. Radiographs revealed a mild interstitial lung pattern and a moderately widened mediastinum (suspected to be secondary to hemorrhage). He was discharged to his owners on continued vitamin K therapy and was reportedly clinically normal 48 hours after discharge.

Case study 2: Post-dental hemorrhage

An approximately 8-year-old female spayed Yorkie named Mini was presented for bleeding in the oral cavity post-dental extractions. She had several canine teeth and a lower premolar removed earlier in the day at her primary care veterinarian's office. The CBC and chemistry panel performed prior to the dental procedure was normal. During the procedure, the site of the premolar extraction was bleeding slowly but continuously even after closure with a gingival flap and application of pressure. Due to continued hemorrhage hours after the dental procedure, she was referred to the Teaching Hospital for further diagnostics and care. The owners reported no other abnormalities aside from a historic exposure to anticoagulant rodenticide and recurrent dental disease. Per the owners, there was no possibility of exposure to anticoagulant rodenticide in the last 2 weeks. Mini was on no medications or supplements.

The CBC performed at the time of presentation revealed a Hct of 30% (normal 40–45%) and a platelet count of 239,000/hpf (normal range 200,000–300,000/hpf). The morphology of the platelets during microscopic examination was normal. A PT/aPTT was also performed. The PT was prolonged at 43 seconds (normal 5.4–9.4 seconds). The aPTT was also prolonged at 27.5 seconds (normal 9.4–13.4 seconds). Both of these prolongations were considered significant as they were greater than twice the upper reference levels. The degree of prolongation of the PT (approximately five times the upper reference interval) versus the degree of prolongation of the aPTT (around twice the upper reference interval) was noted.

The exact cause of Mini's hemorrhage was unclear but suspected to be a secondary hemostatic disorder based on the elevated PT/aPTT and the normal platelet count. She had received both a spay surgery and prior dental extractions in the past that did not cause excessive bleeding, making an inherited thrombocytopathy less likely. Additionally, Mini had not received any drugs that might inhibit platelet function.

Mini was given a transfusion of fresh frozen plasma to provide functional clotting factors. She was also started on oral vitamin K in the event that she had been exposed to anticoagulant rodenticide without the owner's knowledge (see Table 9.2 for rationale). Subsequent oral examination after the transfusion revealed a clot over the site of the tooth extraction. The following morning her PT and aPTT were normal and her PCV had improved to 35%. The owners were offered further diagnostics including liver function testing and/or specific factor testing (e.g. factors VII, V, or X levels) to ensure that there were no other abnormalities causing the clinical signs. The owners declined further workup since her clinical condition had improved and the chemistry panel preoperatively was normal and not indicative of liver dysfunction. She was discharged to her owners on a presumptive 3-week course of vitamin K and was reportedly doing well 2 days after discharge.

Case study 3: It is not the glaucoma…

Maui is a 10-year-old female spayed Chihuahua who presented initially for evaluation of changes to her left eye – squinting, cloudiness, and possible enlargement of the globe. The owner had noted these changes acutely during a flight home from vacation. During the evaluation of her eye by the ophthalmology department, she was diagnosed with uveitis and glaucoma. As part of a workup for uveitis, a CBC and chemistry panel were performed where it was noted that her platelet count was low with platelet clumping noted. An exact number was not available on the analyzer due to the clumping, but there were at least 100,000 platelets/hpf (normal 200,000–500,000/hpf).

Maui was discharged on ophthalmic medications for her left eye and a recheck examination was scheduled for 1 month later during which a repeat platelet count was planned to confirm the thrombocytopenia. At the time of her recheck examination, the owners reported that they had seen some bruising in her left axilla and ventral thoracic region. Two weeks prior to the recheck, Maui had also undergone a dental procedure after the owners noticed bleeding from one of her teeth. Only a cleaning had been performed without any teeth extractions, but no overt dental pathology was noted during the dental procedure to explain the bleeding.

During the physical examination at the time of presentation, besides the abnormalities reported by the owners, peri-umbilical ecchymoses, mild bruising on the left flank fold, and petechiations above the left upper canine tooth and on the right ear were noted. A CBC revealed 6,000/µL platelets (normal 200,000–500,000/µL).

Maui was diagnosed with severe thrombocytopenia. Due to the profoundly decreased platelet count and lack of indications of significant hemorrhage (PCV = 35%; normal 35–45%), she was presumed to have immune-mediated thrombocytopenia. In order to look for an underlying cause of the immune-mediated destruction, radiographs of the thorax and abdomen were taken which were largely unremarkable. An abdominal ultrasound did not reveal any significant abnormalities and a panel looking for underlying Rickettsial disease was normal. She was placed on doxycycline (10 mg/kg/day by mouth for 30 days) in the event a Rickettsial disease that was not identified on the panel was a causative agent for the immune-mediated destruction. Maui also received immunosuppressive steroids (2 mg/kg/day prednisone by mouth) to control the immune-mediated destruction of her platelets. Within 5 days, her platelet count had improved to 132,000/µL on the steroids.

However, 2 weeks later, Maui's recheck platelet count (on the same prednisone dosing) had dropped to 10,000/µL with a few small clumps noted. At that time, the owners saw ecchymoses on her ventral abdomen. She was re-admitted to the hospital for more aggressive immunosuppressive therapy with vincristine 0.02 mg/kg intravenously once and cyclosporine 10 mg/kg by mouth every 12 hours in addition to the continued 2 mg/kg/day of prednisone. Her platelet count initially improved to more than 500,000/µL. This exuberant response was attributed to the vincristine. Vincristine has an undetermined mechanism, but may either cause release of platelets from the megakaryocytes in the bone marrow and/or reduce destruction of existing platelets.

At a subsequent recheck examination 5 days later, her platelet count dropped to 6,000/µL. She was also anemic (19%/6.0 g/dL; normal 35–45%/5.5–7 g/dL). It was suspected that she was bleeding into her gastrointestinal tract secondary to the thrombocytopenia, leading to the anemia. She received intravenous immunoglobulin (IVIG) as a last-ditch effort to stop the immune-mediated destruction of her platelets. She was continued on the 2 mg/kg/day of prednisone and started on mycophenolate mofetil (10 mg/kg by mouth every 12 hours) in lieu of cyclosporine as a secondary immunosuppressive agent. She was also given sucralfate and omeprazole to treat any gastrointestinal ulceration leading to the bleeding.

Three days later, her platelet count was above 500,000/µL. Nine months later it continued to be greater than 400,000/µL on every recheck platelet count performed, despite slowly weaning her completely off the prednisone. During the prednisone weaning, Maui continued to receive mycophenolate at 10 mg/kg twice daily. At the time of writing, the plan was to continue Maui on mycophenolate for the remainder of her life (possibly at a slowly reduced dose) as long as she continued to tolerate the drug.

Further Reading

Ettinger, S.J., Feldman, E.C., Cote, E. (eds) (2017) *Textbook of Veterinary Internal Medicine*, 8th edn. Elsevier, St. Louis, Missouri, USA.

Barr, J.W., McMichael, M. (2012) Inherited disorders of hemostasis in dogs and cats. *Topics in Companion Animal Medicine* 27, 53–58.

Boudreaux, M.K. (2008) Characteristics, diagnosis, and treatment of inherited platelet disorders in mammals. *Journal of the American Veterinary Medical Association* 233, 1251–1259.

Goggs, R., Brainard, B., de Laforcade, A.M., et al. (2014) Partnership on Rotational Viscoelastic test standardization (PROVETS): Evidence-based guidelines on rotations viscoelastic assays in veterinary medicine. *Journal of Veterinary Emergency and Critical Care*, 24, 1–62.

Nakamura, R.K., Tompkins, E., and Bianco, D. (2012) Therapeutic options for immune-mediated thrombocytopenia. *Journal of Veterinary Emergency and Critical Care* 22, 59–72.

Paniccia, R.P., Priora, R., Liotta, A.A., Abbate, R. (2015) Platelet function tests: a comparative review. *Vascular Health and Risk Management* 11, 133–148.

Bibliography

Blair, P., Flaumenhaft, R. (2009) Platelet α-granules: Basic biology and clinical correlates. *Blood Review* 23, 177–189.

Blois, S., Lang, S., Wood, R., Monteith, G. (2015) Biologic variability and correlation of platelet function testing in healthy dogs. *Veterinary Clinical Pathology* 44, 503–510.

Brass, L. (2010) Understanding and evaluating platelet function. *ASH Education Book* 1, 387–396.

Brooks, M.B., Catalfamo, J.L. (2013). Current diagnostic trends in coagulation disorders among dogs and cats. *Veterinary Clinics of North America Small Animal* 43, 1349–1372.

Buttarello, M., Plebani, M. (2008) Automated blood cell counts. *American Journal of Clinical Pathology* 130, 104–116.

Favaloro, E., Mohammed, S., Patzke, J. (2017) Preanalytical issues in hemostasis and thrombosis testing. In: Favaloro, E., Lippi, G. (eds) *Hemostasis and Thrombosis. Methods in Molecular Biology*. Humana Press, New York, New York, USA, pp. 29–42.

Hopper, K., Bateman, S. (2005) An updated view of hemostasis: mechanisms of hemostatic dysfunction associated with sepsis. *Journal of Veterinary Emergency and Critical Care* 15, 83–91.

Hvas, A.M., Grove, E.L. (2017) Platelet function tests: Preanalytical variables, clinical utility, advantages, and disadvantages. In: Favaloro, E., Lippi, G. (eds) *Hemostasis and Thrombosis. Methods in Molecular Biology*. Humana Press, New York, New York, USA, pp. 305–320.

Lippi, G., Favarolo, E.J. (2017) Laboratory Testing for von Willebrand Factor Antigen (VWF:Ag). In: Favaloro, E., Lippi, G. (eds) *Hemostasis and Thrombosis. Methods in Molecular Biology*. Humana Press, New York, New York, USA, pp. 403–416.

Marlar, R.A., Potts, R.M., Marlar, A.A. (2006) Effect on routine and special coagulation testing values of citrate anticoagulant adjustment in patients with high hematocrit values. *American Journal of Clinical Pathology* 126, 400–405.

McMichael, M. (2005) Primary hemostasis. *Journal of Veterinary Emergency and Critical Care* 15, 1–8.

Siegel, J.E., Swami, V.K., Glenn, P., Peterson, P. (1998) Effect (or lack of it) of severe anemia on PT and APTT results. *American Journal of Clinical Pathology*, 110, 106–110.

Sibylle, A., Kozek-Langenecker, M.D. (2005) Effects of hydroxyethylstarch solutions on hemostasis. *Anesthesiology* 9, 654–660.

Smith, J., Day, T., Mackin, A. (2005) Diagnosing bleeding disorders. *Compendium of Continuing Education for the Veterinary Practitioner* 27, 828–843.

Stockham, S.L., Scott, M.A. (2008) Hemostasis. In: *Fundamentals of Veterinary Clinical Pathology*, 2nd edn. Blackwell Publishing, Ames, Iowa, USA, pp. 259–322.

10 Manometer-based Monitoring

ADESOLA ODUNAYO*

Department of Small Animal Clinical Sciences, University of Tennessee, Knoxville, Tennessee, USA

A manometer is one of the earliest pressure-monitoring devices. It measures the difference in liquid or air pressure by comparing it to an outside source, commonly the earth's atmospheric pressure. A water manometer is commonly utilized in veterinary patients to provide critical information on pressures, including intra-abdominal pressure and central venous pressure. In some institutions, electronic pressure transducers are used more commonly, despite their increased cost. Electronic pressure transducers allow for continuous pressure monitoring, as long as they are connected to the patient.

A water manometer, used for intermittent pressure monitoring, is easy to set up and is reasonably inexpensive to utilize for monitoring the critically ill patient. It consists of a plastic or glass tube, marked in centimeters, which is usually filled with a sterile isotonic fluid solution (0.9% NaCl is used most commonly but lactated Ringers solution, plasmalyte, and normosol can all be utilized). A 12–60 mL syringe attached to the plastic tube via a three-way stopcock and extension tubing completes the set up (Fig. 10.1).

10.1 Intra-abdominal Pressure Monitoring

Basic anatomy and physiology

Intra-abdominal pressure (IAP) is defined as the steady-state pressure contained within the peritoneal space that results from the interaction of the abdominal wall and viscera. Abdominal compliance is quite limited because of skeletal structures, the diaphragm, internal organs, and the abdominal wall. Thus when elevated IAP develops, there is interference with tissue perfusion of the intra-abdominal organs, which may lead to ischemia or circulatory changes. Intra-abdominal hypertension (IAH) is defined as markedly increased IAP and is a life-threatening complication that occurs after major abdominal trauma or abdominal surgery. IAH may occur as a result of increased intra-abdominal volume (e.g. hemorrhage or other ascites), inflammation, mass effect, or a combination of these. In human patients, there has been correlation between IAP and organ dysfunction, which ultimately leads to increased morbidity and mortality. As the intra-abdominal pressure rises, a condition called abdominal compartment syndrome (ACS) can occur. IAH is defined as sustained IAP over 20 mmHg, which is associated with new organ dysfunction/failure.

The reason that elevated IAP and ACS can lead to organ dysfunction is due to interference with the abdominal perfusion pressure (APP), which is defined as the mean arterial pressure (MAP) minus the IAP. Abdominal perfusion pressure should be maximized so that there is adequate delivery of oxygen and nutrients to the intra-abdominal organs. In general, APP is compromised when there is IAH and ACS. Maximizing APP usually involves maximizing MAP and minimizing IAP.

Consequences of IAH and ACS include decreases in venous return, leading to decreased cardiac output and hypotension (Fig. 9.2). Affected patients may also develop acute kidney injury, hepatic insufficiency and gastrointestinal signs because of decreased blood flow and poor tissue perfusion. The increased abdominal pressure also pushes the diaphragm cranially, which may result in increased intrathoracic pressure, affecting ventilation and oxygenation. Clinical consequences of IAH may

---

*Corresponding author: aodunayo@utk.edu

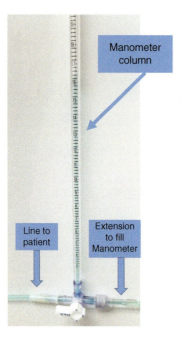

Fig. 10.1. Basic manometer setup. A glass manometer column is filled with fluid to a point above the expected reading. A three-way stopcock is attached to the manometer column. One extension set coming from the three-way stopcock is attached to the patient and a separate extension set is attached to a syringe or bag of fluids to fill the manometer. In this figure, the three-way stopcock is turned off to the patient so the manometer can be filled with sterile fluid.

range from mild effects to life-threatening multiple organ dysfunction. Examples of common conditions that may cause IAH include post-abdominal surgery, ileus (with gradual dilation of the intestines taking up intra-abdominal space), gastric dilatation and volvulus, ascites, abdominal trauma, and sepsis. Animals often develop ileus when there is edema of the walls of the intestines either from fluid overload or leakage of fluid out of the blood vessels. Patients with unexplained causes of hypotension, oliguria/anuria, abdominal pain, azotemia, elevated liver enzymes, or respiratory difficulty, should have their IAP monitored to look for indications of ACS.

Normal IAP in dogs may range from 5–10 cmH_2O, while normal IAP in cats may range from 0–20 cmH_2O. For measurements obtained in mmHg, note that 1 mmHg is 1.36 cmH_2O. It is important to note that IAP varies with physiologic conditions such as phase of breathing, coughing, exercise, or defecation, so small variations are expected to occur. The IAP may also vary with level of sedation, body positioning, body condition score, and bladder instillation volumes during IAP testing (see below). As much as possible, IAP should be obtained the same way every time to minimize variations in the results.

The presence of IAH has been reported in veterinary patients. In one study evaluating intra-abdominal pressures in 20 client dogs after routine ovariohysterectomy, there were significant elevations in the mean postoperative pressure by as much as 15 cmH_2O (Conzemius et al., 1995). This increase in IAP persisted for as long as 24 hours after the elective surgery. However, there was no clinical evidence of significant complications in the group of healthy dogs. Intra-abdominal pressures were also measured in 20 dogs with gross abdominal distension (due to clinical conditions like gastric dilation and volvulus, closed pyometra, hemoperitoneum, and ascites). All of these dogs had severe IAP (>16 cmH_2O) either before or after surgery. Two of those dogs developed anuria, both of which required surgical decompression for management of their IAH (Conzemius et al., 1995).

Grading of IAH and ACS by the World Society of Abdominal Compartment Syndrome is detailed in Table 10.1. Note that there is a slight overlap between normal IAP in dogs and cats and grade I IAH in human patients, so a direct comparison between species is not possible and a veterinarian needs to be cautious of directly applying human information to animals. In addition, it is possible that dogs can tolerate slightly higher IAP before developing negative side effects. It is best to utilize trends in IAP, as well as the patient's clinical picture, in determining how to approach a patient with elevated IAP.

How the monitor works

While there are many methods described for measuring IAP, many of them require complicated and costly equipment. Some of them are also invasive, requiring the placement of a catheter and pressure transducer directly into the abdominal cavity, stomach, rectum, or caudal vena cava. Direct measurements of IAP are impractical under most circumstances, thus surrogate measures of IAP have been investigated. The homogenous transmission of pressure within the abdomen allows IAP to be estimated via either the bladder, rectum, or stomach. Intravesical pressure measurement, using the uri-

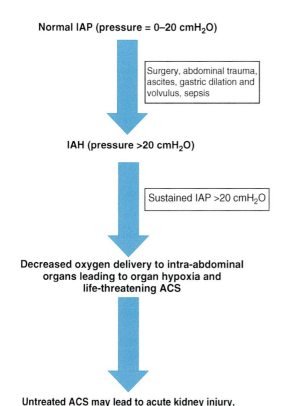

Fig. 10.2. Visual representation of the stages from increased intra-abdominal pressure to abdominal compartment syndrome. ACS, abdominal compartment syndrome; IAP, intra-abdominal pressure; IAH, intra-abdominal hypertension.

Table 10.1. Grades of intra-abdominal hypertension and abdominal compartment syndrome in human patients. Note that normal intra-abdominal pressures in dogs and cats are slightly higher than those reported in humans.

Grade	Pressure mmHg (cmH$_2$O)
Grade I	12–15 (16–20)
Grade II	16–20 (21–27)
Grade III	21–25 (28–33)
Grade IV	>25 (>33)
Abdominal compartment syndrome	> 20 (27) sustained with new organ dysfunction or failure

nary bladder, has been investigated and validated in human medicine and remains the accepted surrogate measure for IAP in clinical use in people. There are no known validation studies evaluating IAP in veterinary patients. However, using intravesical pressure measurement makes it possible to measure IAP in a simpler way with equipment readily available to any veterinary practitioner.

The simplest and most practical method of measuring IAP can be accomplished utilizing the urinary bladder and a water manometer (see Fig. 10.3). The urinary bladder is an intra-abdominal and extraperitoneal organ with a compliant wall. It acts as a passive reservoir of urine and is capable of transmitting abdominal pressure without imparting any additional pressure from its own musculature. The urinary bladder should not be utilized in any patient with pre-existing bladder disease or those with bladder trauma since the bladder should be allowed to heal under those circumstances. Instead, a different organ such as the stomach could be used for those patients. Performing the intragastric pressure is a surrogate for measuring IAP in human respiratory research. However, there is conflicting evidence for the relationship between intragastric pressure and IAP, so using the bladder is preferred if possible in humans (and likely is also preferred in animals).

A commercially available IAP monitoring system (AbViser) can be used in place of a water manometer. This system is directly connected to the patient's urinary catheter and it measures IAP using a pressure transducer after instillation of saline into the urinary bladder.

Items required for monitoring IAP (via urinary bladder):

- sedation for patient if needed and depending on hemodynamic and pain status (butorphanol, methadone, fentanyl, midazolam, dexmedetomidine);
- sterile gloves;
- foley urinary catheter (or red rubber catheter in cats);
- sterile lubricant for placing Foley urinary catheter (or red rubber catheter in cats);
- urinary collection system;
- water manometer;
- three-way stopcocks (2);
- 35–60 mL syringes;
- 1-L bag of sterile saline or any other isotonic crystalloid;

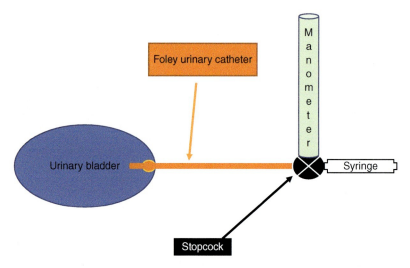

Fig. 10.3. A diagrammatic representation of the setup to measure pressure in the urinary bladder with a water manometer. An extension set can be placed between the stopcock and the syringe or the syringe can be directly attached to the stopcock. If larger volumes are needed to distend the bladder, a bag of fluids can be used in place of the syringe.

- extension sets; and
- fluid administration set.

Steps for obtaining IAP using a water manometer:

1. Ensure patient is comfortable in lateral or sternal recumbency. Administer analgesia or sedation as required. Avoid medications that may affect hemodynamic status in unstable patients (i.e. do not use dexmedetomidine in a cardiovascularly unstable patient). Ensure all subsequent readings are taken the same way, if possible.
2. Place Foley urinary catheter using aseptic technique. Ensure the catheter tip is located just inside the trigone of the urinary bladder by filling the balloon of the Foley catheter with saline, water or air, and pulling the catheter out of the urethra until it can no longer be withdrawn from the bladder (i.e. the Foley balloon is seated in the trigone of the bladder).
3. Empty the urinary bladder into a collection container using a 35–60 mL syringe. Alternatively, the urinary bladder can be emptied into the urinary collection system (see below) before the IAP is obtained.
4. Connect the sterile urinary collection system to the end of the Foley catheter, using both of the three-way stopcock systems connected serially.
5. Attach a 35–60 mL syringe, as well as the water manometer (or pressure transducer) to the stopcock closest to the patient. Attach a 1-L bag of sterile saline to the second stopcock. The second stopcock will be used to fill the manometer and infuse saline into the bladder. Fill the syringe with sterile saline by turning the stopcocks off to the patient and off to the manometer.
6. Instill 0.5–1 mL/kg of sterile saline into the urinary bladder.
7. Zero the manometer (or transducer) to the patient's midline (iliac crest) by holding the manometer in a set location and noting the number on the manometer that corresponds to the midline (see Fig. 10.4). This number is now the zero point. Then close the stopcock to the fluid source and allow the meniscus in the manometer to equilibrate with the pressure in the urinary bladder. Compare the level of the meniscus to the zero number to obtain the actual reading. For example, if the zero point is 6 cmH$_2$O with the manometer on the floor next to the patient and the meniscus settles on 10 cmH$_2$O, the reading will be +4 cmH$_2$O (see Fig. 10.5).

Zeroing the manometer helps establish a zero baseline that is relative to the atmospheric pressure and ensures an accurate measurement of the pressure changes. Please note that there is no 'correct' and validated external landmark in animals to use as the zero point. Some studies use the iliac crest, some studies use the level of the vulva/prepuce, and some studies use the level of the pubic symphysis.

8. Take the measurement about 30–60 seconds after instilling saline into the urinary bladder so that the detrusor muscle is relaxed and there is no active abdominal contraction. The measurement should ideally be taken at the end of expiration.

9. A *clinical decision* needs to be made about the results obtained. If the IAP is high and the patient has clinical signs of ACS, the clinician should make the decision to treat the patient. Repeated measurements after treatment may be used to gage the response to treatment as well as trends in the patient's IAP over time.

10. Disconnect three-way stopcock, syringe, saline bag and extension tubing once finished. Reattach urine collection bag to Foley catheter in a sterile manner.

(This method can be performed in a similar manner using a nasogastric tube in the stomach, in cases where the urinary bladder cannot be utilized. No specific technique has been published or validated in veterinary medicine and the bladder is always preferred.)

Indications for IAP monitoring

IAP should be monitored in any patient with clinical suggestions of IAH or ACS. These signs may include a tense and distended abdomen, oliguria, anuria, hypoxia, hypercapnia, hypotension, acidosis, or ileus. Clinical conditions that may predispose to IAH or ACS are outlined in Box 10.1. It is not recommended that IAP is measured in patients without evidence or clinical signs of IAH or ACS due to over-interpretation of the results.

IAP should be monitored every 4–6 hours with hourly (or continuous) measurement restricted to patients with severe organ dysfunction.

Interpretation of IAP results

Once the IAP has been obtained, it should then be determined if the patient is at risk for IAH, as detailed in Table 10.1. It is important to note that IAH is defined as 'sustained increases in IAP', thus the diagnosis of IAH should be based on *serial* measurements of the IAP. The clinician should make a clinical judgment on the frequency of measurement of IAP based on the clinical condition of the patient, clinical signs of IAH/ACS and severity of IAH/ACS. As a general rule, patients with IAH/ACS should have their IAP checked every 2–4

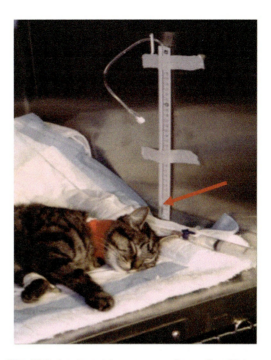

Fig. 10.4. A cat receiving a manometer reading. Note that the manometer is attached to the side of the cage so as to be in a repeatable location each time a reading is taken. In this case, the red arrow marks the zero point for this cat. All measurements are taken in relation to this zero point.

hours. Management of IAH and ACS, typically consists of supportive care initially, and if needed, surgical abdominal decompression. Medical management should be tailored to keep IAP below 15 mmHg.

Surgical decompression is considered definitive management of IAH/ACS. If IAP/ACS is refractory to medical management based on ongoing clinical signs of IAH/ACS and refractory IAH, surgery should be strongly considered for abdominal decompression. In human patients, surgical intervention is considered when IAP is greater than 26 mmHg or the patient's clinical signs cannot be controlled. However, there are no absolute guidelines for when surgical intervention occurs. Surgical intervention typically involves providing decompression by opening up the abdomen. Many of these human patients end up being treated as an 'open abdomen' until the IAP is low enough for abdominal closure. There is sparse information about surgical intervention for ACS in veterinary patients.

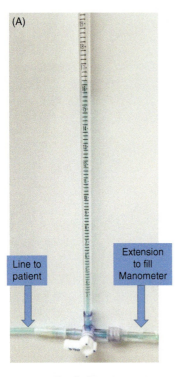 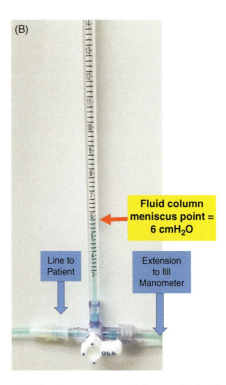

Fig. 10.5. An example of taking a measurement from a manometer. (A) The three-way stopcock is turned off to the patient so the manometer can be filled with sterile fluid to a level of approximately 16 cmH$_2$O. (B) The three-way stopcock has been turned off to the extension for filling leaving the manometer column open to the patient. Note that the fluid column has decreased. The fluid meniscus has settled on 6 cmH$_2$O. Since this patient's zero point was the actual zero number on the manometer, this indicates a IAP of 6 cmH$_2$O.

Supportive care for managing patients with IAH/ACS include the following:

- Reduction of intra-abdominal volume by evaluating intraluminal contents. This includes removal of gastric contents using a nasogastric tube or administration of prokinetic agents such as metoclopramide, erythromycin, or cisapride to move luminal contents out of the body. Enteral nutrition should be minimized until IAP is normal.
- Removal of ascites or hemorrhage in the abdominal cavity. Rectal drainage by placing a Foley catheter into the rectum and aspirating material can also be performed to reduce IAP in patients with bowel distension.
- Abdominal wall compliance can be improved with pain control and sedation to make the abdominal walls less tense. Constrictive bandages should be removed from around the abdomen. Neuromuscular blockers may be considered if mechanical ventilation is required to lessen the chances of breathing against the ventilator and thus increasing pressure within the abdomen.
- Avoid creating tissue edema. This includes limiting fluid administration if possible. Consider judicious use of diuretics, once the animal is hemodynamically stable. Dialysis may be utilized to remove excessive fluids. Tissue edema will not only take up space in the abdominal compartment but also can lead to ileus if the edema is present within the walls of the intestinal tract.
- Maintain adequate MAP using vasopressors as necessary to maintain the APP.

Pitfalls of intra-abdominal pressure monitoring

Intra-abdominal pressure monitoring can provide useful information for critically ill patients. It is important to remember that because many factors

Box 10.1. Clinical conditions that may predispose an animal to intra-abdominal hypertension.

- Abdominal surgery, especially laparotomy closed under tension
- Trauma
- Pancreatitis
- Peritonitis
- Retroperitoneal bleed
- Major burns
- Gross ascites
- Large abdominal mass
- Gastrointestinal obstruction
- Peritoneal dialysis
- Pyometra
- Hemoabdomen
- Diaphragmatic hernia
- Mechanical ventilation with positive-end expiratory pressures above 10 mm Hg
- Massive fluid replacement or blood transfusion
- Pelvic fractures
- Fluid overload

affect IAP readings (anxiety, sedation, recumbency, etc.), serial elevated measurements should be determined before significant therapeutic decisions are made. In addition, normal values of IAP have been determined in different groups of human patients (mechanically ventilated, spontaneously breathing, postoperative patients, post-abdominal trauma). Since these values have not been determined for similar subgroups of veterinary patients, IAP results should be interpreted cautiously. Along the same lines, IAP measurement should only be performed in patients with risk factors and clinical signs of IAH.

Measuring IAP may cause iatrogenic contamination and infection of the urinary bladder, thus patients should be closely monitored for any indications of development of a urinary tract infection.

Case study

Nico, a 12-year-old, male castrated Labrador Retriever was being hospitalized for severe acute pancreatitis. He had been doing well in the hospital on an isotonic crystalloid at 60 mL/kg/day, fentanyl at 3 µg/kg/h and an anti-emetic (maropitant).

On his second day of hospitalization, Nico was laterally recumbent. His vitals were as follows:

- Heart rate: 180 beats/min
- Temperature: 102.8°F (39.3°C)
- Respiratory rate: 28 breaths/min
- Blood pressure: 80 mmHg (systolic)

His abdomen was very tense on palpation and he seemed to be significantly more uncomfortable than he was the previous day. A fluid bolus of crystalloids (20 mL/kg IV over 15 minutes) did not improve his blood pressure. A quick abdominal ultrasound scan (AFAST—see Chapter 7) did not reveal any free fluid or obvious cause for his abdominal discomfort. A urinary catheter was placed and used to measure an IAP, which was elevated at 19 mmHg. Repeat IAP measurement 2 hours later was still elevated at 20 mmHg. Nico's blood work was unchanged from the day of presentation and he did not have any evidence of new organ dysfunction.

Due to the sustained increase in Nico's IAP, he was diagnosed with IAH. Nico was treated with aggressive pain management by increasing his fentanyl dose to 5 µg/kg/h and adding lidocaine and ketamine for additional analgesia. An epidural catheter was inserted to provide additional regional analgesia. A nasogastric tube was placed and about 200 mL of gastric fluid was removed. Nico was also started on a metoclopramide constant rate infusion (2 mg/kg/day) and erythromycin (1 mg/kg via nasogastric tube every 8 hours) to help promote gastrointestinal motility.

About an hour after those changes were made, Nico was significantly more comfortable. His heart rate had decreased to 80 beats/min and his blood pressure had increased to 110 mmHg (systolic). Nico showed remarkable clinical improvement and his IAP had come down to 8 mmHg on the next recheck. Nico's IAP was monitored every 4 hours and his analgesics were slowly tapered over the next 2–3 days, as long as he remained comfortable. Nico was discharged after 5 days of hospitalization, once he started eating on his own and was able to keep his food down.

10.2 Central Venous Pressure Monitoring

Basic anatomy and physiology

The central venous pressure (CVP) is the pressure recorded from the cranial vena cava. Due to the cranial vena cava's proximity to the right atrium, the CVP also represents the right atrial pressure.

The right atrium is unique among the chambers of the heart in that the primary determinant of the pressure within that chamber is the volume in the chamber. Therefore, the CVP (and right atrial pressure) can be used as an estimate of the right ventricular preload (i.e. the volume presented to the right atrium prior to emptying into the right ventricle). The right ventricular preload is largely determined by the venous return and the ability of the right ventricle to eject blood in a normally functioning heart. The venous return is in turn affected by venous tone, venous wall compliance, and circulating blood volume; right-sided cardiac output is determined by the heart rate, afterload, preload, and contractility. Any variables that affect these factors may ultimately affect the CVP.

The CVP has been used historically to assess preload and volume status in critically ill patients, to guide fluid resuscitation, as well as to aid in the diagnosis of right-sided heart failure. The basis for using CVP to guide fluid management originates from the dogma that CVP reflects intravascular volume. It is thought that patients with a low CVP are volume-depleted and need fluids, while patients with a high CVP are volume-overloaded and will not respond to fluid therapy. However, there is a tremendous amount of evidence in critically ill human patients that CVP does not reflect venous volume and that a low CVP does not necessarily mean the patient requires fluid therapy.

The current thought is that CVP is a misleading tool for guiding fluid therapy, although some research in humans does suggest 'extreme' CVP values may be able to guide response to fluids while intermediate values cannot. In human medicine, values below 8 cmH$_2$O (6 mmHg) and more than 20 cmH$_2$O (15 mmHg) are considered extreme values. Typically, approximately twice as many human patients with low CVPs (below 8 cmH$_2$O) respond to fluids (i.e. had an increase in their cardiac output after fluid administration) than those with high CVPs (above 20 cmH$_2$O). Therefore, in a clinical setting it may be wise to refrain from administering fluids when CVP values are extremely high and to give fluids when CVP values are very low. However, besides the fact that there are no similarly determined extreme values in veterinary medicine, the CVP is influenced by many factors, which makes its interpretation complicated (see Comments on CVP Monitoring section). Also, the ability to directly measure cardiac output in a clinical veterinary patient does not exist so the clinician has to rely on indirect measures such as blood pressure and other perfusion parameters (see Chapters 1 and 2).

How the monitor works

CVP is generally measured with a water manometer or a pressure transducer. This chapter focuses on the use of a manometer for the measurement of the CVP. Normal CVP for dogs and cats is generally around 0–5 cmH$_2$O, although values of up to 10 cmH$_2$O can be normal in critically ill patients. If used, a pressure transducer will report values in mmHg. Measurement can be converted to cmH$_2$O by multiplying the mmHg value by 1.36.

Items required:

- a central venous catheter, which can be single-lumen or multi-lumen;
- three-way stopcock;
- 20–35 mL syringe filled with saline;
- a 250 mL bag of sterile saline; and
- specialized noncompliant tubing (extension set) if available.

Steps for obtaining a CVP using a water manometer:

1. Place the patient in lateral or sternal recumbency and place an indwelling central venous catheter using aseptic techniques. The tip of the central venous catheter should be in the cranial vena cava, just before it enters the right atrium (verified radiographically).
2. The central venous catheter should be secured in place, flushed to maintain patency, and lightly wrapped to keep it clean.
3. To obtain a CVP, the patient should be placed in lateral recumbency (ideally, right lateral recumbency but either side is acceptable). Right lateral recumbency places the physical location of the right atrium close to the thoracic inlet for use in zero-ing (see step no. 6). No matter the recumbency selected, as with IAP measurements, CVP should be done the same way every time.
4. The extension set (flushed with sterile saline) should be connected to the central venous catheter. If a multi-lumen catheter is being used, connect the extension set to the central lumen and clamp off the other lumens.
5. The three-way stopcock is connected to the extension set, while the saline-filled syringe is

connected to the other end of the three-way stopcock. Finally, the water manometer is connected to the last connection of the three-way stopcock, ensuring that its orientation is vertical.

6. The water manometer should be zeroed at the level of the patient's right atrium. This involves placing the water manometer in a set location such as attached to the patient's cage, an IV pole, or a wall, to ensure that it does not move during the measurement, and noticing which reading on the manometer lines up with the level of the right atrium – this is considered the zero point. Typically, the thoracic inlet is used as the external marker for the right atrial location when in lateral recumbency.

7. Turning the stopcock off to the manometer, the syringe is used to flush about 5–10 mL of saline into the catheter. The stopcock is then turned off to the patient and the manometer is filled to about 10–20 cmH_2O of saline higher than the patient's expected CVP.

8. The stopcock is finally turned off to the syringe, to allow the fluid in the manometer to equilibrate with the patient's right atrial pressure. The level of the saline in the manometer will fall as it flows into the patient, and then eventually stabilize as the fluid level equilibrates with the CVP. The level in the manometer where the water level stabilizes should be compared to the previously determined zero point to yield the CVP reading. For example, if the zero point was determined to be 4 cmH_2O in the manometer, if the water level stops at 10 cmH_2O, the recorded CVP would be +6 cmH_2O. *Please note that CVP readings can also be negative.*

9. About three to five consecutive measurements should be performed and the average should be recorded.

10. To disconnect the assembly, turn the stopcock off to the manometer and disconnect the extension set from the central venous catheter in an aseptic manner. The CVP measurement setup should be stored aseptically prior to its use again.

Comments on CVP Monitoring

Due to the controversies associated with the value and interpretation of the CVP, many human and veterinary facilities have discontinued the use of CVP in critically ill patients. The author does not recommend using CVP measurements to guide treatment in veterinary patients.

The primary indication historically cited for CVP monitoring is to predict the need for fluid therapy in a critically ill patient (i.e. the patient's predicted fluid responsiveness). The CVP has also been used to determine if fluid therapy should be stopped or altered in a critically ill patient. Even those who currently subscribe to the belief that CVPs can still be used in certain situations to guide clinical decisions limit use of the CVP to when the values are really high or really low. That is to say, a 'really low' CVP reading is a reason to initiate fluid therapy and a 'really high' CVP reading is a reason to stop fluid therapy. There are no real guidelines as to what constitutes high or low enough to dictate alterations in fluid therapy, but the author would typically consider lower than −5 to −10 cmH_2O very low and higher than +15 to +20 cmH_2O very high. Please note that as with IAP monitoring, serial CVP measurements are recommended, in concert with consideration of the clinical condition of the patient. Therefore, one single CVP reading is typically not a reason to change treatments, especially if the patient is not giving any other indications of fluid overload or hypovolemia.

Many factors serve to complicate the ability of CVP to predict the patient's fluid requirements. For example, any increase in thoracic, pericardial or abdominal pressures will be transmitted through the wall of the veins. This can increase the CVP by increasing pressure on the vessels; at the same time, increased pressure on the vessels will also partially or fully occlude them, causing a decreased in volume within the vessels. Since increased CVP readings are supposed to represent *more* volume in the vasculature and eventually returning to the right atrium, in the setting of increased body cavity pressures, the CVP is *not* able to predict the vascular volume. Similarly, changes in sympathetic tone that lead to venoconstriction can increase the CVP but actually reduce the blood volume present in the vessels. Alternatively, venodilation will decrease the CVP but often indicates more volume in the vessels rather than less. Any structural disease affecting the heart will lead to aberrant blood flow through the heart. Hence, more volume can be present in a heart chamber due to regurgitant blood flow or incomplete emptying of the chambers during each cardiac cycle. This can have the effect of increasing the CVP but does not indicate that this increased right atrial volume is also leaving the heart. For example, in the case of the right atrium, tricuspid valve regurgitation or decreased relaxation of the right ventricle will result in more blood retained (or regurgitated) into the right atrium. This can lead to an increased CVP which could be interpreted as the patient being hypervolemic. However, in many cases, the actual blood leaving the heart and being pumped to the tissues is low, making them relatively hypovolemic. Finally, exogenous factors such as general anesthesia and sedatives can also change cardiac function or vessel tone and make interpretation of CVP difficult if not impossible.

At this time, the author believes that CVP does not have a place in the routine clinical monitoring of veterinary critically ill patients. Serial physical examinations and the use of other monitoring techniques described in this book provide more information than the CVP as related to prediction of the need for more or less fluid administration in a patient.

Bibliography

Barton, L., Adams, A. (2012) Peritoneal Evaluation. In: Burkitt-Creedon J.M. and Davis H. (eds) *Advanced Monitoring and Procedures for Small Animal Emergency and Critical Care*. Wiley-Blackwell, Chichester, UK, pp. 449–456.

Chow, R.S., Dilley, P. (2012) Central venous pressure monitoring. In: Burkitt-Creedon, J.M., Davis, H., (eds.) *Advanced Monitoring and Procedures for Small Animal Emergency and Critical Care*. Wiley-Blackwell, Chichester, UK, pp. 145–158.

Collee, G.G., Lomax, D.M., Ferguson, C., Hanson, G.C. (1993) Bedside measurement of intra-abdominal pressure (IAP) via an indwelling naso-gastric tube: clinical validation of the technique. *Intensive Care Medicine* 19, 478–480.

Conzemius, M.G., Sammarco, J.L., Holt, D.E., Smith, G.K. (1995) Clinical determination of preoperative and postoperative intra-abdominal pressures in dogs. *Veterinary Surgery* 24, 195–201.

De Backer, D., Vincent, J.L. (2018) Should we measure the central venous pressure to guide fluid management? Ten answers to 10 questions. *Critical Care* 22, 43.

Fetner, M., Prittie, J. (2012) Evaluation of transvesical intra-abdominal pressure measurement in hospitalized dogs. *Journal of Veterinary Emergency and Critical Care* 22, 230–238.

Magder, S. (2019) Central venous pressure. In: Pinsky, M.R., Teboul J.L., Vincent J.L., (ed.) *Hemodynamic Monitoring*. Springer Imprint, Cham, Switzerland, pp. 223–231.

Marik, P.E., Baram, M., Vahid, B. (2008) Does central venous pressure predict fluid responsiveness?: A systematic review of the literature and the tale of seven mares. *Chest* 134, 172–178.

Milanesi, R., Caregnato, R.C.A. (2016) Intra-abdominal pressure: an integrative review. *Einstein* 14, 423–430.

Pires, R.C., Rodrigues, N., Machado, J., Cruz, R.P. (2017) Central venous catheterization: An updated review of historical aspects, indications, techniques, and complications. *Translational Surgery* 2, 66.

Rao, P., Chaudhry, R., Kumar, S. (2006) Abdominal Compartment Pressure Monitoring – A Simple Technique. *Medical journal, Armed Forces India* 62, 269.

Reems, M.M., Aumann, M. (2012) Central venous pressure: Principles, measurement, and interpretation. *Compendium on Continuing Education for the Practising Veterinarian* 34, E1.

Smith, S.E., Sande, A.A. (2012) Measurement of intra-abdominal pressure in dogs and cats. *Journal of Veterinary Emergency and Critical Care* 22, 530–544.

Way, L.I., Monnet, E. (2014) Determination and validation of volume to be instilled for standardized intra-abdominal pressure measurement in dogs. *Journal of Veterinary Emergency and Critical Care*, 24, 403–407.

Index

Note: Page numbers in **bold** type refer to **figures**
Page numbers in *italic* type refer to *tables*

A and B-lines **135**, 137–142, **139**, 150–152
A–a grad 101–102, 105–108
abdomen 199–208
    intra-abdominal pressure monitoring 199–208, **200**, **204**
    surgical decompression 203
    wall compliance 204
abdominal compartment syndrome (ACS) 199–203, *201*, **201**
abdominal fluid scoring (AFS) system 138, 145
abdominal focal assessment for trauma/triage/tracking (AFAST[3]) 129–138, **134–135**, 145–152, *146*, 205
abdominal perfusion pressure (APP) 199, 204
abdominocentesis 133, 147, 151–152
ablation 60
accelerated idioventricular rhythm (AIVR) 58
acetaminophen 19, 170
acetoacetate 2
acetone 2
acidemia 17, 85–86, 169
acidosis 103–105, 203
    LUKES differentials and high AG 105
activatable fibrinolysis inhibitor (TAFI) 182
activated clotting time (ACT) 187
activated partial thromboplastin time (aPTT) 149–152, 187–188, 192, *193*, 195–196
acute respiratory distress syndrome (ARDS) 101
adenosine diphosphate (ADP) 177
adenosine triphosphate (ATP) 1–3, **4**, 159–160
aggregometry 186, 189, 194–195
albumin 43, 169
aldosterone 29, **161**
    receptor blockers 38
alkalemia 85–86, 99–100, **161**, 170
alkaline 89, 104
alkalosis 86
    metabolic *88*, **89**, 99, 103, 107, *166*
    respiratory 87–88, 99–100, 104, 107, *165–166*
Alpha-2-antiplasmin 182
Alpha-2-macroglobulin 182
AlphaTRAK glucometer **9**, 18–19
altered $P_{(a\text{-}ET)}CO_2$ gradient *118*
alveolar gases 110–112
    exchange 91–93, **91**

alveolar oxygen concentration (PaO$_2$) 92–93, 98, 101
ammonia 152
amperometry 5–7
anaphylaxis 136
anemia 12–15, 19, 76, 93, 145, 148–150, 190–194, 197
    immune-mediated hemolytic 15
    non-regenerative 106
    sickle cell 71
anesthesia 11, 37, 42–44, 58, 74, 80, 83, 108, 117–127, 171, 208
    circuit 112–114, 119–121, 124–125
    mask connector 115
angiotensin converting enzyme (ACE) 29, **30**
    inhibitors (ACEi) 38–39, 42–43
angiotensin receptor blockers (ARBs) 38–39, 42–43
anion gap (AG) 20, 86–88, **90**, 99, 102–105
    use in acid-base analysis 104–105
anorexia 16, 43, 157
anti-thrombin 183
antibody titer testing 43
anticoagulants 169–170, 183–184, **184**
    rodenticide intoxication 190–192, 195
antidiuretic hormone (ADH) 29–30, **30**, 40
anuria 200, 203
arachidonic acid metabolites 29
arrhythmia 12, 44, 50–52, 158–163
    drugs *57–58*
    sinus 52, 56, **56**
arterial blood oxygen content (CaO$_2$) 74
arterial PaCO$_2$ 90–93, 99–101, 106–108, 117–118, 125–128
artifacts 51, 130, **132–133**, 136–138
ascorbic acid 19
ataxia 157
atelectasis 127–128
ATPase pumps 156
atrial ectopy 59
atrial fibrillation (AF) 61–62, **61**, 67–68
atrial standstill 64–66, **65**, 68–69
atrioventricular (AV) node 45–48, 52, **54**, 59–68
atrioventricular block 62–64, **63–64**, 67
atropine response test 64
attenuation 129–130
auscultation 12, 22, 68, 150

209

autonomic imbalance 56
autoregulatory vascular function 30, 38
azotemia 105, 164, 200

base excess (BE) 86–89, 98–100
basophils 19
bat/gator signs 138, **139**, **142**, 149
Beer and Lambert Laws 112
bicarbonate (HCO$_3$) 66, 85–89, **89**, 98–99, 103–107
bilirubin 5, 152
Blastomyces dermatitidis 107
blood 156–158
    osmolality 157–158
    smear review and HPF 184–185, **185–186**
    volume 29–30
blood gas analysis 9, 82, 85–108
    V/Q mismatch **95–96**, 101
    and hypoxemia **92–96**, *93*, 106–107
    metabolic acidosis 3, 85–89, *87–88*, **89**, 99–100, 104–107, *120*, *165–166*
    metabolic alkalosis **88**, **89**, 99, 103, 107, *166*
    non-traditional approach 88–90, *90*, 100–105
    respiratory acidosis 86, **88**, 99–100, 103, 106
    respiratory alkalosis 86, *87–88*, 99–100, 104, 107, *165–166*
    sample collection and handling 93–96
    traditional approach 85–86, 99–105
blood pressure monitoring 26–44, **27–29**, *32*, 151
    diastolic 12, 26, **28**, 30–36, **31**, *32*, 41–45, 150
    mean arterial (MAP) regulation 26–31, **31**, 35, 39–42
    measurement 30–36
    oscillometry 35–36, **35**, 40–43
    pulse 12, 20–21, 26, 30–32, 35, 41
    systolic 12, 20, 26–43, **27–28**, **31**, *32*, 67–68, 127, 140, 151–152, 171, 205
blood urea nitrogen (BUN) 20, 171, **172**
bone marrow disease 15
bradyarrhythmia 40, 50, 62–69, **66**
    differentiation algorithm 66–67
bradycardia 56, 162, 175
bradycardia–tachycardia syndrome 64–65, **65**
buccal mucosal bleeding time (BMBT) 185, 194
buffering 89
    open system 86
bundle branches 45, 49
bundle of His 45

cage-side organ assessment for trauma/triage/tracking (COAST[3]) 129–130
calcium (Ca) 20, 88, **159**
    and coagulation 177–181, 187
    and hypercalcemia 158, **159**, 163, *165*, 169–170, 174–175, *174*
    and hyperphosphatemia 159

and hypocalcemia 158, **159**, 163, *165*, 169–170
    ionized (iCa) 93, 158, 163, 170, *174*, 175
calcium channel blockers (CCBs) 38–39, 42–43, 61
canine infectious disease complex (CIRDC) 195
capillary refill time (CRT) 4, 13–14, 20–22, 149
capnography 110–128
    V/P (mis)matching 110–112
    anesthesia or heavy sedation 117
    capnometry and capnograms, phases/angles 119–121, **121**
    cardiogenic oscillations 123, **125**
    commonly encountered abnormal waveforms 121–124, *122*
    endotracheal tube obstruction/leak 121–124, **124–126**
    feeding tube placement 117
    indications in small animals 117–118
    infrared source and detector 112–117, **113**
    mainstream 113–115, **114**, 125
    mechanical ventilation 117–118
    qualitative and quantitative 112–117
    rebreathing and hypercapnia 110, 117, 121–123, **123**
    sample chamber 113
    sidestream and microstream 115–117, **115–116**, 125–126
    time and lung volume analysis 111–117
    traumatic brain injury patients 118
    upper airway emergencies 117
carbon dioxide (CO$_2$) 75, 170
carbon monoxide (CO) 76
carbonic anhydrase 85–86
carboxyhemoglobin (COHb) 76, 80–83
cardiac output (CO) **29**, 110, 128
cardiac tamponade 141
cardiopulmonary resuscitation (CPR) 111, 117
central nervous system (CNS) 36
    imaging 43
central venous pressure (CVP) 205–208
chest tube site (CTS) 138–140
chloride 20, 102
chlorophyll 71
cholangiohepatitis 136
Clauss assay 187
coagulation 177–197
    endothelium damage 177–179
    glycoprotein receptors and integrin 177–179
    red-top tube test (Lee-White method) 186–187
    specific testing 187–188
    viscoelastic testing 188
complete blood count (CBC) 149–151, 184, 193, 196
congenital heart failure (CHF) 61
continuous rate infusion (CRI) 21, 44, 60
creatinine 20
cyanide toxicosis 80–83
cyanosis 71, 80
cystocolic (CC) view 137

D-dimer assays 188, 195
Dalton's law 91
dead-space gases 110–112, 125–127
dehydration 2, 13–14
demyelination 158
depolarization 45, 52, 64
    atrial 59–61
    cellular 45
    myocyte 48
    SA and AV nodes 45–48, *47*, 61
    spontaneous diastolic 45
    ventricular 45, 48–50, 59, 64–66, 69
diabetes 1–2, 16
diabetic ketoacidosis (DKA) 2–3, 16, 20–21, 146, 161, 164
diaphragmaticohepatic (DH) view 136–137, 140–141
diffusion impairment 93, **94**
diphosphoglycerate (2, 3 DPG) 160
distal renal tubules (DRT) 29, 30
Doppler flow detection unit 32–36, **32–34**, 40–43, 152
doxycycline 192
drugs 56
    anti-arrhythmic *57–58*
    immunosuppressive 191, 196
    non-steroidal anti-inflammatory (NSAIDS) 190
    sympathomimetic 44
ductus arteriosus 12
dyshemoglobinemias 81–82

ecchymosis 188, **189**, 191, 196–197
echogenicity 130, **131**, 136
ectopy, ventricular 56–58
edema 204
EDTA 184, 193–194
effusion 136–137, 145–152
    abdominal 15, 145, 190
    cavitary 17, *18*
    joint 190
    pericardial 136, 140–141, **141**, 150–152
    pleural 13–15, *119*, 136, **139**, 140–142, 149–150, 190
electrocardiography (ECG) 12, 45–69, 133
    analysis and interpretation 50–51, *53–55*
    atrial fibrillation (AF) 61–62, **61**, 68
    augmented unipolar leads 47
    ballpoint pen method 50
    bipolar leads 47–49, **48**, 63–67
    bradyarrhythmias 62–69, **66**
    cardiac conduction physiology 45–46, **60**
    deflection, positive/negative 46–48
    electrode placements 46–49, 52
    machine operation 46–49, **47**
    measures of length and time 48, **49**
    SA and AV nodes 45–48, **47**, 52, 59–68, **63–64**
    standard calibration 48
    ventricular and supraventricular tachyarrhythmias 56–61, **59–60, 65, 67–68, 67**
    waveforms and diagnosis *53–55*
electrodes 45–52, **48**, 98, 102, 162, 168–170, 186
electrolytes 21, 89, 93, 97–100
    abnormalities *166–168*
    monitoring 156–176
emphysema 149
end tidal (ETCO$_2$) 110–128, *119–120*
endolithium damage 177–179
enzyme-linked immunoassay (ELISA) 185
enzymes 18
    amperometry 5–7
    flippases 177
    floppases 177
    scramblases 177, 180
eosinophils 193
epinephrine 2
epistaxis 190
erythrocytes 184
extrinsic/intrinsic factor tenase complex 180–183, 187

failure (heart) 15, 136
famotidine 171
ferric iron (Fe^{3+}) 71–72, 75–76
fibrin **178**, 180–183, **183**, 187–190
    crosslinked 182, 188–190
fibrinogen 177–182, **178**, **181–183**, 187, 194–195
fibrinogen degradation products (FDPs) 182, **183**, 188, 195
fibrinolysis 182–183, **182–183**, 187
fibrosis 64
flame atomic emission spectrometry 162, 168
flame photometry 162, 168
fluid analysis 136
fluid overload 15
fluid therapy 22, 40, 43, 206–207
focal assessment for trauma/triage/tracking (FAST) 129–152
    abdominal (AFAST^3) 129–138, 145–152
    cage-side organ 129
    thoracic (TFAST^3) 129–142, 145–152
    veterinary bedside lung (VetBLUE) 129–131, 135–136, 141–152
Foley catheter 201–204
free fatty acid (FFA) 2
free water deficit 104
frozen plasma 192, 195
fusion beats 58

Gamblegrams 88, **89–90**
gas scavenger 115
gastric dilation 200
glaucoma 196
glide signs **135**, 136–142, **139, 142**, 150–152

glomerular filtration rate (GFR) 38–39
glucagon 2
glucose 1–5, *2*, 9, 16–21, 102
    testing 1–5, *2*, 9, 16–21
glucosuria 2
glycolysis 3
glycoprotein 177–179
guided vascular access technique (UST) 143–145, **143**, *144*, *149*

halogen ions 102
heartworm test 43
hematocrit 19, 171, 194
    tubes 5, *8*
hematuria 188
hemoglobin (Hb) 20, 71–76, 80, 92, 110
    alterations 80–82
    deoxygenated (DeOxyHb) 14, 71–73, 76, 81–82
    oxygenated (OxyHb) 71–73, 76, 80–82
    relaxed state (RHb) 72
    tensed state (THb) 72
hemolysis 158, 169–170
hemoptysis 195
hemorrhage 4, 36–37, 110, 117, 137–138, 145, 150, 158, 189–192, 195–196, 204
hemostasis 150, 177–195
    disorders 188–195
    phases 177–182
        primary 177–179, 184–186, 188–194, **189**
        secondary **178**, 179–182, **180–181**, 186–187, 190–195
Henderson–Hasselbach equation 86, 98
heparin sulfate 183
hepatic failure 16
hepatic insufficiency 199
hepatic lipidosis 2, 16
hepatorenal (HR) view 137–138
high powered field (HPF) 185
hydrogen ion (H⁺) 75, 85–87, 98, 161
hydrogen peroxide (H_2O_2) 5–7
hydroxybutyrate dehydrogenase 7
hydroxylase 160
hyperbilirubinemia 169
hypercalcemia 158, 163, *165*
hypercapnia 110, 117, 123
hyperglycemia 2, 161
    clinical signs and causes *16*
hyperkalemia 38, 65, **65**, 69, 160–162, 165, *166–167*, 169–171
hyperlactatemia 17, 104
hypernatremia 156–158, **157**, 161–163, *163*, **167–168**, 170–171, *172*, **172**, 174
hyperphosphatemia 104, 159–160, **159–160**, 160, 164, *165*
hyperproteinemia 168–170
hypertension 30, 36–43, *37*, *38*

hyperthermia 11, 98–99
hyperventilation 86, *87*, 91, **94**, 99–100, 104–107, 110, 118, *122*
hypervolemia 208
hyphema 188, **189**
hypoadrenocorticism 65
hypoalbuminemia 90, 104, 136, 169
hypocalcemia 149, 158–160, **159**, 163, *165–167*, 174–175
hypochloremia 104
hypoglycemia 2, 14–16, 40, 151
    clinical signs and causes *16*
hypokalemia 21, 40, 58, 161, **161**, 165, *166*
hypomagnesemia 58
hyponatremia 2, 38–40, 156–158, **157**, 163–164, *163*, 168
hypophosphatemia 159–160, 164, *165*
hypotension 37–44, *39*, 56, 200, 203
hypothermia 11–14, 42, 98, 171
hypothyroidism *174*, 175
hypoventilation 80, *81*, 86, *87*, 91, **92**, 100–110, 118, 121–123, *122*
hypovolemia 10, 15, 52, 166, 190, 192, 208
    shock 37
hypoxemia *17*, 37, 71, 79–82, 87, 92–93, **92–96**, *93*, 99–101, 106–108, 127
    anatomic shunt **95**
    diffusion impairment **94**
    low and high V/Q mismatch **95–96**
    lung function assessment 106–108
hypoxia 3, 82, **201**, 203
    tissue 37, *93*

i-STAT lactate monitor 7, 20
icterus 170
idiogenic osmoles 158
ileus 200, 203
immunosuppressive drugs 191–192, 196
inflammation 14–15, 106–107, 163, 179
    leukogram 151
    pyogranulomatous 107
    systemic response 37
inotropy 27
    positive 40, 44, 68
inspired oxygen content (FiO_2) **94**, 100–101, 106–108
insulin 1–2, 21, 66, 164, 170–171
international normalized ratio (INR) 187
intervertebral disk disease (IVDD) 105–106
intra-abdominal hypertension (IAH) 199–200, *201*, 203–205
intra-abdominal pressure (IAP) 199–207, **202**
intravenous immunoglobulin (IVIG) 197
ion-selective electrodes (ISE) 162, 168–169
isotonic crystalloid 21–22, 205

juxtaglomerular (JG) cells 29, **30**

ketone 2, 5–7, **12**, 16–21, 88
ketonemia 6
ketonuria 6
ketosis 16
kidneys 3, 36–39, 86, 156–160, 164, 165, 173–174, 199

lactate 3, 7–9, *13*, 17–19, 82–83, 88, 100, 149–151
    blood testing 3, 7–9, *13*, 17–19
    as disease severity biomarker 17, *18*
Lactate Plus monitor 7, **12**
lactic acidosis *17*
Lambert-Beer law 76
latex-enhanced immunoassay (LIA) 185
left atrium:aorta (LA:Ao) ratio 140, **141**
leukocytes 5, 184
    phagocytic effects 159–160
leukocytosis 169–170
leukogram 106
lipemia 169–170
lung point (pneumothorax) 140–141, **142**, 145
lung rockets 138–139

magnesium 88, 170
manometer-based monitoring 199–208
mean arterial pressure (MAP) regulation 26–31, **28**, 34–35, 41–43, 199, 204
megakaryocytes 177, 189, 192
mentation 4, 9–10, 21–22, 36, 68, 103, 151, 157–160, 171, 175
metabolic acidosis 3, 85–89, **87–88**, **89**, 99–100, 104–107, *107*, *120*, 165–166
metabolic alkalosis *88*, **89**, 99, 103, 107, *166*
metabolism 1–2, **4**, 100
    aerobic 1–2
    anaerobic 3, 19, 104, 150
metabolites, arachidonic acid 29
methemoglobin (MetHb) 75–76, *76*, 80–82
microhematocrit tube 5, *7*
mitochondria 2
monocytes 179
mucous membrane (MM) 4, **14**, 76, 102, 151
    color 14, 20–22, 43, 67–68, 81, 150–151
mycophenolate mofetil 192, 197
myocardial distension 26–27
myocytes, cardiac 45, 56, 65–66, 69
myoglobin 71

Nafion tubing 116
neoplasia 14, 192
neuroglycopenia 2
neurologic signs 157
neutrophils 193
nodule signs **135**, 138–142, **139**, *148*

normosol 199
Nova Prime Plus Vet **10**

oliguria 200, 203
oscillometry 35–36, **35**, 40–43
osmolality 156–157, 169
oxidative phosphorylation 80
oxyhemoglobin curve **73–75**, 80, 92

P waves 45, 50–51, **52**, *54*, 58–69, **59–66**
P/F ratio 100–102, 107–108
packed cell volume/total protein (PCV/TP)1 5, 9, 14–15, 22, **23**, 102, 145, 149–151, 195
pancreatitis 136, 205
parasympathetic nervous system (PNS) 46, 52
parenchyma 190
partial pressure of oxygen (PO$_2$) 71, 80, 97–98
patient positioning (recumbency) 131–138, **134–135**, 206
pericardial sites (PCS) 138–141, 140–141, **141**
pericardiocentesis 148
petechia 102, 188, **189**, 191, 196
phentolamine 39
phosphatidylserine 179
phospholipids 187
phosphorus (P) 159–160
    and hyper/hypophosphatemia 159–160, **160**, 163–165, *164*, *165*
piezoelectric crystals 129, 132
plasma (PaO$_2$) 5, 19, 80–83
plasmalyte 199
plasminogen activator inhibitor (PAI-1) 182
Platelet Function AnalyzerR (PFA)-100® 186
platelets 177–197
    aggregometry 186, 189, 194–195
    analysis *178*, 183–185, **185–186**, 192–194, **193**
    blood smear evaluation 185, **185–186**
    clumping 183–184, 192–193
    count 183–184, 192–194
    factors and integrin 177–183, **181**, **184**, 187–194
    function tests 185–186, 194
    granules contents and function *178*
    plug formation and phases 177–179, **179**
    von Willebrand's disease 177–181, 185–186, 189–191, 195
polydipsia/polyuria 158–163
polymorphic ventricular tachycardia **59**
porphyrin 71–72, **72**, 76
Possey Cufflator™ 122
potassium (K) 20
    bromide 102, 169–170
    and hyperkalemia 160–162, 165, *166*, 169–171
    and hypokalemia 161, **161**, 165, *166*
    intracellular 158
PR interval 45
prednisolone 150, 197

procainamide 58
protease inhibitor 183
proteins 5, 15, 100, 183
proteinuria 43
prothrombin time (PT) 149–152, 187–188, 192–196, *193*
prothrombinase complexes 180–181, **184**
pulmonary fibrosis 93
pulmonary–pleural line (PPL) 138, **139**, 142
pulse oximeter (SpO2) 71–74, 80–83, 127
pulse oximetry 71–83, 127
Purkinje fibers 45
pyometra 200
pyrexia 43
pyruvate 3, **4**

QRS complex 45, 48–51, **52**, 56–62, **59**, **63–65**, 66–69

R-R intervals **52**, 61–64, 67–68
rate/rhythm/pressure (heart) 12, 20–21, **29**
  calculation and analysis 50–51, *51*, **51**
re-entrant loops 59
rebreathing 120–122, **123**
  causes 120–122
red blood cells (RBCs) 5, 18–19
renin-angiotensin-aldosterone system (RAAS) 29–30, **29–30**, 38–39
repolarization 45
  ventricular 45, 50
respiratory acidosis 86, 88, 99–100, 103, 106
respiratory alkalosis 86, *87–88*, 90–100, 104, 107, *165–166*
retina 36
return of spontaneous circulation (ROSC) 125
rhabdomyolysis 161
rickettsial disease 197
  polymerase chain reaction 43
Ringers solution 169, 199
rodenticide intoxication 190, 195
rotational thromboelastometry (ROTEM) 188

salicylates 170
Sanz electrode 98
saturation of oxygen (SaO$_2$) 71–76, 81–82, 92, 98
Seldinger technique 145
sepsis 16, 179
serotonin 177
serum chemistry (CHEM) 149
serum chloride (Cl) 156
shock 9–11, 13, 39–43, 50, 69
  hypovolemic 37
  septic 37
shred signs **135**, 138–142, **139**
shunt fraction 112

sick sinus syndrome (SSS) 64
sinoatrial (SA) node 45–46, *47*, 52, 56, 59–68
sinus, arrhythmia 52, 56, **56**
sinus node dysfunction (SND) 64
sinus rhythms 52–56, **52**, **56**, 62
sodium (Na) 29, 66, 89, 156–158, 162–164, 168–169
sphygmomanometer 33
splenic contraction 15
splenoral (SR) view 137
step signs 138–140, **139**
sulfur dioxide (SO$_2$) 98
supraventricular ectopy 59
supraventricular premature complex (SVPC) 60–61, **65**
sympathetic nervous system (SNS) 46, 50, 56
systemic vascular resistance (SVR) 28–29, **29**, 37–38

T waves 50–51, **52**, **59–61**, 65, 68
tachyarrhythmia 40, 50, 67–68, **67**
  differentiation algorithm 62
tachycardia 43, 62–64, 190
  sinus 56, **56**, 64
  supraventricular (SVT) 59–64, **60**
  ventricular (VT) 56–58, **59**, 62
tachypnea 22, 79, 99, 106, 146, 195
target organ damage (TOD) 36, 39, 42–43
temperature 10–11
thoracentesis 148
thoracic focal assessment for trauma/triage/tracking (TFAST[3]) 129–142, **134–135**, **139**, 145–152
3betahydroxybutyrate (3-HB) 2, 7, 16
thrombin 179–183, 187
thrombocytopathia 184, 189–191
thrombocytopenia 106, 184, 188–193, **188–189**, 196–197
  immune-mediated (ITP) 188, 191
  pseudo- 192
thrombocytosis 169–170
thromboelastography (TEG) 188
thromboembolism 102, 128
thrombomodulin 183
thrombosis 195
thromboxane 190
tick-borne diseases 188, 192
tissue, perfusion 14, 31, 200
tissue factor pathway inhibitor (TFPI) 183, **184**
tissue factor (TF) **135**, **139**, 142, *148*, 179–180, **180**, 187–188
tissue plasminogen activator (tPA) 182
toxins 9, 52, 88, 105, 192
Trauma Score 13
tricarboxylic (TCA) cycle 1–3

uremia 105
urinalysis 20, 43
urinary collection system 201
urine protein-to-creatinine (UPC) ratio 43

urobilinogen 5
urokinase plasminogen activator (uPA) 182
uveitis 196

vagal tone 62–64
    maneuvers 60
vascular contraction 15
vascular function, autoregulatory 30, 38
vasoconstriction 13, 30, 42–44
vasodilation 13, 37
vasomotor tone 14, 37
vasopressin 29, 40–44
venous admixture 92
venous occlusion 182
ventilation 112, 127
    manual 117

ventilation/perfusion (V/Q) (mis)match **95–96**, 101, 110–112
ventricular ectopic complex 56–58
ventricular escape rhythm 62–64
ventricular premature complex (VPC) 56–58
Veterinary Bedside Lung Ultrasound Exam (VetBLUE) 129–131, 135–136, **135**, 141–152, *148*
vincristine 196
vitamins, C/K 19, 192, 195–196
volvulus 200
von Willebrand's factor (vWF) 177–181, **179**, 185–186, 189–191, 195

World Society of Abdominal Compartment Syndrome (WSACS) 200

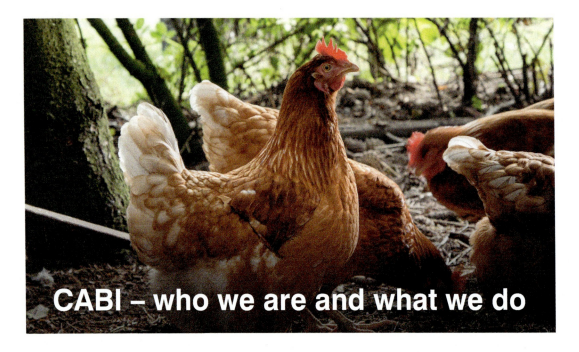

CABI – who we are and what we do

This book is published by **CABI**, an international not-for-profit organisation that improves people's lives worldwide by providing information and applying scientific expertise to solve problems in agriculture and the environment.

CABI is also a global publisher producing key scientific publications, including world renowned databases, as well as compendia, books, ebooks and full text electronic resources. We publish content in a wide range of subject areas including: agriculture and crop science / animal and veterinary sciences / ecology and conservation / environmental science / horticulture and plant sciences / human health, food science and nutrition / international development / leisure and tourism.

The profits from CABI's publishing activities enable us to work with farming communities around the world, supporting them as they battle with poor soil, invasive species and pests and diseases, to improve their livelihoods and help provide food for an ever growing population.

CABI is an international intergovernmental organisation, and we gratefully acknowledge the core financial support from our member countries (and lead agencies) including:

  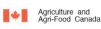

Discover more

To read more about CABI's work, please visit: **www.cabi.org**

Browse our books at: **www.cabi.org/bookshop**,
or explore our online products at: **www.cabi.org/publishing-products**

Interested in writing for CABI? Find our author guidelines here:
www.cabi.org/publishing-products/information-for-authors/